Inventory Management for Veterinary Professionals

Nicole I. Clausen, CSSGB, CCFP
Founder, Veterinary Care Logistics

WILEY Blackwell

Published by John Wiley & Sons, Inc., Hoboken, New Jersey.
Published simultaneously in Canada.

For general information on our other products and services or for technical support, please contact our Customer Care Department within the United States at (800) 762-2974, outside the United States at (317) 572-3993 or fax (317) 572-4002.

Wiley also publishes its books in a variety of electronic formats. Some content that appears in print may not be available in electronic formats. For more information about Wiley products, visit our website at www.wiley.com.

Library of Congress Cataloging-in-Publication Data Applied for:
Paperback ISBN: 9781119717928
ePDF: 9781119717935
ePUB: 9781119717966
oBook: 9781119717959

Cover Design: Wiley
Cover Images: © uchar/Getty Images, Courtesy of Nicole Clausen

Set in 9.5/12.5pt STIXTwoText by Straive, Pondicherry, India

SKY10085009_091824

Dedication

This book is dedicated to anyone who has ever shaken a bottle and wanted to cry.

To anyone who felt like they didn't belong.

And, of course, to the greatest dog who ever lived, my sweet Tank.

Contents

Preface

To my dear reader,

This book is the culmination of my life's work: a collection of stories, strategies, tactics, and references on how to manage inventory in a veterinary practice. I know what a struggle and a challenge it can be, whether you're a first-time inventory manager or a seasoned professional striving to be better. I think inventory management is an interesting part of your practice. It's full of puzzles and obstacles, lack of appreciation and backorders, successes, and roadblocks (and often all in the same day!). Sometimes, it feels like you're on top of the world, and sometimes it feels like you can't do anything right. But at the end of the day, you're enabling patient care to thrive. You are the one who makes sure your team has everything they need to care for your patients.

So, this book is for you. Whether you're a receptionist, a veterinary assistant, a veterinarian, or anything and everything in between, this book is for you to learn and grow with. I wrote this book to be a long-lasting resource and reference for managing inventory in your practice. Throughout the book, you'll find stories of my journey from a baby inventory manager to an inventory consultant and educator, strategies that are time-tested that can be adapted to your unique practice, best practices to keep top of mind, real-world scenarios for how you can apply this knowledge, and examples of how other veterinary professionals have set up their inventory.

How to Use This Book

Throughout this book, "Best Practice" is referenced to help you identify the most important takeaways from each protocol of the inventory management methods that I teach. Inventory is not "one size fits all" and so these questions can guide you as you learn and develop what works best for you. While some of this information is stuff that I learned in books eons ago, most of it was learned by necessity in the real world, and I faced real consequences when I got it wrong.

I wrote the book I wish I had when I started. I wrote the book I wish I had when I found my footing and wondered "What next?"

Here's how it's laid out: Chapters 1–9 contain all the strategies, theory, and know-how that you need to create an inventory ecosystem that can evolve and adapt alongside you and your practice. Then, Chapters 10–13 focus on other ways to implement your new inventory knowledge and systems into your practice. While I know some of you are short on time and want to skip right ahead to implementation, I really encourage you to spend some time studying the first half of this book. Not every strategy will work for every practice, and understanding the foundational concepts and inner workings of inventory management will help you identify what will and won't work for you. A big lesson I've learned and reiterated to all of my clients is that "inventory management is a practice, not a destination."

I hope this book not only inspires you in your practice but also reminds you that you are not alone in this. If you're struggling to find your footing or feel like you have an impossibly long road ahead of you, this book is here to help guide you along the way. There aren't a lot of resources or training available for inventory; it's often passed down from "generation to generation" like a game of telephone (remember that from grade school?). This book was inspired by you; to give you a resource that you can use and learn from over and over again. Thank you for reading. Thank you for taking on the often thankless role of managing inventory in your practice. Even if they don't realize it, you mean so much to your patients and clients.

Forever for the oceans and always cheering you on,

Nicole

Acknowledgments

My heart is filled with immense gratitude as I write this. First and foremost, I want to thank my friend and writing coach extraordinaire, Ash Wylder, for your support, guidance, and belief in me. Without you, this book would not have been possible.

Thank you to my wonderful family for believing in me and being a sounding board. To my sister, my best friend, the one who believed in me when I couldn't, for every adventure, every laugh, who helped me heal from every heartbreak and injustice I (and we) have faced, thank you. There are no words to describe fully how much you mean to me. And, of course, thank you for creating my two favorite tiny humans on the planet.

Thank you to Tank, Ollie, Hei Hei, and my other creatures for dutifully being by my side as I wrote this.

Thank you to the waters that cover our planet and clean our collective souls. You house not only my hope for the world but also the sea creatures that initially captivated my imagination. Without you, there is none of us. I'm eternally in awe and gratitude.

Thank you to my very dear friend Sarah Coffield, for encouraging me to share my knowledge with others.

Throughout my time in vet med, I've had the incredible privilege and opportunity to meet some of the most amazing people. Thank you to my clients and students turned friends who've been on this journey with me. Thank you for the opportunity to be a part of your inventory. Thank you to Nicole Harvey, who was my very first remote client and who has been an unwavering supporter since. Thank you to Dr Garry and Nicole Gotfredson, two of the kindest and most hard-working people I've ever met and my very first client. From the bottom of my heart, thank you to every single client for trusting me to help with your inventory.

Thank you to Brandy for your help and guidance as a brand-new inventory manager. You sparked a love and passion for inventory that will last a lifetime. Thank you to all the inventory educators that came before me and paved the way for this book to be possible.

Thank you to Emmitt Nantz for your kindness and unwavering support of me and my work. You are a truly exceptional co-founder and an even better friend.

I am eternally grateful to Erica Judisch, Merryl Le Roux, Vallikkannu Narayanan, and the entire team at Wiley for taking a chance on me and for your kindness and patience as I brought this book to life.

And finally, there are so many people who have shaped my life and have shown me how to embrace my neurodivergence, my weirdness, and my gentleness. Your unconditional support means more to me than words can describe.

About the Companion Website

This book is accompanied by a companion website:

www.wiley.com/go/clausen/inventory

This website includes:

- Self-Assessment Questions
- Back order tracker
- Circle dot challenge
- End of year checklist
- Inventory Evaluation worksheet
- Inventory habit & Routine Inspiration Worksheet
- Standard Operating Procedure template
- Large Re-order tag template
- Mini Re-order tag template-narrow, mini re-order Tag template
- New item request form worksheet
- Product Evaluation worksheets
- Re-order checklist worksheet.

1

Introduction to Inventory Management

A long time ago, in a galaxy far, far away, I was freshly tasked with managing inventory. At the time, I was brand new to the practice. I always wore several hats and was the "Jane of all trades." Need help fixing this piece of equipment? I'm your gal. Need someone to put together a custom mailing list? I've got you. Need someone to calm down a grumpy client? Sure thing! So, as a "yes person," when I was asked to manage inventory, I happily agreed to a fun new adventure. I was in for a surprise.

In what feels like a different lifetime, the previous inventory manager was leaving the practice and trained me very briefly before leaving. As she was reviewing the current processes, she said, "When you shake a bottle, and it feels low, order it." I vividly remember standing in the pharmacy, unable to wrap my head around it. I kept thinking (and asking), "What does that even mean? What does 'low' mean?" For me, it was much too subjective and could be interpreted so differently.

I kept asking the question in a few different ways, hoping to get a more concrete answer, but it never came. That was the bulk of my training on how to manage inventory. To say that I struggled in the beginning is a giant understatement. I did not order things because I did not even realize the practice carried them. I ordered things at the wrong time because "low" to me was not the same as low for the practice. I also ran out of things because no one told me it was low.

Now, to give you a little context, I have always considered myself a high achiever, and I care deeply about how well I'm performing and doing in my role (think Hermione in class). Not only was doing well vital to me personally, but I knew that my challenges were affecting my team. I wanted them to be happy with me, and I did not want them to be frustrated that items were running out. Coming into this experience and struggling right off the bat really shook the confidence I had in myself. I did not know how to improve and I struggled emotionally, knowing I wasn't doing a great job. No one at the practice had managed inventory before, and I was really on my own little island.

The problems and challenges seemed to compound. My anxiety got a jump start pulling into the parking lot; my mouth would go dry, I'd feel a little queasy, and then I'd soldier on because I did not know what else to do. At the time, I had no idea how to use the practice management system (PiMS) for inventory and before me, they had not really used it much at all. I did not have a grasp on when something needed to be ordered or even what to order. I remember just walking around the pharmacy, shaking bottles, wondering, "Is this low? Should I order this? What about this?" I had way more questions than I had answers.

Every time we ran out of something, it pained me inside. Every time I forgot to order something, I would be so embarrassed that I wasn't doing a better job. After this happened a few times,

Inventory Management for Veterinary Professionals, First Edition. Nicole I. Clausen.
© 2024 John Wiley & Sons, Inc. Published 2024 by John Wiley & Sons, Inc.
Companion website: www.wiley.com/go/clausen/inventory

I thought to myself, "There has to be a better way. This just does not seem right and is not sustainable in the long term (or really even in the short term)."

So, I started learning everything that I possibly could. I poured over supply chain management books, went over every inch of the AVImark® software manual, read everything I could about veterinary and human hospital inventory management, and asked around at different local practices. I was on a mission to learn as much as I could. Slowly but surely, I started to get my feet under me.

I now had hope – hope that things could get better, that it would not always feel this way, and that change was possible. A lot of trial and error, time, and constant brainstorming went into trying to find what worked. Before starting this process, I did not realize what was possible; I just knew there had to be a better way. Looking back, I put so much time, energy, and effort into setting up inventory systems and fixing the PiMS that I could have written this book years ago. After years of helping other clinics implement what I've learned, finally, this book is here.

The emotional highs and lows of the process of learning and fixing inventory for that practice were really the catalysts for where I am today. Not only did I realize how much I enjoyed managing inventory and more of the operational aspects of a veterinary practice, but I also realized how few resources are out there on inventory management. When I made the transition from working in a practice to inventory consulting and training, I had one main goal. I thought to myself, even if one person feels like someone is in their corner and does not have to struggle alone, I've accomplished what I set out to do.

As I've shared my story over the years, I've come to realize just how common an experience it is. Often, the only training for inventory management is, "When you shake a bottle and it feels low, order it." This method of inventory management is passed down from generation to generation because "this is how it has always been done'" feels safer than the risk of implementing new systems that are easier and less time-consuming. Managing inventory does not need to be so stressful. You can enjoy this work by finding the right methods for you and your practice.

It can be scary to lean into challenging conversations with your care and leadership teams. It takes bravery to say "Wait, this is not right" or "We could be doing better," especially if something is the way it's always been done. But you are the person who is uniquely skilled to help pave a profitable, practical, and more peaceful way forward for the practice.

I remember the first time I did a complete, practice-wide inventory count at the end of the year. The practice had opened over eight years earlier and nothing had ever been counted. I embarked on this count all by myself. It took me weeks. I am so grateful for that process because of what I learned from it. I got to see the belly of the beast, as they say. But it took me HOURS of counting, fixing, adjusting, and changing quantities, codes, and item setups. There were so many inventory codes to update and change. So many items where the on-hand quantity needed to be adjusted by thousands or even tens of thousands. But, every year after that, it got exponentially easier. What took me over three weeks the first year took about two days the next.

I think that's a common story in a veterinary practice. Inventory can be a bit like an overgrown garden. There are weeds everywhere and you are not really sure what's growing, what's thriving, and what is decomposing. Pulling the weeds, cutting through the overgrowth, and removing unnecessary plants and invasive species takes a lot of time and effort. But once you do, your garden begins to thrive and healthy plants shoot up. It can be easily maintained with a small pair of pruning scissors and a pair of gloves (plus some extra weeding time during spring). The garden, or what we'll begin to see as our coral reef ecosystem, is similar to our inventory; it might take some time and effort to fix and adjust all the outdated and old information but once you put that work in, your new inventory systems are vibrant flowers and bountiful vegetables.

I find it helpful to think about inventory and practice operations like an ecosystem. All the systems or pieces work together to form a symphony of structure that allows your patients to have everything they need and your practice to generate revenue so that patient care can continue for years to come.

Throughout this text, we'll be exploring inventory management and each of its parts. Within inventory management, there are important foundational principles and concepts that we'll explore together. But I invite you to consider how you might adjust or adapt these to your own unique practice. There is no one-size-fits-all approach or solution to inventory. The good news is that there are some best practices and guidelines to follow, but there is wiggle room to be curious and creative about what works best for your practice. Harking back to the garden metaphor, how you tend to a vegetable garden in the Pacific Northwest is very different from how you'd tend to a flower garden in the Southeast. My best advice? Trust yourself. This book is a guidebook but it is also just a tool. You're the one pruning things that do not work and introducing systems that do. And if you want extra help, I'm here.

I've experienced that when inventory feels overwhelming and chaotic, people will grasp and cling to *anything* that seems like it will make it feel easier and help the practice not to run out of pharmaceuticals and supplies as frequently. But I think we can get caught up in the trap of seeking blanket advice and forget to be intentional about how and where we apply it. As a result, because we might not have fully considered our unique practice, the tactic or strategy does not stick and we realize it is not sustainable. We start running out again (or more often), and expired products start appearing (like someone got them wet after midnight). Maybe our PiMS goes wildly off track. Then we are right back where we started *and* we lose a bit of hope that our inventory can ever be better.

With each of the concepts and principles that you'll learn in the following chapters, you'll also find "Best Practice" questions to help you apply them to your unique practice so that you can implement lasting and sustainable change that positively impacts your feelings about work, the clinic's cycle of inventory, and the ecosystem of the entire practice.

1.1 What No One Told You During Your "Training" as an Inventory Manager

When you think of inventory management, what comes to mind? Is it scrambling to place an order in between appointments? Is it trying to find a makeshift "desk" or workspace to receive your orders? Is it unpacking a seemingly never-ending amount of boxes? Is it a veterinarian asking you in a desperate tone where (insert important medication) is? While some of that can be true, inventory management is so much more than that. Not only is inventory much more encompassing but it also does not have to feel like a drag. There are many veterinary professionals (myself included) who truly enjoy inventory. It's a perfect blend of zooming out to look at the big picture, examining the granular details with a monocle perched over one eye, and an incredible amount of problem solving in between.

"Best Practice" Questions to Consider
- How do you view inventory management?
- How does your practice view inventory management?
- Do you wish the role was respected or valued more in your practice (and maybe even by you)?

Before we dive in, let us begin with some common definitions so that we have a shared language throughout this book. First off, what is "**inventory**"? I like to think about inventory as essentially a list of all the items in your practice related to caring for a patient. This includes pharmaceuticals, prescription or retail diets, injectables, in-house reference lab supplies, white goods, syringes and needles, and more. Items like office supplies, pens, toilet paper, and other janitorial supplies aren't included in this category as they are considered more of a facility expense. Equipment is also a completely separate category; even though, technically, an anesthetic machine helps to care for a patient, an anesthetic machine is not considered an inventory item but rather an asset.

Now, what does it mean to manage inventory? Managing inventory is much more than just placing orders and hoping that things aren't on backorder. It's about creating sustainable, simple systems (your inventory ecosystem) that help you effectively have what you need for patient care and support the profitability of your practice.

A hairy truth about this field is that the tasks involved in managing inventory are often unseen work and go unnoticed by the rest of the team. But without inventory, we cannot care for our patients. We could not even take a patient's temperature because we would not have thermometers! Often, I'll hear of inventory managers referred to as just the "purchaser" or the "order person" but there is so much more involved.

If you got dropped into inventory (or volun-told this was your new role and responsibility) without much training, I'm sorry. Sadly, it's a common scenario in our industry to just "get on with the job, shake the bottles, and do not take up too much space." If you are struggling, frustrated, or overwhelmed, you are certainly not alone and I'm so glad that you are here. It's my mission in my work to change this paradigm.

1.2   Inventory Can Be Hard But It Matters. Here's Why

Managing inventory is interesting. There are two main goals: to have what you need on hand for patient care and to maintain or improve the profitability of your practice. What's interesting about that is that those two goals are in complete opposition to each other. If you only cared about having what you need on hand, you would have tons and tons of inventory. You would never, ever run out of anything and you would have a wonderful assortment of options for your care team. On the flip side, if you only cared about the profitability of your practice, you would have an extremely lean inventory. You'd likely often run out and have a very limited inventory overall. You'd also be stressed with emergency orders and likely have a very frustrated team on your hands.

As an inventory manager, finding the delicate balance between **too much** and **not enough** is part of your role.

1.3   What is the Impact of Inventory Management on Our Practice?

"Best Practice" Questions to Consider
- Take two to three minutes and think about your "Why."
- Why is being in vet med so important and meaningful to you?
- Why did you want to be in vet med?
- What or who inspired you to enter this field?

Let us start with the impact on patient care and our team. Before we do, though, I invite you to take two or three minutes and think about your "why." Why is being in vet med so important and meaningful to you? Why did you want to be in vet med? Maybe you wanted to be a veterinarian for as long as you can remember. Maybe you wanted to be a veterinary technician after learning you could have a career caring for animals. Maybe, like me, you fell in love with vet med, and it's your "home."

Coming into the vet can be stressful for folks, and I enjoy doing what I can to make it a better, more comforting experience for clients. Community and family are so important to me, and our pets and creatures are a part of that. It's shifted a little but now, it means so much to support veterinary professionals who care for others in so many wonderful ways.

Now, let us look at the impact of inventory management on patient care and our team. Whatever your "why" is, inventory probably supports it. For many veterinary professionals, I imagine their "why" is to care for patients. To give a voice to those who do not have one. To help animals live long, happy, fulfilling lives with their families. To make that happen, it's critical to have what we need in stock to care for our patients. Otherwise, we are not able to care for them as we'd like to.

I remember once (before I discovered the power of reorder points) that someone had used the IDEXX stain pack for the complete blood count (CBC) machine and did not tell me. It was such an infrequently used item that I had also forgotten to check and see if another one needed to be ordered. Long story short, the stain pack needed to be changed and we simply did not have one in our inventory. That meant we were unable to run CBC for any of our surgeries that day. Let me tell you, I moved mountains to make sure those pets were able to get their labs run and surgeries performed that day. That's what happened externally. Internally, I realized just how important my role in the team is. That experience sparked my quest to figure out a solution, a better system to make sure that nothing like that would happen again. It's an experience I'll never forget.

Around that same time, someone had put an empty box of Antisedan® behind the open vial. I did not even check to see if the box was full or empty; I just assumed we had another completely full vial in stock. So when the open vial ran out and we discovered there was no more Antisedan in the practice, it was gut-wrenching. For those of you who do not know, Antisedan is an injection often used to reverse the effects of sedation, so you can see what a big blow that was.

Both of those scenarios showed me firsthand how important inventory management is to our practice. Not only does it affect patient care but it affects our team. Not having what they need in stock is a giant roadblock and a source of frustration. They want to treat their patients but they are not able to (and it's out of their control). These situations really add up and can affect your team's morale, compounding stress and tension between team members.

Not having what we need in stock also jeopardizes the trust that our clients have in us. Let's imagine that a client comes in and we are out of a number of products or supplies needed for that appointment. The client might then start to question our practice's integrity. "If they are constantly out, maybe they aren't operating smoothly. What else might be getting missed? What is really going on back there once my pet leaves the exam room?"

I cannot tell you how often, after explaining what I do (to nonveterinary professionals), people say, "Oh, my vet needs you! They seem to always be out of something." Obviously, this is not a great cultural sentiment. And who can shift the paradigm from chaotic to reliable trust? You. That's why your role as an inventory manager is so important. You're not just the "order person," you hold the key to patient care.

We've talked about the impact good inventory management practices can have on our patients and teams, but we should not forget the impact it has on the person actually managing inventory! If you do not have systems in place or did not receive adequate training, it can be lonely and disheartening to swim against the current of all this chaos, stress, and mental load. You might realize you are struggling and want to do better, but you are not quite sure how. In the back of your mind, you might feel that you should already know this, so asking for help seems silly. It's not.

Do any of these feel familiar?
- Maybe you feel like you can barely keep your head above water and spend most of your time putting out fires, reacting to things that have run out.
- Are you getting panicked texts and phone calls on your day off that the practice is out of something?
- Maybe you do not feel like a valued member of your team.
- What is your experience like?

To feel that going to work is such a heavy burden impacts our lives both professionally and personally.

Besides the impact of having what we need in stock, there is a huge financial component to inventory in any practice. **Inventory is the second largest expense in a veterinary practice, second only to labor and compensation expenses.** Although it can be the number one expense on some occasions. It affects the cash flow of a practice and can influence profitability. Think of all the bottles in your pharmacy as if they are filled with dollar bills. If any of your products are just sitting on the shelf, not selling, that's money "locked" on the shelf.

If you are spending too much money or your margins are razor thin, it's likely having (or going to have) a negative impact on your financials.

Helpful Definitions
- **Cash flow**: the amount of money moving in and out of a business.
- **Margin**: the amount of money a business makes after subtracting all its costs and expenses from the revenue it generates.
- **Profitability**: how well a business is making money or earning a profit. A profitable business is one that ends up with money left over after paying all expenses.

Let's look at a quick example. Consider that if a $2,000,000 practice has a cost of goods sold (as a percentage of revenue sold) of 30%, then they likely spend roughly $600,000 annually on inventory. Similarly, a $5M practice with a cost of goods sold of 25% will spend roughly $1.25M every single year on inventory. That is a significant expense, so mismanagement can be extremely costly.

On a bigger scale, because inventory impacts the profitability of the practice, it also affects how valuable a practice is when it's time to sell. Michael Hargrove, DVM, MBA, CVA, a valuation analyst at Summit Veterinary Advisors, explained that during a practice valuation, "the more profitable a business is, the more valuable it will be from a valuation standpoint. The higher the cost of goods go, the more it detracts from the bottom line and the more it has a negative impact on value" (M. Hargrove, personal communication).

"Best Practice" Tip
It's important to get a very accurate picture of your inventory costs. Work with a trusted, veterinary-specific accountant to ensure that your cost of goods data and information are as accurate as possible, especially if considering selling the practice or planning for long-term goals.

At this point, your heart may be beating faster than it was at the beginning of the chapter. I know that inventory management comes with a lot of pressure to get it right. There is a lot of responsibility in this role, and you are one of a team. If you use this book as the tool it is designed to be, you will learn how to balance the pressures with foundational systems and practices that take the guesswork out of the equation.

While not everyone is a good fit for inventory management, anyone can learn to do what needs to be done to have a functioning veterinary practice where the team rely on each other and help their patients daily. In a well-functioning system, even when mistakes happen, they can be easily mitigated. A little reminder here: I LOVE my work. My hope is that you do too. If you do not love inventory, that's okay, too. I want to help make it easier so you can get back to your patients more quickly. Okay, back to it.

Helpful Definitions
- **Valuation**: the estimated value of the business. During a valuation, a specialist looks at things like revenue, profit, assets (like buildings or equipment), debts, and other factors. The number can change over time, just like the value of a car or a house.

1.4   When Do People Look to Reassess their Inventory System?

Many of my clients and students fall into one of three main categories: either they are tired of feeling like they are barely treading water and just constantly fighting "inventory fires," they have recognized their inventory costs are too high and want to reduce them, or they are considering retiring or selling within the next five years. Sometimes, our inventory feels "good enough" until it does not. It might seem like "it's fine" until our goals or priorities shift and then all of a sudden, the status quo needs to change.

Alternatively, you might be reading this book because you are just getting started on your veterinary medicine educational journey and have not worked in a practice yet. If that's you, I'm so glad you are here. Throughout this book, many of the "Best Practice" questions or quizzes are geared toward someone who is currently working in a practice. If you are not yet in practice, do not skip these. Think intentionally and critically about what you might do in practice. If you are on the road to becoming a veterinarian and want to own a practice one day, use these questions to help guide your vision.

"Best practice" for using this book as someone new to the industry is to craft a "mock practice" for yourself and apply the examples and questions to the veterinary practice you have imagined. Take a moment now and dream up your clinic. What patients will you see? What is your role in the practice and how involved are you with inventory management? How many veterinarians do you envision? Are you a general practice or do you have a specialty focus? Is your practice metropolitan or in a rural area? Does your practice have any unique services or offerings for patients and clients? Who is on your team? Who helps with inventory management? Thinking through these questions while imagining a mock practice can help make the strategies and tactics presented throughout this book more tangible.

For readers who want to make inventory easier and less stressful or reduce their inventory costs without the intention to sell, the strategies in this book can help to streamline your systems and reduce how often you run out, as well as the amount of time spent managing inventory. It also frees up money for team bonuses, new equipment, and business capital to open a new location, expand your practice, remodel, or add new team members.

It's important to remember that high inventory costs can have a negative impact on the practice, but when you reduce the costs, that freed-up capital can open up a world of possibilities for your practice. Are you starting to see what an important role this is? I hope so.

"Best Practice" Exercise

- Whether you are currently working in a practice or hope to one day, I invite you to brainstorm a list of your top 10 products. As you are reading through different situations and scenarios presented in this book, you can refer back to this list to consider how you might implement this in your current or future practice using one of these items.
  - If you are currently working in practice, think about your top-selling items (in terms of units and revenue generated).
  - If you are in the learning process and have not worked in a practice yet, what do you think might be the top or most common product in a veterinary practice? Alternatively, make a list of the top 10 medications or products you are most familiar with.
  - Tip: The common top-selling products I've noticed in a small animal general practice facility are (in no particular order):
    - gabapentin 100 and 300 mg
    - trazodone 50 and 100 mg
    - Apoquel® 16 mg
    - Flea/tick prevention
    - heartworm prevention
    - cephalexin 250 and 500 mg
    - vaccinations
    - prednisone 20 mg
    - doxycycline 100 mg
    - Convenia® injectable
    - carprofen 75 and 100 mg
    - Cerenia® injectable and tablets.

Lastly, one of the topics that is often widely discussed in our industry is the low wages in comparison to credentials, experience, education, skill level... basically everything. One of the things I love about setting up your inventory is that creating those systems and reducing inventory costs is something you can do today that creates a positive impact on your practice almost immediately. Lowering the practice's inventory costs can give us the opportunity to invest more in our teams by paying them fair wages.

Inventory management affects almost every aspect of a veterinary practice, from patient care to the mental well-being of the inventory manager, the morale of the team, the financial viability of our practice, and everything in between.

1.5 Inventory Goals

"Best Practice" Quick Quiz

1) What are the two main goals of inventory management?

   When it comes to managing inventory, there are two main goals. First and foremost, we want to have what we need on hand for patient care. Second, we want to balance that with the goal of improving (or even maintaining) the profitability of our practice. Essentially, we want to find the balance between too much and not enough. Depending on your practice, you might have other goals nestled within these two main overarching goals.

   Your goals will probably change and adapt over time. Let's say you are just getting started focusing on your inventory. Your main goal might be to have what you need and minimize expired items but as your experience and expertise grow, your goals may widen to include tracking and monitoring key performance indicators (KPIs) and/or regular margin analysis. So, although all of these goals are important to consider, they do not have to be perfectly executed right away. It's actually helpful to prioritize only a couple of the most impactful goals at a time.

Here's an example: Let's say you are baking a cake. You know that to make this cake, you need to mix the dry ingredients in a separate bowl from the wet ingredients, turn on the oven, grease the pan, combine everything, and then wait. You cannot do that all at once. It's literally impossible to simultaneously add and mix all the ingredients at one time unless you have help, and if you have ever tried cooking with your niece, you know that help does not always mean things will move quicker. So, what do you do? Well, you start with preheating the oven. Then you move to mixing all the dry ingredients, then the wet, then greasing the pan, then pouring it all in.

Breaking these chunks down into doable parts (collecting all the dry ingredients and then mixing them) is important to ensure you do not forget a step or get ahead of yourself and end up with a cake without any eggs (sorry, Rebecca). It's the same with inventory. Also, it's important to note that while cake plates and forks are nice to have at the table when it's time to dig in, it does not make sense to set these out unless there is a cake to dig into. Focus on the most important pieces first.

Side note: Some people do best when they have an "ending" metric for success. My book coach almost always puts out the empty plates on the table before starting to make dinner so that while she's whipping things together in the kitchen, she can visualize how it will look on the plate and make decisions that match the end goal. There are ways to trick yourself into success but those techniques will be introduced later. For now, know that you should choose the most important goals first. I'll show you how.

Sustainable and lasting strategies are *always* preferred over perfection! Here are some examples of sustainable, lasting strategies.

- Your PiMS or other electronic inventory software program is well utilized, and you are able to track your inventory, view accurate financial and inventory reports, and help sell/dispense inventory.
- The number of stockouts and expired products is minimal. There will be some (like emergency medications), but you have systems in place to reduce the frequency and friction of dealing with them.
- Processes are in place for adding new products and controlling the number of items and products carried.
- Inventory is managed through a proactive (rather than reactive) approach, and there are guidelines for when, what, and how much to order; this includes regular orders as well as promotional or bulk purchases – all while minimizing the "oops" orders.
- Everyone in the practice, including the practice owner and management team, supports the inventory process and understands how important inventory management is for the practice.
- There is ongoing compliance with the Drug Enforcement Administration, OSHA, State Pharmacy Board, and other regulatory bodies.
- There are Standard Operating Procedures (SOP) for all phases of inventory management so that all processes can be executed with ease and minimize the risk of theft, diversion, or misuse.
  - A quick note on SOPs: I do not view SOPs as something that is written down and then forgotten (or ignored when it gets busy). I like to think of SOPs as a supportive framework that helps guide systems and processes so nothing gets missed or forgotten. They are also a great policy in case someone "wins the lottery" and they (along with their knowledge and know-how) are no longer with the practice.

Helpful Definitions
- **Stockout**: running out of a product or item.
- **SOPs**: a set of rules or instructions for doing something the same way every time. Essentially, they are guidelines that explain how to perform tasks or handle certain situations consistently and efficiently.

"Best Practice" Questions to Consider
If you are reading through the list thinking, "We're nowhere even close to this," I invite you to think about the following issues.

- What is the biggest roadblock in our inventory right now?
- What goal feels most important to work toward first?
- What are we doing well now?
- What are my short-term and long-term goals for the practice, and how does that relate back to our inventory goals?

1.6 The Three Mindsets for Inventory Management

After spending years managing inventory and helping thousands of other veterinary professionals, I've come to realize that there are several key mindsets when it comes to managing inventory. But first, what is a mindset? A mindset is a set of beliefs, notions, or assumptions that shape how you view yourself and the world around you. A mindset can influence how you view, think, or feel about certain situations. Whenever you are attempting something new in your practice, remember these mindsets and come back to them any time.

Inventory managers are valuable. Sometimes, as an inventory manager, when you are counting things or trying to place an order, it might feel like you aren't as valuable because you aren't directly caring for a patient. It's easy to fall into the trap of feeling less important than the veterinary care team because you aren't actively working with clients or patients. It's possible your team gets frustrated because you cannot hold a dog or call a client back. But always remember how incredibly valuable the inventory manager's role is. They are responsible for keeping what the care team needs in stock so they can care for the patients. Just because you aren't actively working with an animal doesn't mean you are any less important or valuable!

Be curious and try stuff. Occasionally, in veterinary medicine, it's easy to get caught in the trap of "we have always done it this way." Other times, it's hard to think about attempting something new when you are short-handed and just trying to make it through the day. But there is incredible power in being curious and trying new things, new systems, and different processes. Look for the friction in your system. Could a particular area of your inventory run more smoothly, can something tedious be automated, or is the current way the best way for you?

One of the things I've come to realize over the years is that not every method will work well in every practice. Reorder tags might work excellently for one clinic but not for another. On the flip side, one practice might utilize its PiMS to its fullest potential while for another, it is just extra effort with no payoff. As you are reading through this book or learning about inventory from other sources, I invite you to look at them through the lens of curiosity and think: How might this benefit my practice? How might this method or process serve us?

If you try something and it does not work, that is okay! It just means you are one step closer to finding something that does work, and you learned valuable lessons about your practice and your team along the way. If something is not working as well as you'd like, think about how you might be able to pivot. Could the team get involved? Could they offer feedback? What about another fellow inventory manager or practice owner?

Be a detective, not a perfectionist. When something runs out or otherwise goes wrong in an inventory system, as an inventory manager or other team member who assists with the inventory process, it can be hard not to blame yourself. If you run out of something, it's easy to think, "I'm horrible at managing inventory. I should not be doing this!" or "The practice should just have someone else manage inventory." Instead of striving for perfection, try examining what went wrong through the lens of a detective instead. Think: "I wonder why this product ran out. I wonder what processes or double-check system I could put in place so this does not happen again." Rather than getting down on yourself, pick out a cool monocle at a vintage store, take a deep breath, and start investigating. Perfectionists blame themselves for shortcomings. Detectives investigate the cause-and-effect cycle. That's what I'm inviting you to do: Look at the situation as if you are a detective.

Change and experimentation can be challenging, especially when you are trying to do the best you can. Imposter syndrome can start to creep in and make you question if you are doing the right thing and if you are even suited for the job. These little second-guessing "thought gremlins" are our brain's way of trying to keep us safe and in our comfort zone. But once we step out of our comfort zone, we must pass through the fear zone to reach the growth zone. Now, that is where the magic starts to happen! Think about stepping out of your warm clothes in a cold room so that you can get into bed. It's just a hurdle, but we can really get hung up on wanting to stay warm at that moment.

I also hope that this gives you permission to release a few negative beliefs that are holding you back or getting in the way. I did not just become an inventory consultant overnight. I had to put in the time, work, and effort to become a master at inventory. When I first got started, I continuously struggled with thoughts of, "I should know how to do this. I should be able to, but I just cannot get it right."

There were days when I felt like I could not do anything. Everything felt like pulling teeth. Everything felt exhausting. And that is when those thoughts would creep in.

"Why could not I just 'do it?'"
"Why does this feel so hard?"
"Am I actually just incompetent and should let someone else take over?"

I did not want anyone to know I was feeling this way because I did not want them to validate this very negative, gut-wrenching stuff I truly believed about myself. But here's the reality: I wasn't bad at managing inventory. I had taken over an inventory that was in really rough shape and I had not given it enough time for things to straighten out. If you are in this thought spiral, I can almost guarantee that the same is true for you.

1.6.1 Mindset Exercise

When you are an overachieving, goal-oriented person, it's easy to get sucked into this never-ending cycle of hustle and go, go, go. We want to do better and we want to do what's best for our practice. We see the gap between where things are and where they should be (or we want them to be). Here's what I invite you to do: Say the false belief out loud.

"I'm bad at managing inventory."

Say it in the mirror if you need to. Release it. Let it go. And then I want you to turn it into a true belief.

"I'm not bad at managing inventory. I wasn't trained, but I can (and will) turn this ship around."

You can write it on a sticky note and stick it on your mirror, your desk, or wherever you'll notice it. I hope that in your quest to improve your inventory and improve your practice, you are also kind to yourself in the process!

"Best Practice" Mindset Summary
1) Inventory managers are valuable.
2) Be curious and try stuff.
3) Be a detective, not a perfectionist.

Add two mindsets of your own to this list that will help you remember who you are, who you want to be, and how you want to show up.

1.7 The Role of an Inventory Manager

What is the role of an inventory manager? The short answer is, it depends. In one practice, the inventory manager might be in charge of order replenishment, receiving, and vendor relationships while the practice manager handles pricing, the PiMS, and all other responsibilities. The inventory manager may be in charge of the entire process. Or, in some situations the inventory manager is also a veterinary technician and has certain times carved out throughout the week for inventory. It will vary from practice to practice, which is why it is so important for you to trust your instincts and make the choice to implement the techniques that are best for you and your practice while learning the strategies in this book. Just because it's in these pages doesn't mean it's the right option for your practice at this time.

As an inventory manager, it's imperative that your role and responsibilities are clear to you, your supervisor, and all other key stakeholders. Not only that but it's so important to have dedicated, uninterrupted time throughout the week to devote to managing inventory properly. Most inventory managers are responsible for hundreds of thousands of dollars of inventory every year. With that level of investment, it's critical to the success and profitability of the practice that proper time and resources are allocated to managing it.

I remember when I did not have any dedicated inventory time and would try to fit things in between my roles as a client service representative and a veterinary assistant. I recall being at the front desk with one computer for checking patients in and out and a completely different workstation for receiving purchase orders into AVImark. I would place an order, enter the packing slips, and then the phone would ring. I'd have to switch gears mentally and get to the other workstation to assist the client. It's hard to switch tasks like this so frequently, especially when each role requires so much focus. A lot of research is coming out about the negative aspects of multitasking and the decrease in productivity when interruptions are present during focused blocks of time. Consider this your permission to set boundaries. I did.

I found that I used a different part of my brain for inventory than for other responsibilities in the practice. So, having to switch back and forth between tasks constantly, I wasn't ever able to get into a focused rhythm. Once I had dedicated time for inventory, it felt like a breath of fresh air to only have to worry about client service or inventory and not both at the same time. I got to be present with the task at hand.

In the day-to-day rush of running a veterinary practice, managing inventory can often become an afterthought, something that's done in between appointments, in between checking clients in and out, or whenever something has completely run out. One of the most common questions I get asked is, "How much time should I spend managing inventory?" The short answer is, it depends! There are many factors to consider when calculating how much time should be spent.

How often should one spend managing inventory in any given week? As with most things, that depends on your situation. It will vary depending on the size of your practice, how many veterinarians are on staff, how well established your inventory system is, the type of practice, how many locations there are, and other factors. The more work that needs to be done to fix an inventory system, or if not many systems have been established, the more time and effort will be required to either fix or maintain it. The more established and efficient the inventory system, the less time will be required for management and upkeep.

If you are working to fix, establish, and create an inventory system, your week will look very different from that of someone who is in maintenance mode.

One of the biggest variables to examine is the quality of the time spent managing inventory. Spending one hour of uninterrupted, dedicated time is more productive than one hour spent bouncing around between client phone calls, holding patients, and trying to manage inventory. With that being said, other factors include:

- the number of veterinarians in a practice or the size of your inventory
- the number of helpers or inventory assistants available to you
- the capabilities of the inventory module in your PiMS or other inventory software
- your current inventory systems and how streamlined they are
- the amount of time and effort needed to "fix" or improve your inventory systems.

If you are putting a lot of time and effort into "fixing" or getting your inventory straightened out, you are going to be spending more time than if your inventory system is streamlined and generally well established. I recommend, at the very least, starting with dedicated, uninterrupted time each week to manage your inventory. The next step is to determine what tasks you'll need to complete on a regular basis, what you'll be delegating, and what schedule and tasks you'd like to work toward.

"Best Practice" for Fixing Your Inventory
1) Schedule dedicated, uninterrupted time each week to manage your inventory.
2) Determine the tasks you need to complete on a regular basis.
3) Determine what tasks to delegate.
4) Map out the schedule and tasks you are working toward.

Tip: If you are not sure exactly what this looks like yet, that's okay! We'll be diving more in-depth into fixing your inventory system in Chapter 10.

It's vital to remember that managing inventory is much more than just placing orders and order replenishment. It's also about developing systems and processes to ensure efficiency, proper control, and profitability of the inventory department. For inspiration, here are some potential roles and responsibilities of an inventory manager.

- Oversee and maintain inventory of pharmaceuticals, hospital supplies, dietary and nutritional products, retail items, and any other products related to patient care.
- Forecast demand by calculating and setting reorder points and reorder quantities for each product.
- Create and maintain reordering systems for all items and train team members on how to use the inventory system, if applicable.

- Place orders in a timely manner, keeping in mind any shipping charges or minimum shipping amounts.
- Develop policies and procedures and an inventory tracking system that minimizes theft and diversion by team members and clients.
- Calculate and monitor key inventory performance indicators, such as cost of goods sold as a percentage of revenue, inventory turnover, value of inventory on hand, and total variances.
- Calculate product markup, selling price, and overall gross profit margin. Oversee strategic inventory pricing.
- Set up an effective purchasing and turnover tracking system to eliminate waste and help the practice balance inventory costs and storage space.
- Cultivate and maintain positive relationships with vendors and suppliers.
- Discuss new products, any relevant promotional periods, and rebate progress with reps. Meet with the care team or management team to discuss.
- Communicate with the team on any product changes, backorder or supply chain issues, and any important recall information.
- Create and maintain cycle count schedules and evaluate any significant variances or shrinkage.

Helpful Definitions
- **Inventory turnover**: a measure of how quickly an item(s) comes in and leaves a business; it is a great measure of inventory efficiency. A high turnover means items are not just sitting on the shelf, whereas a low turnover means they are on the shelf for long periods before they are used or sold.
- **Diversion**: when someone with authorized access to medications misuses them for personal gain or nonmedical purposes. Motives for diversion can include personal use or selling the drugs.
- **Variance**: the difference between the actual amount of a medication or item and what was supposed to be there according to records or expectations.
- **Shrinkage**: a term used to describe when an item goes missing without a clear explanation and cannot be accounted for. This can be due to theft, errors, or other causes.

In addition, here is an outline of regularly occurring tasks that an inventory manager should complete to inspire you when brainstorming and creating your own unique task schedule.

Biennial (every two years)
- Count and create a biennial controlled substance report. As of March 2024, the Drug Enforcement Administration requires a count every two years. For more information on controlled substance regulations, see Chapter 12.

Yearly
- Provide an accurate end-of-year count and value for all inventory in the hospital. Tip: Lean into your PiMS or other inventory software for this; many PiMS/software systems have a report that will calculate and total the value of inventory on hand without having to hand calculate this in a spreadsheet program.
- Create a dashboard that lists all the KPIs and metrics that are tracked. This should be updated monthly and quarterly. A dashboard can be created in Excel or another spreadsheet program. This can even be as simple as a piece of paper!
- Perform an ABC analysis; use this report to identify the high-, medium-, and low-value items in your practice. This will help to allocate your time so you spend more time and effort on higher value items and less on lower value items.

Quarterly

- Update the KPI dashboard with the most recent KPI calculations.
- Review and update reorder points; these should be recalculated at least every quarter to every six months or after a veterinarian joins or leaves the practice to ensure order levels update as the practice grows or changes.
- Review categories and clean up the PiMS as necessary; lean on reports from your PiMS to help with this process. Use this time to make sure your inventory does not "backslide." This time could be used to inactivate any items no longer carried, recategorize anything that does not make sense, or update any inventory items as necessary.
- Review any duplicate SKUs or medications; look for any particular categories that have more than a primary and secondary product. For example, if there are seven different types of ear cleansers or four types of joint supplements, these should be noted.
- Monitor current promotions and rebates for cost savings. Your representatives are a great resource for this and can identify if there are any upcoming promotions that would financially benefit the practice.

Monthly

- Create and update a budget. Note: I do not recommend creating a budget by specifying that XX% of last week's revenue is this week's budget. It can be a very reactive way to manage a budget and puts the practice at risk of not generating future revenue due to stockouts.
- Review the previous month's budget. Tip: Add the projected versus actual budget to your KPI dashboard.
- Update the KPI dashboard with the new monthly calculations.
- Monitor expiry dates and identify products that are either expired or will expire within three months.
- Perform the monthly cycle counts and adjust the quantity on hand in the PiMS.

Weekly

- Place an order; this might be twice weekly if you are a high-volume practice, i.e., Tuesday and Friday.
- Create purchase orders in your PiMS once the order has been placed to help communicate what was ordered.
- Enter and monitor any variances or on-hand adjustments. Tip: Watch for any significant or large adjustments or note if adjustments continue to rise month on month. For example, if adjustments in month one were $2,000, the second month was $3,500, and the third month was $7,000, this is valuable information and should be addressed with an internal investigation of some degree.
- Count controlled substances and reconcile controlled substance logs. Note: This may need to be done more frequently, every day or at the end of the shift, to ensure the controlled substance logs are accurate and complete at all times.
- Count "AA" and "A" or high-turnover items. More time and effort should be allocated to high-value and high-turnover items than low-turnover or low-value items. For example, the same amount of effort should not be expended managing tongue depressors as vaccines.
- Adjust any hospital usage items to reflect the accurate quantity on hand, if your practice keeps track of hospital supplies and consumables.

As Needed

- Enter/receive invoices as they come in (ideally within 24 hours).
- Stock and organize inventory.

- Review the wants and needs list, reorder tags or other reordering systems for additions to the inventory purchasing worklist.
- Visually check inventory is in the proper location and it is stocked by product dating.

"Best Practice" How to Plan Your Time

When planning out the amount of time spent managing inventory each week, start by brainstorming the various factors listed above.

1) Will you have dedicated time to manage inventory?
2) How many veterinarians do you have?
3) How much effort will you need to put into "fixing" your inventory rather than managing it?

1.8 Qualities of an Inventory Manager

Who and what an "inventory manager" is in veterinary medicine can vary wildly. Some practices might have a dedicated inventory manager, others might have multiple team members who share different responsibilities, and sometimes the practice manager can be the inventory manager. Throughout this text, for simplicity, I'll be referring to a veterinary professional who is tasked with inventory management in some way as an inventory manager.

What makes a good inventory manager? What traits can help you succeed in your role? There are several characteristics of a successful inventory manager. Often, they are detail orientated, organized, and have a passion for seeing the practice succeed. They take ownership of their role and are excited about their "zone" and how they contribute to the practice. They are not only detail oriented but can look at the bigger picture and serve as a visionary for the inventory department.

It's also helpful for this person to be comfortable with spreadsheets, formulas, and calculations. There are a number of important things that should be calculated on a regular basis, both simple formulas as well as more advanced ones. Being comfortable with technology is also important so that the inventory manager can adapt as PiMSs and ordering platforms evolve.

Communication skills are essential in this role. As an inventory manager, it's important to relay information about backorders and product availability to the team. The inventory manager will likely need to discuss new products and alternative medications and provide guidance to the veterinarians about expiring products, duplicate items, or stock-keeping units (SKUs) while feeling confident about engaging in those conversations. It is also important for this person to cultivate and maintain relationships with different supplier and vendor representatives.

There are other helpful skills that may not be as obvious as the aspects mentioned above. One of the interesting parts about managing inventory is that the end goal is an ever-evolving, constantly moving target. There will always be products that need to be replenished, items to organize, and inventory flow to track and control. There are often backorders, new products, discontinued products, vendor changes, and a bazillion other shifts that occur on a regular basis.

As a result, I often find that having an open mind and a certain level of comfort with change is beneficial. I often seen inventory managers excel when they are willing to try different things, explore what works, and recognize patterns that others may not see. Ultimately, the people that thrive in this role learn to get comfortable in the question and feel okay not knowing exactly what the answer is.

Inventory management may not be the best fit for everyone, but a talented inventory manager is worth their weight in gold!

Over the years, throughout my journey working with other inventory managers, I've experienced a range of veterinary professionals who love inventory and others who would love never to place another order in their lives. Occasionally, during these conversations, it will come up that they do not feel as valuable a team member because they aren't directly involved in patient care. They feel that their role is not as important or their team gets frustrated because they do not understand how much inventory managers actually influence the success of the practice, and all they see is someone sitting at a computer.

If that resonates with you, I know exactly how you feel. I have certainly been there myself. I want to not only give you permission that it's okay to love inventory, enjoy creating systems, and really thrive in the more operational aspects of your practice, but I also want to remind you how valuable and important your role is. Even if you aren't directly working with patients or struggle because you are not on the floor as much, you are enabling patient care to thrive. Because of you, your team is able to provide excellent care with all the supplies and medications necessary.

I use this affirmation with my clients. Perhaps it will help you, too.

- I belong.
- My gifts are needed in my practice.
- There is space for my talent and skills.
- There is space for me.

When I first got started in veterinary medicine, I never thought I would love inventory management, let alone be an inventory consultant and educator to other veterinary professionals.

I got my first start in vet med while I was in high school. I was looking for my first job and applied to a number of different businesses. I had never really thought about becoming a veterinarian or working in a veterinary practice; it never crossed my mind as a career path. I was too interested in marine biology and working with whales to consider a long-term career in vet med.

When I started working as a receptionist in a local clinic, I thought it would just get me through high school and maybe college. As time passed, I really got excited about patient care and the medical aspect of interesting cases. As a high school student without experience (my training at the time was very limited), I found myself gravitating toward "the back" treatment area. At the time, I did not comprehend how important the front desk role was and wanted to be a part of the "cool" stuff that happened in the back.

I unwrapped all the IDEXX slides in the morning to make presurgical lab work a bit easier on the team, watched our traveling orthopedic surgeon perform surgery from the viewing window, and sneaked to the treatment room to watch an abscess be drained. I was so interested and curious about everything. Well, except standing in the dark room manually processing radiographs from a barium series for what felt like a decade. I'll admit that wasn't my favorite.

As time passed, I graduated high school in Washington State, moved to Montana, and started at another practice as a receptionist/vet assistant while I was in college. More and more, working in vet med felt like home. I felt like I belonged. I enjoyed the patient care, connecting with clients, and watching puppies turn into adults. I got to be a small part of the family's lives. For me, it felt like a natural fit to become a credentialed technician. I even thought I wanted to be a veterinary technician specialist (VTS) in emergency medicine.

At the time, I was wearing three different hats, splitting my time between inventory manager, receptionist at the front desk, and veterinary assistant. When you think of the cool kids of the vet office, who springs to mind? The vet techs, right? Me too, but as I leaned deeper into becoming a credentialed technician, something felt off. There was something missing for me but I had trouble sorting through it. Becoming a veterinary technician felt like what I *should* do. I'd think, "Everyone else loves patient care. Shouldn't I? It seems like the best job in the building."

At the time, it was hard for me to admit I actually loved working at the front desk. I still miss it to this day! It was even harder to admit that I really enjoyed inventory management. But, as I leaned into that role more and began to process what I truly enjoyed over what I thought I should like, I recognized how much joy I found in connecting with others and being an operator. I got to create systems and structures that served others.

I enjoyed connecting the dots that no one else sees. I enjoyed setting up AVImark, using formulas to calculate reorder points, analyzing margins, and unpacking boxes. I restructured and reorganized almost every single area of that practice. I could not get enough of improving processes, systems, and spaces. I was hooked. It felt so fulfilling to solve puzzles and uncover and improve challenges while also setting my team up for success by making sure they had everything they needed.

Throughout my life, I've always felt like a bit of an outsider – like I was weird. Growing up, I enjoyed doing homework; I liked to learn and was often buried in a book or covering the kitchen table with a craft project. I started a newsletter about shells for my family when I was in elementary school, took a marine biology class at the University of Washington before I could even drive, and my sister remembers me taking apart computers just to put them back together. Sadly, I was bullied growing up. I often felt like I was "too much" or too weird. I felt like I had to hide my interests and joys to be accepted.

So, to admit to myself (and to others!) that I actually enjoyed inventory management and that I loved systems, processes, and continuous improvement felt vulnerable and scary. Sitting at my makeshift desk crunching numbers and building a spreadsheet while the team prepped for surgery, thinking "Wait, this is fun, and I actually enjoy it," as I got a little queasy thinking about admitting it and trying to take up as little space as possible in the room.

What did it mean for me to actually enjoy what other people detested? The stuff that the cool kids did not want to do? To me, inventory had always been the part of the practice that no one wanted. Everyone seemed to cross their fingers and hope they would not have to do that. Admitting that felt like a defining moment in my life. To plant my flag in the ground and say, this is me. This is who I am. I'm good at this. It felt like I stepped into my power (if only a little) and was the start of a journey back to myself and who I really am.

If you had told me at that time that someday I would be an inventory management consultant and educator, write a book, teach others how to manage inventory and create training courses, I would have thought you were from another planet. I probably would have laughed at you; it went against all my beliefs about myself. Now, do not get me wrong, I would not pass up studying and learning about (and from) whales if given the opportunity, But I'm so thankful to the part of me that admitted I loved inventory all those years ago.

"Best Practice" Questions to Consider
- Do you enjoy managing inventory? Why or why not?
- Would you like to see your role evolve or change?
- What skills do you think it would be helpful to develop?

1.9 Creating an Inventory Team

Depending on the size of the practice, it might be vital to have others involved in the inventory process. Their roles and responsibilities may vary depending on the goals, size, and culture of the practice. Ultimately, even with an inventory team, there should be one person who is the lead and responsible for the entire inventory department.

Tasks that could be delegated include the following.

- Cycle counts or end-of-year inventory counts – another team member could be delegated the responsibility of counting throughout the week for cycle counts and then giving the data to the inventory manager for adjustments.
- Department leads could be in charge of monitoring the hospital supply or specialty items within that department and alerting the inventory manager when a particular stock is running low.
- The role of unpacking boxes could be delegated to any available team member to assist with the receiving process.
- Ordering in-house laboratory tests and necessary supply items could be delegated to the laboratory technician.
- The responsibility of compiling an order could be delegated to an inventory team member, and the practice or inventory manager would be responsible for verifying and placing the order.
- For practices with multiple locations, a team member at each location could be in charge of identifying any items that are running low, performing cycle counts, and then reporting the information back to the inventory director.
- A particular team member could be in charge of replacing reorder tags or adjusting reorder bins as the product arrives back in stock.

There are a number of possibilities for delegating inventory management tasks and other responsibilities throughout the practice. If you are considering delegating, think about what absolutely must be done by you and cannot be completed by anyone else. Then, brainstorm any tasks that you love and any that you would prefer not to do. If it's feasible, delegate the tasks that are drudgery for you to complete; someone else might enjoy that task!

It's also helpful to determine your most valuable skills and talents. For example, if you are a veterinarian and practice owner, it might make more sense to step into either a CEO-type role or focus on your patients and delegate managing inventory to another team member. If you are a practice manager or hospital administrator, your time and effort might be better spent on other tasks than performing cycle counts or unpacking boxes, which can be delegated to another team member.

1.10 Getting Your Team on Board

Inventory is definitely a team sport. Although there might be one or two people who are ultimately responsible for inventory, inventory management in your practice will be much more successful when the entire team understands the importance of inventory, follows any applicable processes or procedures, and can extend grace and empathy toward the inventory team. This will be especially important when we first start to manage inventory, as significant time and effort are needed to move the needle forward. This is also the time that the work is most likely to feel thankless. The needle may not move quickly, and it's important for the inventory manager and the entire team to have patience with themselves and each other during this process.

Let's take a look at some situations or scenarios in which getting your team on board with inventory would be helpful.

- You're a practice owner who is learning about proper inventory management and looking at your long-term goals and wants to engage your team and get their buy-in for improvements.

- You're a new practice manager who has a lot of ideas you'd like to try, and getting your team on board is necessary for success.
- You're an inventory manager wanting to implement reorder tags into your inventory, and you need your team to understand and follow the process.

Whatever this might look like for your particular situation, effective communication is key. Over the years, I've developed a conversation framework that I've found to be helpful, especially when having challenging conversations. The MRI-P framework can be used in any conversation, from conveying micro-decisions to high-stakes discussions.

"Best Practice" The MRI-P Framework

M – stands for Mutually Important: what is mutually important? Connect to the "why" and the ultimate vision.

R – stands for Rationale: state the facts, current situation, boundary, or rationale.

I – stands for Insight: offer a solution (for example: "What I can do for you is...") or get them involved in the decision-making process ("Would you like A or B?").

P – stands for Plan: explain the plan or future cast your vision. It can also be helpful to establish a next step or check-in (for example: "We're going to try this for X time, and then I'd love to check in and see how you are feeling").

The first step in this process is to lay the foundation and convey what's mutually important. Help others to understand any context of why you feel changes are necessary and ensure that you are bringing them along on the journey. The key is to really include them in the process and help dispel any negativity that might come up. An example of what this might look like could be as follows.

"I've recently started reading a book on improving our inventory, and I've noticed a few things about our inventory that I think could go better. I've also been learning that managing inventory appropriately is important because ____(explain a few reasons that might resonate with them). With all that I'm learning, there are some areas that I want to work on."

Every person on your team might have a different "why" and it's important to learn more about them and what motivates them. This can help align their "why" with your goal and mission. For example, if you are speaking to the practice owner, maybe their "why" is so they can retire soon and spend more time with their family, maybe they want to make an impact on the veterinary or local community, or maybe they just want to see patients and not worry about the business side.

For other members of the team, maybe their "why" is to care for patients, maybe it's that they want to build a career in veterinary medicine, and maybe it's a job so they can take care of their family. Each person has a different "why" so it's important to understand this on a deeper level; otherwise, this conversation will likely not be as impactful.

The next step of the process is to share the rationale and reasoning behind your conversation. This is a great opportunity to provide context to the conversation and explain the facts and details to the person you are speaking to. Some team members might need more information than others. As an example, if they are a more analytical personality type, they would likely appreciate more details on the situation.

After sharing the rationale, the next step is to provide insight. Depending on the conversation, this might be offering a solution or getting them involved in the decision-making process. I have found that the team is much more engaged when you bring them with you and they feel like they have a voice.

The final step of this process is to share your vision. The key to this is to share your excitement with others about what is possible (if that's appropriate for the conversation). How will this change impact them? How will it improve the practice? This is your opportunity to shine as the advocate and visionary for your inventory and the practice in general.

Now, let's put it all together and see how this might look in your practice.

Situation: an important product has gone on backorder and there is no estimate for when it might be available again. You are currently relaying this information to your veterinarians.

M – Mutually Important: "Ultimately, we are here for our patients, and all of us care deeply about the care we provide..."

R – Rationale: "Unfortunately, XYZ has gone on backorder, and it's not available to purchase right now. I spoke with the distributor and there is no estimated availability. Apparently, there was a material shortage, and both human and veterinary medicine are experiencing the effects of the backorder."

I – Insight: "I was able to find a similar product. For the time being, either ABC or MNO are available. Here's some information I put together on the two different products, along with cost and pricing data. Would you rather I purchase product ABC or product MNO?"

P – Plan: "In addition to ordering the new alternative product, I'll add us to the backorder list for the original product, so as soon as it's available, we will get a shipment of it. I'll keep watch for any additional information as well. In the meantime, I'll add this product to our 'backorder list' and put a note where the product normally is on the shelf."

Here is another example.

Situation: due to the Food and Drug Administration (FDA) Guidance for Industry (GFI) #256, certain compounded medications are no longer available for purchase. An important medication that you stock is no longer available in the strength you normally purchase. After discussing this with your practice owner, you are conveying the information and decision to your team.

M – Mutually Important: "Our patients' safety is our highest priority here, and our clients' trust in us means everything. With that being said..."

R – Rationale: "Recently, the FDA issued some guidelines that impact our compounded medications, so the strength will be changing for XYZ and ABC. I know this is frustrating, but these regulations were put in place to protect our patients."

I – Insight: "What we can purchase is now 50 or 100 mg/ml. Our PO opted for the 50 mg/ml. So starting on (this date), we'll be carrying this new strength moving forward."

P – Plan: "What I'm going to do is create a new code in our system with an alert for the team and create a client handout to tell owners the amount may be changing. Let's plan on reviewing this at our next team meeting to check in. Is there anything else you think might be helpful for the team?"

This last example will hopefully bring this lesson home for you.

Situation: after reading this book, you feel inspired to make some changes in your inventory and want to discuss your ideas and vision with your management team.

M – Mutually Important: "I've recently been reading a book on improving our inventory, and I've noticed a few things about our inventory that could go better. I've also been learning that straightening out our inventory can have a lot of positive effects for our practice. Not only can it reduce the chance of running out and therefore make care easier for our team, but it can also reduce our inventory costs and have a positive impact on the practice's finances."

R – Rationale: "Right now, in our inventory, we order something when it's written down in the 'want book'. It works okay but often things are missed, or our team has to stop what they are doing to write it down."

I – Insight: "What I'd like to do is start calculating reorder points and adding those into our inventory. I'd like to start using a PiMS to monitor low levels and use reorder tags for hospital supplies and white goods. It would benefit us because we would have better inventory tracking, we can actually use the reports in our software, and it would keep us from having too much inventory and reduce the risk of running out."

P – Plan: "With all that I'm learning, there are some areas that I want to work on. I know there will be a time investment upfront for me to make this happen, but here are the goals that I envision for our practice: we aren't running out of things, our inventory costs will go down, and we feel like we have control over our ordering. Normally, I spend ____ hours a week on inventory, but it would be helpful to have an additional ____ hours on Monday. I'd also like to check in with you on my progress and review what I'm working on together. Would that be possible?"

"Best Practice" Questions to Consider
- Are there any important conversations that you'd like to have?
- How does this framework differ from how you would normally have conversations?
- How would you like to adjust your communication with your team moving forward?
- How will you prepare yourself to have these conversations?

It might also be helpful to provide a summary and an action plan for your team members at the end of these meetings. This could include the following.

- What your ultimate vision is for the inventory.
- The goals you'd like to work toward.
- How you'll accomplish your vision and any milestones you'd like to meet along the way.
- Your action plan and how team members can help or support you moving forward.

If it's necessary or would be helpful, I also recommend setting up regular follow-up meetings to check in about progress with your inventory.

Here's a list of fun strategies for getting your team on board and engaged in managing inventory.

- **Create some (friendly) competition**: nothing quite pulls a veterinary team together like food and a little competition. So add in a little contest! If your practice (or a specific department) does not run out of an item in XX number of days, they get a pizza party! You could extend this to controlled substance logs, missed charges, inventory counts – really anything!
- **Add in a fun sign**: do you recall those safety signs from construction sites? The ones that state "This jobsite has experienced XX days since a time-loss incident." You could add a silly version of this sign in your practice as a way to bring awareness and as a lighthearted reminder to keep inventory top of mind. Think: "This practice has not missed a reorder tag in XX days."
- **"Command™ strip" reorder tag bins in convenient locations**: use Command strips to attach little bins to put reorder tags in throughout the practice. You can attach bins to various spots like the storage closet, on the outside of the refrigerator, central supply, inside the cabinet where hospital supplies are stored, etc.
- **Surprise your team with a tasty treat**: Kelly K, one of the wonderful members of the Veterinary Inventory Strategy Network, randomly puts a fun-size piece of candy in a reorder bin so that when someone puts a reorder tag in the bin, they find the tasty treat!

- **Wear a colorful vest**: to help alert your team that you are on "inventory-only" time, wear a neon safety vest as a signal that you cannot be interrupted and it's your time to work on inventory only.
- **Get your team involved**: another helpful strategy is to involve your team so they are invested and take a personal interest in making sure the strategies work. For example, let your team provide input on what products should have reorder tags, and delegate part of the project to someone who shows a lot of interest. Basically, involve your team and make it a fun process!

1.10.1 Co-creating an Inventory Improvement Plan

It can be beneficial to work with your inventory manager or management team, depending on your role, to co-create what I like to call an "inventory improvement plan." Creating a plan of action on how you want to improve your inventory can provide a roadmap and "guiding compass" for your journey. Not only that but when you feel like you are "in the weeds," this document or plan can remind you of the positive direction you are heading in.

Mentorship can be so beneficial for an inventory manager and veterinary professional. When your manager is not only your supervisor but your mentor as well, it opens the door for them to:

- support you through the learning and growth process
- assist you in your professional growth
- understand the elements and learning path that you'll be on
- advocate for you and the improvements to your practice you are working on.

"Best Practice" Inventory Improvement Plan
To kick start creating an "inventory improvement plan," I invite you to schedule a 20–30-minute meeting with your supervisor, management team, or inventory manager. During this meeting you can cover the following points.

- Discuss your current inventory systems. What is working well? What's not working so great? What other observations do you have about your current inventory?
- What goals do you have for the "future state" of your inventory? What would you like to see improved or changed?
- What goals do they have?
- Brainstorm together any ideas you might have for activities that will help reach your inventory goals.
- Keep in mind that you'll be learning many best practices and systems throughout this book, so it's okay if you do not have the answers now.
- Discuss your vision and anticipated outcomes after reading this text. What do you hope to learn? What do you hope to accomplish?
- Set up a regular 1:1 brief check-in to review progress and walk through any challenges or other obstacles that might come up.

1.11 Best Practice Recap

Throughout this chapter, we introduced inventory management, what it means to be an inventory manager, how to involve your team, why inventory management matters in a veterinary practice, and strategies for getting your team on board. Before we dive deeper into the tactics, strategies, and best practices in the following chapters, I want to commend you for taking this on. This process takes so much courage. You are going against the industry status quo of "shake the bottle" training and claiming responsibility for the flow of inventory through your practice. Transforming your inventory can be a massive undertaking, depending on your current situation. Even if they do not say it, everyone in your practice thanks you for doing this work. It simply needs to be done.

I invite you to celebrate your wins, no matter how small or seemingly insignificant! There is no "finish line" for our inventory; unless we change roles, there will always be another order to place or something to improve on. So, knowing that there is not a firm end goal, how can you celebrate what you are accomplishing along the way?

Another thing I invite you to remember is that your inventory will not be fixed overnight. This is an iterative process! If your practice has not had any inventory systems in years (and maybe even decades), it's going to take some time. Small baby steps will start to snowball and all of a sudden, you'll be much further along than you ever thought possible. You can do this!

2

Your Inventory Ecosystem and the Flow of Inventory Through your Practice

To me, helping practices manage inventory is so much more than a job. It's very interesting, very fulfilling, and very rewarding. Helping veterinary professionals and inventory managers feel empowered and confident feels like one of my purposes in life and always "fills up my cup." This work does not just feel like my job; it's bigger than that. So, when I started writing this book, I thought about how I could separate who I am from what this book aims to teach you, but I could not figure out how to do that. There was no way to keep these worlds separate because much of what I share has also shaped who I am, how and why I manage inventory, and informed my path to the place where I am now: an inventory consultant and educator.

Throughout this book, you'll see references to the things that make me, me. You'll read ocean and other creature metaphors. You'll see references to Tank's Animal Hospital in many of the examples. You'll also see references to Heather and other important people in my life. Before we dive deeper into the book, let me share a little bit about them with you.

Let us start with Heather, my younger sister (Figure 2.1). She is my very best friend and I cherish our relationship deeply. She has helped me so much throughout the years that it's hard to put into words the impact that she's had (and continues to have) on me and in my life. She has two kids, Alton and Georgia, who are just the light of my life and are included in different examples throughout the book.

There will also be plenty of ocean references and metaphors. I love the oceans; that's where my soul feels at home. I always feel peace there. I grew up in Washington State, north of Seattle. My grandparents lived on Whidbey Island in a house right on the water of Puget Sound (Figure 2.2). If you aren't familiar with Puget Sound in the Pacific Northwest, it's a body of water that's connected to the Pacific Ocean. The water is fairly cold and although it's connected to the ocean, there aren't any huge waves; the water stays relatively calm and consistent. I grew up swimming in the Puget Sound year-round – I'd get in the water as often as I could.

My dad, sister, and I spent our days digging through tide pools, examining all the tiny sea creatures, searching for the *perfect* shells, flipping over rocks, and looking at crabs, seaweed, and all sorts of species. That precious time is where my love for the oceans began. As I've gotten older, it's the place that I always come back to; the saltwater spray, chilly wind, and wild underwater world – experiencing those things are soul-deep signs that I'm home. I am fascinated by the creatures in the ocean, so do not be surprised if you find a hidden sea creature metaphor tucked away in the caverns of this book.

When I started in practice, I had no idea I was neurodivergent but looking back now with my diagnosis, it makes so much sense. I'm not saying that you have to be neurodivergent to love

Inventory Management for Veterinary Professionals, First Edition. Nicole I. Clausen.
© 2024 John Wiley & Sons, Inc. Published 2024 by John Wiley & Sons, Inc.
Companion website: www.wiley.com/go/clausen/inventory

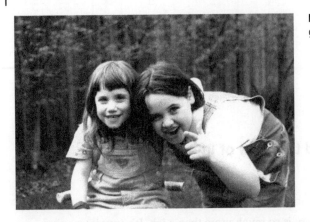

Figure 2.1 Heather (left) and me (right) growing up. Nicole Clausen.

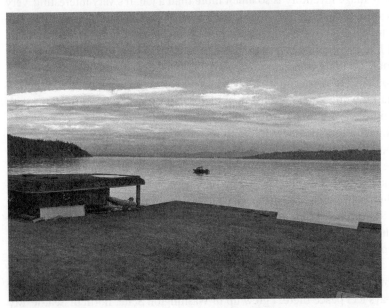

Figure 2.2 The view of Puget Sound from my grandparent's house on Whidbey Island, Washington. Nicole Clausen.

inventory. Still, after taking inventory of my personality, I can see where my neurodivergent traits have helped me align with this role. I enjoy puzzles and investigating categorizations, especially when something is off or does not make sense. I love numbers, calculations, and spreadsheets. My brain is able to quickly pick up on why something is not working and identify what needs to happen to correct it. Patterns, patterns, patterns. Are you sensing a pattern?

But, with some of the superpowers that come with being neurodivergent, there are also challenges. I can get lost in hyperfocus mode, which comes in handy sometimes (see finishing this book) but it wasn't so great when I had big projects that I hyperfocused on *and* other tasks to be responsible for at the same time. My brain just works differently in a lot of ways. I have not always been aware of these factors and because of that, I used to struggle (maybe even in things that I was good at).

I've never had the experience of working with managers or supervisors who were familiar with or understood neurodivergence, and I have not always been good at advocating for myself. I'm sharing this with you for two reasons. First, I hope it gives a little insight into my brain as you read

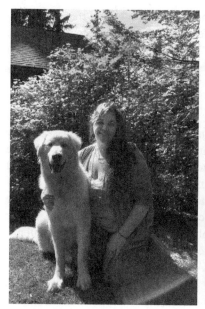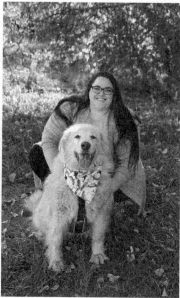

Figure 2.3 A picture of Tank and me as we grew up together, taken 11 years apart. Tank passed away in my arms four months after the image on the right was taken. Nicole Clausen.

my strategies and theories on inventory management. But also, if you are neurodivergent, I hope you know that you are not alone. There are many skilled inventory managers who also have neurodivergent superpowers.

As for Tank? I've saved the best for last. Throughout the book, you'll see references to Tank's Animal Hospital in honor of my sweet Tank. Tank was my heart and soul dog; he was there through so many difficult and beautiful moments for nearly 13 wonderful years. He was always by my side (except when it snowed, he'd go play and lounge in the cold while I stayed warm indoors). From the day he came home to the day he passed, he was big, fluffy, mischievous, silly, and kind (Figure 2.3). He lived an incredibly full life and made friends with everyone he met. He passed away by my side shortly before his 13th birthday. I wanted to include him in this book as a tribute to the greatest dog that ever lived.

For me, helping veterinary professionals is a job that allows me to make use of these other important parts of myself. It feels like more than just the work I do: It's a thing that's allowed me to learn and integrate parts of myself that did not always feel like they fit. All these different pieces of me have shaped and informed how my brain works, how I set up inventory systems, and ultimately, how I teach others to set up their own systems and structures.

2.1 Your Inventory (and Practice) is an Ecosystem

I like to think about inventory, or really our practice, as an ecosystem. Every aspect, every team member, and every function is essential and serves a purpose in the role of caring for our patients. Whether you are a veterinarian, a kennel attendant, a client service rockstar, a practice administrator, or any role in between, what you do matters and impacts your clients, patients, and, ultimately, your community. The same is true for our inventory.

Inventory has different moving pieces, different functions, and different tasks that ultimately come together to support patient care. As I shared earlier, I feel at home and at peace in the ocean. It's full of life and teeming with systems, structures, and organisms. Our inventory is like an ecosystem, much like a thriving coral reef.

2.1.1 Understanding Inventory as a Coral Reef

We have very foundational systems, like ordering, replenishment, receiving, organizing, selling, or using our inventory, etc. These are at the very core and heart of inventory management; they are the rock formations that support the entire coral reef ecosystem. Without these, our ecosystem and inventory would start to crumble or, at the very least, not function well.

Then, we have our ancillary systems. Although not absolutely critical to our inventory, they serve a vital role and function. These are like all the diverse species of fish and coral in a reef. In our inventory, these systems or structures might be like a policy on adding new inventory items. Although not critical, it's helpful to make sure your pharmacy does not balloon. Another might be a system for auditing medical records or limited discounts. Although it's not absolutely necessary, auditing our records helps ensure we are selling inventory appropriately. Our ancillary systems, just like the fish and coral in a reef, help to support the overall ecosystem.

The technology in our practice, the practice management system (PiMS), or other software that you use are the sharks of the reef. They are crucial to the balance of the ecosystem and provide benefits including helpful reports, functions to track the sales or consumption of items, functionality to know when an item should be reordered, and many more. But they are also a predator and eat things. Technology is wonderful when it's working but if your tech is not behaving, it can cause a lot of stress and problems. Also, I totally believe that printers can "sense fear" when you are in a hurry or a rush.

Our patients and the people in our practice (including you!) are like the sun. Coral reefs depend on light for photosynthesis. It provides energy and nourishment for the coral; that's why coral reefs are often in shallower waters to be closer to the much-needed sun. Without you, the inventory manager, or our patients, our inventory systems would cease to exist. Proper inventory management requires people and patients to sustain it. Plus, if you are ever having a tough day, just remember you are the sun. You bring much-needed light to your practice!

Finally, we can think about the flow of microorganisms, nutrients, and algae throughout the coral reef as the flow of inventory in our practice. The flow of nutrients is much-needed food for an incredible array of diverse species of plants and animals in coral reefs. In a similar fashion, the cycle or flow of inventory in our practice is what enables patient care to thrive. The movement of inventory through the foundational systems, like ordering, replenishment, and beyond, is ultimately what effective inventory management is.

You can also think about the flow of water and the tides as the pace at which inventory flows through your practice. If you have a fast flow of inventory, you'll be replenishing the nutrients (products and supplies) much more often than if you have a slower pace. These paces may change with the different seasons: summer and spring versus fall or winter. You might have a different flow or pace during different seasons, and even different items might fluctuate through the year.

Inventory, as with most things in life, is a cycle. It comes into our practice through purchasing and receiving and leaves the practice in a variety of ways, such as consumption, administration, or dispensing to patients or clients. Within that over-arching cycle of inventory, there are also natural ebbs, flows, and cycles on a smaller scale. You might also experience the natural ebb and flow of demand as your practice gains or loses a doctor or sees a quick dip in appointments as families are gearing up for the start of the school year.

Just like a coral reef, our inventory is an ecosystem. There are critical foundations, key systems and structures, people and patients, technology, equipment, and the flow of inventory through your practice. Each piece works together, intertwined. If one starts to struggle or have challenges, it will affect the rest of the ecosystem. For example, let's say that as the inventory manager, your practice is short-handed and you need to spend more time than normal at the front desk. Because your "inventory time" is now limited, you might start noticing more inventory challenges (if you don't have structures of support or processes that you can delegate).

"Best Practice" Understanding the Ecosystem
- Foundational systems: rock formations that support the entire coral reef ecosystem.
  - What are the foundational systems or structures in your inventory?
- Ancillary systems: fish and coral in the reef that help to support the overall ecosystem.
  - What are the ancillary systems in your inventory and practice?
- Technology, software, and PiMS: sharks that balance the ecosystem but can also wreak havoc.
  - What technology, software, and PiMS do you currently use in your practice?
- Patients and team members, including you: the sun that allows coral reef ecosystems to exist.
  - What is your practice's patient population? Who is involved in your inventory?
- Microorganisms, nutrients, and algae: flow and cycles of inventory through the practice.
- The flow of water and tides: the pace of flow of inventory.
  - At what pace does inventory flow through your practice? Are you in a busy season for your practice?

2.1.2 Another Way to Think About Inventory

It might also be helpful to think about what I like to call the **PETS acronym**. P stands for people and patients, E is equipment, T is technology, and S is systems and structures. When it comes to your practice and your inventory, you can think about PETS overall.

"Best Practice" Using PETS Acronym
Consider the following questions while mapping out your practice's coral reef system. The PETS acronym plugs in nicely, so addressing these questions can help you understand where the weak spots in your inventory ecosystem might be.

P – Who are the people involved in inventory management? Who are our patients? What type of patients does our practice serve?

E – What equipment do we have? How is it maintained? Who is in charge of that?

T – What technology do we use in our practice? Does it function like it should? What are the challenges?

S – What inventory systems do we have set up? What systems would be helpful to implement?

You certainly do not need to have all the answers right now; we are just getting started in this book, my friend! But it can be helpful to think about the acronym both from the viewpoint of an inventory system as a whole and within each aspect of the cycle or flow of inventory in your practice. In the next section, I'll introduce the flow of inventory and how you can utilize each component for your unique practice.

As a reminder, you know your practice the best. You are your own best answer! I am going to be reviewing strategies that I've developed and taught to hundreds (maybe even thousands) of other practices. What is incredible to witness is how these clients add their own unique twists in order to adapt them to their practice. I invite you to be curious about what would work best and how you can add your own razzle-dazzle flavor.

2.2 Introduction to the Flow of Inventory in Your Practice

When I was a brand new inventory manager and learning everything I could, I studied human healthcare inventory management and supply chain management. I realized that healthcare and veterinary inventory have a similar "path" in the facility but, of course, there are plenty of differences as well. As I grew as an inventory manager, I adapted and defined the flow of inventory through a veterinary practice and refined and fine-tuned my systems.

Fast forward to today (after teaching inventory to countless practices), and I've broken down the flow of inventory through your practice into six different parts. Each part of the overall flow has systems and structures of setup, tactics to consider, and important action steps to take on a regular, recurring basis. This flow of the "nutrients" or inventory throughout your practice as a whole depends on each of these six parts acting like a mini ecosystem. If one of these parts does not have systems or is not considered, the flow will start to falter.

The six different "buckets" of inventory management activities and parts of the cycle or flow of inventory in your practice are as follows.

1) Forecasting + purchase planning
2) Efficient ordering + replenishment
3) Receiving + organizing
4) Strategic inventory pricing
5) Appropriate inventory sales + consumption
6) Inventory optimization

Throughout this book, each part of the flow of inventory is discussed in much more detail and depth in a corresponding chapter. Within each chapter, I'll outline various strategies and systems that you can implement in your own practice in order to set up your inventory. In the following section of this chapter, we'll look at an overview of each part of the inventory cycle.

2.2.1 Forecasting + Purchase Planning

Demand forecasting and identifying what's low is what happens prior to ordering and replenishment. This is our "starting point" where we find that something is low and anticipate how much we'll need to order to meet the demand of our practice. Rather than just guessing or relying on a whiteboard to tell us what's running low, we use our previous data in our practice to estimate what we'll need in the future.

Not only can we quantify what "low" means, but we can set up a variety of flags to know exactly when it's low (without relying on someone writing it down), and we can calculate exactly how much to order. It's a very intentional process that uses data to guide our decisions. If your goals for your inventory include running out less, ordering less frequently, or keeping stuff in stock feeling less chaotic, using demand forecasting can help you get there!

"Best Practice" Exercise

Let's explore the PETS model for the "forecast + identify" part of the flow of inventory. You may not know the answers to these questions now, but as you read through this chapter, start to think about and consider these aspects.

- **People and patients**: who will be in charge of this aspect of the cycle and ultimately responsible for it? Will anyone else from the team assist in any of the processes? How will patients impact this part? (Hint: for the "forecast + identify" part, patients affect everything! The type of patients that you see and your hospital's unique demand will significantly impact this part of the cycle.)
- **Equipment**: what equipment will you utilize in this part? What equipment in this part of the cycle requires regular maintenance? What does this look like?
- **Technology**: what technology (software, applications, websites, etc.) will you use to "forecast + identify"?
- **Systems and tasks**: what systems and structures need to be created, set up, and established in this part of the cycle? What tasks need to be completed on an ongoing and regular basis?

2.2.2   Efficient Ordering + Replenishment

Replenishing and ordering your inventory happens once you have discovered an item is low. If you aren't using reorder points in your inventory or relying on someone on your team telling you an item is low, you are probably ordering much more often than you'd like to! The more often that you order, the more time (and indirect labor costs) is spent unpacking and receiving all those orders. Plus, as more and more vendors are adding shipping costs and order minimums, efficient ordering is more important than ever.

In this part of the cycle of inventory, we'll review:

- best practices for ordering
- replenishment techniques
- ordering workflows
- tactics for budgeting
- tips for promotional and bulk ordering.

Now, consider the PETS model for this part of the cycle of inventory. Who are the people involved in these processes or tasks? Is there any equipment that will be necessary? What will this look like? How can you utilize and leverage technology or software to make any processes easier? What systems and tasks will need to be set up or improved?

These strategies can take the guesswork out of ordering and help you feel more confident with exactly what to order. Intentional inventory ordering and replenishment can make it feel much less reactive and chaotic.

2.2.3   Receiving + Organizing

Receiving and organizing your inventory is an important (and sometimes overlooked) aspect of managing inventory. It can seem as though it's "just" unpacking boxes and putting items away, but it's more than that. It's the gateway, the first stop inventory makes in your practice. It's the first step in making sure that the new inventory is not damaged, has an appropriate expiry date, is not short-dated, that temperature-controlled items are handled properly, and that overall, each item is safe for patient care. It's important to organize your inventory when it arrives so that everyone can find what they need and you know exactly what you have on the shelves.

Next, consider the PETS model for this part of the cycle of inventory. Who are the people involved in these processes or tasks? Is there any equipment that will be necessary? What will this look like? How can you utilize and leverage technology or software to make any processes easier? What systems and tasks will need to be set up or improved?

2.2.4   Strategic Inventory Pricing

Strategic pricing ensures that each item is intentionally priced with the profitability of your unique practice in mind. How you price your inventory and your services is a highly personal decision and should be based on your practice's goals, values, and vision. Ideally, not only should they be priced appropriately, but prices should be increased as costs go up or at regular intervals to account for inflation. Additionally, it's helpful to routinely review the pricing on services with inventory items involved (such as anesthetic services, injectables set up by weight class, or chemotherapy administration) and pricing for competitively shopped items.

Now, consider the PETS model for this part of the cycle of inventory. Who are the people involved in these processes or tasks? Is there any equipment that will be necessary? What will this look like? How can you utilize and leverage technology or software to make any processes easier? What systems and tasks will need to be set up or improved?

2.2.5   Proper Inventory Consumption

Selling or consuming the inventory appropriately involves ensuring there are no missed charges, clients are being charged appropriately, and inventory items are linked to their corresponding treatment/service codes. If items are not dispensed appropriately, then counts in the PiMS will not reconcile, and a snowball effect of errors in reports and the PiMS happens. As inventory is sold or used, the amount on the shelf decreases and eventually reaches the minimum reorder point, and the cycle can begin again. Additionally, if inventory is not sold correctly, it could negatively affect the profitability of the practice.

Next, consider the PETS model for this part of the cycle of inventory. Who are the people involved in these processes or tasks? Is there any equipment that will be necessary? What will this look like? How can you utilize and leverage technology or software to make any processes easier? What systems and tasks will need to be set up or improved?

2.2.6   Continuous Inventory Optimization

Optimizing should be done on a regular basis. The Oxford Dictionary states that optimizing means to "make the best or most effective use of (a situation, opportunity, or resource)." When reviewing our costs, we do not want to spend less; we want to make the most of our spending. When stocking our practice, we do not want to stock every item possible; we want to stock intentionally based on what's best for our patients. We do not want to order based on shaking a bottle to "see when it's low," we want to use demand forecasting to make the best use of our inventory investment. One of the foundations for continuously improving your inventory is to evaluate your items regularly.

"Best Practice" Questions for Regularly Evaluating Inventory Items
- Does it make sense to carry this?
- Is it still selling?
- Do I have way too much inventory on the shelf?

Sometimes, we can get caught up in the day-to-day "busyness" of our practice. This aspect of the inventory cycle really focuses on pulling back and looking at our inventory to say, "Where can we improve? How can we make things easier or more efficient?" Carrying out this process along the way, rather than waiting until it feels like the wheels are coming off the bus, can help our inventory and practice run more smoothly.

Now, consider the PETS model for this part of the cycle of inventory. Who are the people involved in these processes or tasks? Is there any equipment that will be necessary? What will this look like? How can you utilize and leverage technology or software to make any processes easier? What systems and tasks will need to be set up or improved?

In each of the chapters related to a part of the inventory cycle, we'll review it much more in-depth, as well as providing insight and strategies for implementing best practices in your unique inventory. If you are feeling a little overwhelmed and thinking, "Where do I even start? My anxiety (and my imposter syndrome) is creeping in!" remember that is completely normal. Then, take a deep breath. I recommend just starting with one project or improvement first rather than trying to tackle them all at once. Just one. If you are not exactly sure where to start, if you do not have reorder points set up or have used them before, that's always an excellent place to dive in first.

It might seem all overwhelming and slightly impossible at first but I invite you to focus on just taking one baby step at a time. Eventually, your baby steps will start to snowball and your inventory will run more smoothly than you ever thought possible. On that note, do not forget to give yourself a pat on the bank and celebrate each win and baby step!

"Best Practice" for Dealing with Overwhelm
1) Take a deep breath.
2) Remind yourself that small steps lead to a big impact. There will always be another order to place, a puzzle to put together, or another goal to work toward, so do not forget to celebrate yourself along the way!
3) Ask for help, take a break, or both!

2.3 Communicating with Your Team

> An ecosystem is sustainable when it is able to adapt to environmental changes, which is made possible by its biodiversity ... Biodiversity has to do with the richness of diverse biological resources and the integration of these resources into a resilient ecosystem. By analogy, we suggest that the complexity of resources is the foundation for the functional capacity and consequent sustainability both in organizations and employees. (Docherty et al. 2008, p. 234)

How we interact with our team in this ecosystem is central to not only the practice's success but our success as an inventory manager. Your team members might not understand the value or importance of managing inventory. It's understandable, as much of what goes into inventory management is unseen by the rest of the team. But there are many instances where the success of our role depends on our ability to communicate with our team.

Thinking back to our coral reef ecosystem, as the nutrients (inventory) flow through the practice nourishing different aspects of our "reef," important information must be distributed amongst the team. Depending on your practice, you might need to:

- discuss with your veterinarians or practice owner when a new product is released
- communicate about products that are backordered or in limited supply

- discuss product or formulation changes
- update your team on products that have been ordered
- review any other policy or workflow changes.

There can be lots of reasons why you'll need to communicate with your team. What might these be for you and your practice? What would be the best way to convey information?

Here are a few ideas to give you some inspiration.

- Create an inventory "command station" with a whiteboard or bulletin board with spots for backordered products and other important information.
- If your practice uses Slack or another similar platform, create a "Backorders" channel or an inventory channel. You could even have a "Want List" channel for team members to add products that need to be ordered.
- Give short updates or relay policy changes during team meetings.
- Use project management software (like Notion, Asana, or ClickUp) to connect specifically with your inventory team. You can also use the system to delegate tasks, monitor project progress, and more.

With this in mind, we need to discover how we fit into a well-functioning whole alongside other individuals. This does not necessarily mean sharing everything with your co-workers. It does mean understanding that everyone in your practice comes with various skills, knowledge, mental models, beliefs, and perceptions. As an author, I'm also trying to support this diversity in you, the reader. I hope that by showing you what I've found works over the years, you'll be able to design and thrive in a healthy ecosystem that works for your unique practice, too.

2.4 Inventory Manager Spotlight

Meet Bree Henry, CVIP!

"When it comes to managing our inventory, it's always at the forefront of my mind! However, understanding that the rest of my team does not always prioritize the inventory process due to their diverse responsibilities and workload has been a realization. It's unrealistic to expect them to focus on inventory as much as I do.

To address this, I've adopted a communication strategy with constant dialogue in various forms. Recognizing that everyone absorbs information differently, we utilize a Group Me inventory chat thread, tasks in our PiMS, a whiteboard with current backorder information, a Google sheet on every desktop dedicated to inventory wants/needs, and reorder tags. Through these channels, I consistently relay information to keep my team updated on inventory developments.

This multifaceted approach not only saves them time in seeking answers but also aims to alleviate stress by ensuring they are well informed without having to actively seek out information from me. It's about creating a streamlined and accessible flow of information regarding inventory, acknowledging and respecting the different ways team members prefer to receive updates."

Inventory has different moving pieces, different functions, and different tasks that ultimately come together to support patient care. Our inventory ecosystem, just like a coral reef, functions to help move inventory efficiently and effectively throughout our practice.

3

Introduction to Demand Forecasting and Reorder Points, the Foundation of Our Ecosystem

3.1 Author's Note/Story

I remember very vividly when I first discovered reorder points (ROPs). Prior to using ROPs, I would wander around the pharmacy and other storage areas, literally shaking bottles and trying to guess "Is this low?" or "Should I order this?" That's how I placed my weekly order. I walked around, physically shook containers and bottles, and guessed if they should be ordered. It certainly was not an exact science by any stretch of the imagination! Not only that, but it took a long time because I had to inspect every single item in the practice. It was a huge guessing game, and I constantly worried that I was forgetting to order something or that I guessed wrong and we were about to run out.

Turns out, I would forget to order things often. I would realize the following day "Shoot, I forgot to order metronidazole injectable. Let me order it today." Or I would get a text on my day off letting me know that we had run out of something, or a team member would call to ask if something was ordered and when it was supposed to come in. Needless to say, the entire process did not work well for me or my team. So I took matters into my own hands.

As I started calculating and implementing ROPs, it revolutionized the way I managed inventory. Right away, I realized the demand (how much was used or sold) was fairly consistent for most items. It was even predictable. As I viewed the sales history for particular items, I saw that, on average, we sold a relatively similar amount each month. That applied to pharmaceuticals, hospital supplies, in-house reference laboratory supplies, and basically anything that was either consumed or sold. There were only a very tiny number of items that did not follow suit.

For the first time, I was able to quantify what "low" meant for each item, and I was no longer constantly guessing "Is this low? Is that low?" I knew.

I'll bet if you ask each of your team members "What does low mean for gabapentin 100 mg?" you are likely to get a different answer from each person. Low is subjective, so using previous sales or purchase data to quantify what low means can change the game in your inventory.

Now, fast forward quite a few years. What's even more meaningful and memorable is teaching other inventory managers and veterinary professionals about the power of ROPs. I remember working with a very dear client of mine, one of my very first, and she had a similar experience to me. She shook bottles to see what was low, and up until our work together, she did not have much training but wanted to do better for her practice.

As we were working together, I introduced the concept of ROPs and showed her how to find the information using sales data and how to calculate what she needed based on those numbers.

Inventory Management for Veterinary Professionals, First Edition. Nicole I. Clausen.
© 2024 John Wiley & Sons, Inc. Published 2024 by John Wiley & Sons, Inc.
Companion website: www.wiley.com/go/clausen/inventory

I could see the lightbulb go on. Her whole demeanor changed. I could see the confidence start to settle in as she realized "I can actually do this! There is hope!" My career path as an inventory consultant was solidified at that moment.

"Best Practice" Reorder Points Guiding Principles
- Do not wait for it to be perfect.
- Let it be easy and do not overcomplicate it. Overcomplicated does not necessarily mean better!

Since then, one of my favorite things to teach other inventory managers is calculating and using ROPs. They are fun to calculate, and I enjoy seeing the enormous impact that just one calculation can make!

Over the years, I've seen several different ways to calculate ROPs. As with most things in life, there is no one best way; there are pros and cons to each option. Something else to note here is that **it does not have to be perfect**. There is no perfect way. I find that occasionally if I cannot do it perfectly, I would rather not do it at all. I want to wait until it can be absolutely perfect before moving forward with it, but that does not actually help

Using ROPs is a dynamic and iterative process. You might calculate a ROP for rabies vaccine this month and in eight months, you'll need to calculate it again because you have gained two veterinarians. As you explore this chapter, think about what a "good, better, best" scale would look like in your practice and just start, even if it's your top 10 items or just your vaccinations. Something is better than nothing, and waiting on such a game-changing tactic until it is perfect will be a waste of time.

My second invitation is to remember it can be easy. I've seen veterinary professionals, consultants, accountants, and other speakers in vet med really overcomplicate order points over the years. It does not have to be complex in order to be impactful. I tend to find the opposite is true: **The more complex it is, the less helpful it is**. Complexity is not sustainable and it's often not a lasting solution. If we remember our two main goals, to have what we need on hand for patient care but also to keep profitability in mind, that's what is most important.

"Best Practice" Inventory Goals Reminder
- Keep what we need on hand for patient care.
- Keep profitability in mind.

In this chapter, you'll be introduced to several different methods for calculating ROPs. I recommend trying the different calculations and seeing what works best for you and your practice. Is there one method that makes sense to you? Is there another way you'd like to try as you get more familiar and comfortable with ROPs? We do not have to overcomplicate anything in our inventory just because all we have seen are complex, challenging, or confusing systems.

I prefer my inventory to be simple, intentional, and sustainable over complicated and complex any day.

3.2 Introduction to Demand Forecasting

Demand forecasting is the process of using data and information to predict how much inventory you'll sell or use in the future. Essentially, it's looking at the past to make an educated guess about what's coming. Calculating ROPs is a large part of demand forecasting, where we use previous purchase history or sales/consumption data to predict what you'll use in the future. It tells us what to order.

I like to compare demand forecasting with holiday baking and grocery shopping. Let's say you want to whip up a beautiful spread of home-made cookies for your loved ones. You pore over recipe books to find exactly what you want to make. You find delightful chocolate truffles, delicious triple ginger cookies, yummy frosted sugar cookies, and you want to try your hand at making English toffee. Would you write down what you want to make and then run to the grocery store without a list of what you'll need? "Hmm ... let's grab a package of butter, some chocolate, and some eggs" ... and you throw some other things in the cart that look good.

Probably not.

Before heading to the grocery store, you'd likely create a list of all the ingredients you need and the exact amounts you'll need after comparing what's currently in your pantry. Then, when you got to the store, you'd know exactly what and how much of each item to purchase.

That's the goal with our inventory! We can use our previous sales information (our "recipes") to predict what we'll likely need in the future. As an example, let's say that in the past three months, you have sold 2000 capsules of gabapentin. It's likely (unless another veterinarian joins your practice) that in the next three months, you'll sell a similar amount of gabapentin. The concept of demand forecasting creates the foundation of our inventory strategy and purchasing within our practice.

You might be thinking "There is no way we could try and predict what we use! Everything varies so much!" This might be the case, but I invite you to explore the concept of demand forecasting. In my experience, I've found that, generally speaking, 90% of our items have predictable sales or consumption patterns. I remember as I was calculating ROPs for hospital supplies, I realized that every month, without fail, I would order about 20 sleeves of gauze squares. I could order the item multiple times throughout the month but in the end, I always ordered around 20 sleeves. Armed with this realization, I started digging more into my hospital supply purchases and found similar results.

As a result, I was able to calculate ROPs and develop order flags so that I knew when something was low without having to go digging through cabinets and drawers. Purchasing hospital supplies became much more streamlined and systematized, and my sleep got better as a result. Plus, I like doing things less often with bigger results. I saved a lot of time purchasing for the month rather than randomly ordering a few sleeves of gauze here and there.

Let's explore demand forecasting together.

3.3 Demand Forecasting and Purchase Planning

Demand forecasting is the process of using historical sales and usage data to develop an estimate or forecast for what your practice will use or need in the future. It helps to shift practices from reactive ordering ("Oh no! We ran out, let us order a bunch") to proactive ordering. It really allows you to thoughtfully plan what you purchase.

Before I discovered ROPs, so much of my day was taken up by the mental weight of tracking our inventory in my brain. It did not matter how much effort I put in, I'd still fall short. I'd often forget to order something, which meant returning to the closet, shaking bottles, and placing another order. What I needed was a better method. Enter ROPs. Suddenly, I felt confident that we'd be well stocked and in control of the inventory. Because my mind wasn't always partly focused on inventory, I was able to be more present with the patients, clients, and team throughout the day.

You deserve to feel in control of your ordering; demand forecasting can help you get there.

Demand forecasting is the cornerstone of your inventory management strategy. It builds the foundation for what we need to order and when, so we do not have to rely on someone to guess what's low. It does not feel great when someone took the last of something, didn't tell you, and now is mad that you do not have it. Estimating how much we'll use in the future can help us step away from that uncomortable situation.

"Best Practice" Ultimate Goals of Demand Forecasting
- Understand how much you are using or selling of each item in your practice.
- Know when you should order something (without the "want book").
- Calculate how much of something you should order and plan what you'll purchase.

Many veterinary practices rely on team members to write it on "the list" if they think it's running low. Trying to manage inventory that way does not set anyone up for success. First and foremost, it requires teammates to guess what's low. Second, they are likely focused on patient care and will not understand the needs of the practice. If you are currently leaning on this method, you are in for a treat with ROPs!

3.4 Determining When an Item Needs to be Ordered

The first part of demand forecasting is about recognizing when something needs to be ordered and answering the question "What does low mean?" There are a number of different ways to answer this question, so be curious about what method might work best for you and your practice.

Methods that aren't reliable for knowing what's low.

- The "bottle shaking method."
  - Definition: shaking bottles or digging through cabinets to see what is low.
  - The problem: it's subjective. Every team member has different definitions for "low" for different items. Plus, there is often a disconnect between what a team member thinks is low and the needs of the whole practice.
  - The fix: use demand forecasting to quantify and standardize what "low" means.
- The "want book."
  - Definition: relying on the fact that other team members will write an item in the book when it's "low."
  - The problem: it's subjective, like the "bottle shaking method," and if someone does not write something in the book, it does not get ordered and the practice might experience a stockout. It can also be a point of frustration for the team.
  - The fix: set up reorder flags and utilize ROPs for a more proactive approach.

Let us dive in. **A ROP is the level of inventory at which a particular item should be ordered**. This is also considered the **minimum inventory level**. An easy way to remember this is the point at which something should be ordered. A ROP is unique to that particular item and can vary depending on the season, the growth of the practice, the addition of new veterinarians, and more. Once ROPs are calculated and implemented, I recommend recalculating them quarterly to biannually (at a minimum), and whenever a veterinarian joins or leaves the practice.

Most items in a veterinary practice have a fairly consistent demand or usage. About 5–10% of your products might have some seasonal shift or other reasons for swings in demand. Surprisingly enough, I've also found this to be true for emergency practices. However, an ER practice might have a slightly higher percentage of items with inconsistent demand than a clinic that focuses mostly on general practice. So, if you are an emergency or specialty practice, you still benefit from ROPs!

Some products that might not remain steady throughout the year include seasonal products like flea/tick medication and heartworm prevention for cold winter areas. Warmer, humid climates might see an increase in allergies and the need for dermatology products in the springtime. Practices that treat large animals like livestock and equine will likely see an increase in demand during foaling, calving, and herd health management seasons.

Other products include emergency medications for smaller or GP locations. As an example, you might not order epinephrine when it's "low" but instead when the bottle is about to expire. For large emergency practices, you might use this product much more frequently, and ROPs might make more sense for maintaining the correct inventory.

As we explore ROPs and demand forecasting, I invite you to think about your top products (that we identified in Chapter 1) and how you might use ROPs for these items. I would also suggest thinking about items that might need special care (like seasonal products) or items that your practice cannot function without.

3.5 Utilizing Your Sales and Usage to Forecast Demand

At the very core and foundation of your inventory management strategy is using your practice's usage or sales history to estimate and forecast your demand. Returning to the metaphor of our inventory as a coral reef ecosystem, ROPs are the rock formations that uphold the entire coral reef. They are an integral part of our inventory and are the backbone of the whole flow and cycle of inventory in our practice.

It's so helpful (and important!) to use the information for your unique practice from your practice management system (PiMS), software, or other reporting processes when developing your inventory strategy. Utilizing usage and sales history allows you to make data-informed decisions and strategically order, stock, and manage all phases of inventory. Using data can help us find the delicate balance between having what we need in stock for our patients and keeping the financial performance of our practice in mind.

Sometimes when we are working day to day in our practice, we might have some assumptions about how much we are using or selling. We might think "Wow, we never use this product" or "We go through these items like water," but once we review our sales reports, a more accurate picture is painted and it might turn out to be the opposite of what we expected. That's why bringing in sales or purchase information for our order point calculations is so beneficial.

Historical sales data can typically be found in your PiMS. Even if you have not used the inventory module in your software system, most practices use their practice management software system to invoice clients and maintain accurate medical records. As a result, there is often data available to calculate ROPs and reorder quantities.

There are a few cases where the information from your software or similar reports might be inaccurate. First, if you sell a particular injection as a flat charge (for example, sedation <50 lb or vitamin B injection) and your software does not track or pull from inventory how many units were administered, your sales information might be incorrect. Another example is for products that are both sold and used in-house (like an ear cleanser). You will be able to identify how many units have been sold but not necessarily how many have been consumed and used in-house.

"Best Practice" Questions to Consider
- Are there any products or items where the sales history or information might be inaccurate or not show the full picture?
- How can you keep these items in mind as you start to calculate your ROPs and forecast your demand?

If sales or usage information is not available from your PiMS or similar reports, your purchase history from your distributors or vendors can be helpful.

For products that aren't sold, like hospital supplies, syringes, needles, and other white goods, you'll want to use the purchase history from your distributor for calculations.

The downside of using purchase history, rather than sales history, for items that are dispensed is that if any overordering has happened, it will be perpetuated with the ROP calculations. If you suspect that you have had instances of overordering in your inventory before, I strongly encourage you to use as much sales data as you have available to you and make informed decisions. Try to take the guesswork out as much as possible, and when it's not possible, remember that this is a practice. It might take a couple of cycles to sync up with your specific practice's ordering needs

For pharmaceuticals, injections, vaccines, diets, and other things that are dispensed in your software and have sales data available, most PiMSs have reports that calculate the total usage or sales for a particular time period. This can be very helpful. Using the data from these reports, ROPs and reorder quantities can be calculated. Once this information is calculated, you can identify what "low" means for that specific item. You can add a flag in your software to alert you when the "low" threshold is reached, and the reorder quantity tells you how much to order for the next cycle.

3.6   Methods for Calculating Reorder Points

Helpful definitions
- **Lead time**: lead time is the time between when you realize a product is low and when it's received and ready to be sold. It's essentially the waiting time after you have discovered it's low.
- **Safety stock**: a backup supply or extra "cushion" of inventory just in case. It's additional inventory beyond what you would normally keep as "insurance" against any unexpected situations.
- **Average daily use**: the amount that your practice uses or consumes in a typical day. For example, among all my dogs, they eat about four cups of food a day. Their average daily use of dog food would be four cups.

There are several different methods for calculating ROPs, but there are two main ways I find most helpful. The first method is more precise and uses your average daily use, lead time, and safety stock preferences to determine reorder levels. Your average daily use for an item is calculated, and then that is multiplied by the lead time.

Typically, lead time is the number of days it takes for an order to be delivered after it has been placed. But in the case of ordering in veterinary medicine, it's also important to take into account the number of days between when something becomes "low" and when it will be ordered next. Here, the lead time is the number of days between when an item is flagged low and when it has arrived and is ready to sell to clients. The goal with the "lead time" method is to have enough stock on hand so that you will not run out between when an item is low and when it arrives.

Safety stock should also be factored into this equation. Safety stock is a level of inventory that is maintained for "just in case" situations and acts as a buffer. Having a buffer can be helpful in situations like delayed shipments, backorders, or other unexpected events. Have you ever kept a few IV primary lines or a backup box of syringes hidden away in your office? Likely without realizing it, that's an example of safety stock.

As an example, I live in Montana and the winters can be frigidly cold with consistently negative temperatures. For anything that has strict temperature controls (like for in-house laboratory analyzers), I would have an extra buffer of safety stock just in case that item froze and a replacement needed to be ordered. The extra safety stock helped me not run out a number of times when there were shipping delays or replacement products needed to be ordered.

The second method for calculating ROPs is based on what you would use in a specific time frame, such as a two-week supply. I've found that setting your ROP or minimum supply to order when you have a two-week supply left is a great place to start. This is helpful because, let us say, you order once a week on Monday, and then on Tuesday or Wednesday, you find that you are running low. You would not reorder until the following Monday, so you would need enough stock on hand to last until you place your next order, time for the shipment to arrive, and a little extra buffer stock.

Using the **time-frame method** is an excellent way to get started with ROPs and get comfortable with what works in your practice and what does not. If your practice is growing rapidly, I often suggest trying a three-week supply as your ROP because your three-week supply becomes a two-week supply very quickly.

There are pros and cons to each method. The lead time method is helpful because it allows you to be more precise and customize the safety stock or lead time. This can be helpful for items where the lead time is longer (such as Class II controlled substances or specialty products that may take longer to ship). The downside is that it is more complex and harder to calculate the ROP for an item in your head. Since this method is a bit more complicated, that can be a barrier to getting ROPs set up and implemented.

The specific time-frame method is helpful because it's an easy and relatively quick calculation. The downside of using this method is that it is not as flexible and customizable, although you can make it more adaptable by using different time periods for different categories. As an example, your pharmaceuticals that come from your distributor could be a two-week supply, but specialty items that take longer to ship could have a ROP set to order when there is a three- or even four-week supply on hand.

Both of these order point methods are tools for forecasting your demand. Both methods will use your sales or purchase history to give an idea of how much you'll use in the future. In most cases, I help people use the time-frame method first and then add the lead time method if they want to refine and add more precision to their ROPs. I suggest and recommend practice calculating order points for your top five products using both methods and consider your unique practice before making a final decision on which formula to use.

At the end of the day, calculating and implementing ROPs will be a game-changer for your practice. I recommend starting with whatever method you feel most comfortable with. You can always iterate and improve on this process later, so try not to let the fear of it not being perfect keep you from getting started.

Throughout this process, it's important to remember the inventory mindsets. Do not be afraid to try new and different things in your practice! Be curious; see what works well and what does not work so well for your unique situation. I've seen different types of ROPs and different ROP calculations work differently in practices across the country. Be a detective. Sometimes it's easy to get frustrated when something does not work and think "Ugh, I'm bad at managing inventory," but it's more productive and kind to think like a detective. Think to yourself "This did not work as well as I'd hoped. Why did that happen? What can I do moving forward to improve it?"

3.6.1 Calculating Reorder Points: Time-frame Method

Generally speaking, a good guideline to use is this: when you have two weeks' worth of stock on hand, that item is considered low and it's time to reorder. The concept of setting your "low" or minimum level for a two-week supply is that, in an effort to order weekly, you would have enough stock to get through another ordering cycle, plus a small buffer.

As mentioned earlier, this time period can be adjusted from two weeks to another time period that makes more sense for your practice.

$$Reorder\ point = \frac{units\ sold\ or\ purchased\ in\ time\ period}{number\ of\ two\text{-}week\ periods\ in\ time\ period}$$

Generally, I recommend calculating ROPs using your annual usage. This gives you a solid average over the course of 12 months. But there are some cases where it makes sense to shorten that time period. Is your practice going through a high-growth phase or has a veterinarian recently left or joined your practice? Consider a shorter time-frame. Typically, I do not recommend calculating ROPs with anything less than three months' worth of data.

The first step in this process is to find an item's annual (or another time-frame that makes the most sense) usage. This information can be found in your PiMS for items that are sold and dispensed. Typically, most software systems will have a report that shows the quantity sold over a time period for each item in your inventory.

For items that are consumed or used but not sold, like hospital supplies, white goods, syringes, etc., this information can be found by using the purchase history from your distributor. Many distributors have previous purchase information displayed for each item on their ordering platform.

The second step is to divide the annual (or other time-frame) usage into two-week segments (or other time periods that you'd prefer) (Table 3.1).

- Step 1: find your annual usage.
- Step 2: calculate your two-week supply by dividing the annual usage by 26. The reason the annual usage is divided by 26 is because there are 26 two-week periods in a year.

$$Two\text{-}week\ supply = \frac{annual\ usage\left(or\ purchases\right)}{26}$$

At this stock level, this particular inventory item is now considered low, and once the threshold has been reached, it's time to reorder. As mentioned previously, the two-week "rule" is a guideline and, depending on your unique practice, can be increased or decreased depending on the goals of the practice.

If you are using a short usage duration (such as three months), the process will be the same; you'll just want to adjust your variables. Let us examine an example of finding the two-week supply over a three-month period.

$$Two\text{-}week\ supply = \frac{units\ sold\ or\ purchased\ in\ three\ months}{6.5}$$

Table 3.1 Two-week periods in different numbers of months.

Number of months	Number of two-week periods
3	6.5
6	13
12	26

Let's try an example: Tank's Veterinary Hospital recently added a new veterinarian to the team. They were also voted the "Best Veterinarian in the PNW," so they have been much busier lately and are seeing more patients. They almost ran out of rotors so Georgia, the inventory manager, wanted to recalculate the ROP. Since their practice is in a high-growth phase, she decided to calculate the ROP using the last three months of sales data. Their practice has used 87 in-house chemistry rotors in three months. Let us calculate the two-week supply to find the ROP.

$$Two\text{-}week\ supply = \frac{units\ sold\ or\ purchased\ in\ 3\,months}{6.5}$$

$$Two\text{-}week\ supply = \frac{87}{6.5}$$

$$Two\text{-}week\ supply = 13.38 \approx 13$$

When Tank's Veterinary Hospital reaches 13 in-house chemistry rotors, they are low and should be reordered.

If, while calculating your ROP, it results in a very small number (i.e., four capsules), there are a couple of things to keep in mind. First off, a ROP that low means that the annual usage is very low. Should this product continue to be stocked? If so, then with a low ROP, I recommend increasing it to an average-size dose for that prescription. For example, if an antibiotics ROP was calculated at five capsules, I would increase it to a seven- or 14-day course.

3.6.1.1 Reorder Point Example: Rabies Vaccines

In this example, Tank's Animal Hospital has used 1476 vials of rabies vaccine in the last 12 months. To find the average two-week usage, divide 1476 vials by 26.

$$Two\text{-}week\ supply = \frac{annual\ usage}{26}$$

$$Two\text{-}week\ supply = \frac{1,476}{26}$$

$$Two\text{-}week\ supply = 56.8 \approx 57\ vials$$

In this example, once Tank's Animal Hospital reaches the inventory threshold of 57 vials of rabies vaccines, it's now considered low and time to reorder.

3.6.1.2 Reorder Point Example: Boxes of Syringes

In this example, Tank's Animal Hospital has purchased 71 boxes of 3 cc syringes in the last 12 months. To find the two-week usage, divide 71 boxes by 26 (the number of two-week periods in 12 months).

$$Two\text{-}week\ supply = \frac{annual\ purchases}{26}$$

$$Two\text{-}week\ supply = \frac{71}{26}$$

$$Two\text{-}week\ supply = 2.7 \approx 3\ boxes$$

In this example, once Tank's Animal Hospital reaches the inventory threshold of three boxes of 3 cc syringes, it's now considered low and time to reorder.

If you have not calculated ROPs before, I invite you to calculate ROPs for five different products using the "two-week supply" method and see what the result is.

"Best Practice" Questions
- How do these ROPs compare with how you are purchasing now?
- Is there anything that surprised you?
- Are there any challenges or roadblocks you anticipate when it comes to order point calculations?

3.6.2 Calculating Reorder Points: Lead Time Method

Let's move on to the lead time method, which is a multi-step process. The first step in this method is to determine your average daily use. Once this has been calculated, it can be multiplied by the lead time, or the number of days between an item being flagged as low and when it has been received and is ready to sell. In addition, it's essential to include any safety stock or buffer in this calculation.

Even if you decide that the lead time method is not the best for you or your practice, I invite you to consider the concept and be familiar with the average daily use of your products and how this can help you. Knowing how much you sell or use in a day, a week, or even a month can help provide context when ordering and encourage data-informed ordering decisions to be made.

- Step 1: find your annual usage or purchases.
- Step 2: calculate the average daily use.

To calculate the average daily use, you'll divide your annual usage or purchases by the number of days the practice is open in a 12-month period (Table 3.2).

$$Average\ daily\ use = \frac{annual\ usage\ or\ purchases}{number\ of\ days\ open\ per\ year}$$

3.6.2.1 Average Daily Usage Calculation Example

In this example, Tank's Animal Hospital has sold 9512 capsules of gabapentin 300 mg in a 12-month period. This practice is open five days a week (260 days open, a total of 365 days).

$$Average\ daily\ use = \frac{annual\ usage}{number\ of\ days\ open\ per\ year}$$

Table 3.2 Breakdown of the number of days open per year based on the number of days open during the week.

Days open in the week (d)	Days open in the year (d)
4	208
5	260
6	312
7	365

Table 3.3 Example calculation of the lead time (in number of days) for Tank's Animal Hospital.

Sunday	Monday	Tuesday	Wednesday	Thursday	Friday	Saturday
		AM: Order placed PM: Item flagged low	*Day One*	*Day Two*	*Day Three*	*Day Four*
CLOSED	*Day Five*	*Day Six* Order placed	*Day Seven*	*Day Eight*	*Day Nine* Order received	

$$Average\ daily\ use = \frac{9,512\ capsules}{260\ days}$$

$$Average\ daily\ use = 36.58 \approx 37\ capsules\ per\ day$$

- Step 3: calculate the lead time.

In this step, calculate the lead time for this particular product. The easiest way to do this is to count the number of days between when an order could be flagged low and when that order would be received and ready to sell.

Let's examine an example; in Table 3.3, Tank's Animal Hospital places an order once weekly and the supplier has a three-day shipping time. If an item were flagged low on Tuesday afternoon or Wednesday, it would not be ordered until the following Tuesday. Then, the order would not arrive until Friday.

In this example, the lead time for this particular product is nine days. This can vary slightly depending on whether the order was placed before or after the cutoff time. I prefer to calculate the lead time as if I were to place the order after the cutoff.

Table 3.4 is an example from Ollie's Veterinary Hospital, which orders twice a week and is open five days per week. This particular item has a two-day shipping time and the lead time is five days.

Once the lead time has been calculated, the average daily use should be calculated by the lead time. Products that are purchased from the same supplier will have the same lead time. A helpful tip for this process is to calculate the lead time based on each supplier.

- Step 4: multiply the average daily use by the lead time.

In the fourth step, multiply the average daily use by the lead time to find the ROP. Keep in mind that there is no safety stock or cushion in case there is a high demand week or there are any shipping delays.

$$Reorder\ point = average\ daily\ use \times lead\ time$$

Table 3.4 An example from Ollie's Veterinary Hospital, which orders twice a week and is open five days per week. This particular item has a two-day shipping time.

Sunday	Monday	Tuesday	Wednesday	Thursday	Friday	Saturday
	AM: Order placed PM: Item flagged low	*Day One*	*Day Two*	*Day Three* Order placed	*Day Four*	CLOSED
CLOSED	*Day Five* Order received					

From previous steps, it was calculated that Tank's Animal Hospital uses 37 capsules of gabapentin 300 mg per day and has a nine-day lead time for this particular product.

Reorder point = average daily use × lead time

Reorder point = 37 capsules × 9 days

Reorder point = 333 capsules

In this example, the ROP for gabapentin 300 mg is 333 capsules. That means once the on-hand amount reaches that threshold, it's considered low and should be ordered. **I HIGHLY recommend adding a buffer or safety stock into this calculation**, which we'll review in Section 3.6.3.

As you saw in one of the above examples, if a practice orders twice per week, their ROP is only five days' worth of stock. I often find that for many practices, that is too "lean" and causes extra stress for the inventory manager and increases the chance of running out. In the following section, we'll review the concept of safety stock, how it's helpful, and how you can layer that onto your ROPs.

"Best Practice" Concepts Check
- When is it best to use the lead time method?
- When is it best to use the time-frame method?
- Which method do you feel most comfortable with so far?
- Which method best fits your practice's needs?

3.6.3   Calculating Safety Stock in the Lead Time Method

Safety stock is a level of extra inventory or buffer to safeguard in case of backorders, delayed shipping, or any other unexpected events. A safety stock cushion can be added to the ROP to give extra leeway for those circumstances or items that you do not want to run out of.

You might already be adding safety stock to your inventory without even realizing it! Some examples of safety stock that you might not realize: the extra bottle of euthanasia solution kept in the safe, the extra bottle of isoflurane kept in the practice manager's desk, or an extra stash of intravenous catheters, needles, and syringes tucked away in a drawer. I've found that many inventory managers will have some degree of safety stock built into important items, perhaps without realizing what they are doing.

Safety stock is important to consider for items that are critical to your practice, such as any "A" or top-selling items, anesthetics, vaccinations, in-house laboratory supplies and tests, euthanasia solution, or anything that, if there were a stockout, would severely impact the practice and well-being of the patients (Figures 3.1 and 3.2).

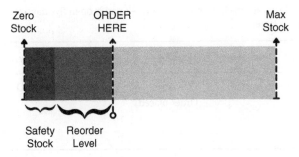

Figure 3.1 Breakdown of different stock levels for a particular item.

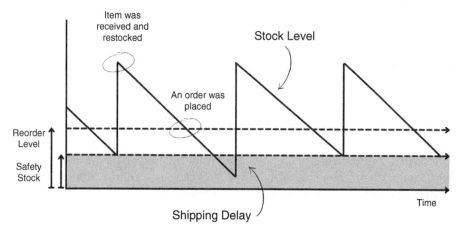

Figure 3.2 Timeline of different stock levels. Note the reorder point level and safety stock level. Also shown is the point when an order was placed and received. Additionally, when there was a shipping delay, the stock level dipped into the safety stock and allowed for unforeseen circumstances without running out of stock. Safety stock level not to scale.

3.6.3.1 Safety Stock: Instincts and Experience Method

Safety stock levels can be calculated in a multitude of different ways, ranging from simple to incredibly complex. Let's examine several different ways that are the most realistic for veterinary practices.

The first method is based on your experience as an inventory manager. For example, you know you want to have an extra bottle of euthanasia solution at all times. The key thing to remember is to watch for any potential overstock or "creep" of inventory on hand. There is a difference between establishing a safety stock level and having "a bunch" on hand, leading to overstock. This method is preferred for things that would be detrimental to a patient outcome if this item ran out. Examples include isoflurane, any anesthetics, euthanasia solution, etc.

"Best Practice" Exercise

Make a list of items that would be detrimental to patient outcomes if they ran out in your practice.

3.6.3.2 Safety Stock: Daily Use Method

The second method for calculating safety stock is to determine how many extra days' worth of stock you want to have on hand. As an example, let us say that for all your vaccinations, you want to keep an additional four days' worth of stock on hand. To calculate this, you would multiply your average daily use by the number of days.

$$Safety\ stock = average\ daily\ use \times number\ of\ days$$

As with most tactics and concepts in your inventory, there is no one right way to do this. Generally speaking, I find the second method of calculating safety stock to be a great balance between being helpful and being overly complicated.

3.6.3.3 Tank's Veterinary Hospital Example: Daily Use

Tank's Veterinary Hospital has decided to keep an additional four days of safety stock for all vaccinations. Their average daily use for the leptospirosis vaccine is three vials.

$$Safety\ stock = average\ daily\ use \times number\ of\ days$$

$$Safety\ stock = 3\ vials \times 4\ days$$

$$Safety\ stock = 12\ vials$$

In this example, the leptospirosis vaccine safety stock level was calculated to be 12 vials.

3.6.3.4 Safety Stock: Maximum Use minus Average Use Calculation Method

The third method involves using an equation to look at the difference between the maximum quantity used/lead time and the average quantity used/lead time. Using the formula method calculates the safety stock levels more precisely and reduces the chance of overstock levels and the "creep" of inventory on hand. When calculating your safety stock, it's important to keep in mind that this formula does not take into account any seasonal changes or swings. So, if you are calculating a product that tends to have seasonal demand changes (like medications and products that help with peak allergy season in the spring), this formula might not be the best option.

If safety stock has not been historically calculated in your practice, start small. Start with either your "A" products or those you absolutely never want to run out of.

$$Safety\ stock = \left(maximum\ daily\ usage \times maximum\ lead\ time\right) - \left(average\ daily\ usage \times average\ lead\ time\right)$$

3.6.3.4.1 Safety Stock Calculation Example In this example, Product A has a maximum daily usage of 67 capsules and a maximum lead time of 10 days. It also has an average daily usage of 51 capsules and an average lead time of eight days.

$$Safety\ stock = \left(maximum\ daily\ usage \times maximum\ lead\ time\right) - \left(average\ daily\ usage \times average\ lead\ time\right)$$

$$Safety\ stock = \left(67\ capsules \times 10\ days\right) - \left(51\ capsules \times 8\ days\right)$$

$$Safety\ stock = 670 - 408$$

$$Safety\ stock = 262\ capsules$$

In this example, the safety stock level was calculated to be 262 capsules.

Using this method, if there is wide variability in your maximum daily usage or maximum lead time, your safety stock number has the potential to be excessive. Often, our first instinct is to eliminate stockouts altogether, but having too high a safety stock level or having too much on hand "just in case" might result in too much money being tied up in inventory, which can cause problems in other places.

This is a good example of the opposing goals of inventory management! Ultimately, we want to have what's needed for patient care without it negatively impacting the practice financially. Having too much "just in case" can have negative effects on your profitability.

"Best Practice" Concept Check
- Which safety stock method seems like it will work the best for your practice?
- If you were going to combine safety stock methods, which two make the most sense?
- What is your primary concern when considering how to calculate your safety stock?

3.6.4   Revisiting the Lead Time Reorder Point Calculation

Now that we have reviewed the concept of safety stock, let's explore how we can layer this onto our ROPs that have been calculated with the lead time method. As you recall, to calculate with the lead time method, you'll multiply the average daily use by the number of days in lead time. As we discussed, the time-frame method already naturally has a buffer built in, but the lead time method does not.

Without an extra buffer of safety stock, the ROPs might be "too lean" and have an increased chance of running out. Let us add the lead time method and the concept of safety stock together.

$$Reorder\ point = \left(average\ daily\ use \times lead\ time\right) + safety\ stock$$

Returning to Tank's Animal Hospital, Dr Tank wants to calculate a ROP for cephalexin 250 mg using the lead time method, adding in three days of safety stock. To calculate the ROP, we'll need the following information.

- Annual sales: 13,890
- Days open per year: 260
- Lead time: eight days
- Days of safety stock: three

The first step will be to calculate the average daily use.

$$Average\ daily\ use = \frac{annual\ usage}{number\ of\ days\ open\ per\ year}$$

$$Average\ daily\ use = \frac{13,890}{260}$$

$$Average\ daily\ use = 53.4$$

Once the average daily use has been determined, Dr Tank can use the lead time and safety stock formula to find the ROP.

$$Reorder\ point = \left(average\ daily\ use \times lead\ time\right) + safety\ stock$$

$$Reorder\ point = \left(average\ daily\ use \times lead\ time\right) + \left(average\ daily\ use \times days\ of\ safety\ stock\right)$$

$$Reorder\ point = \left(53.4 \times 8\right) + \left(53.4 \times 3\right)$$

$$Reorder\ point = 427.2 + 160.2$$

$$Reorder\ point = 587.4 \approx 587$$

In this example, when Tank's Animal Hospital reaches 587 capsules of cephalexin 250 mg, they are low and need to be reordered.

3.6.4.1   Example: Time-frame Reorder Point Versus Lead Time Reorder Point Calculations

Now, let's explore a side-by-side example of the two different ROP methods to demonstrate the differences between what's involved and what the outcome is.

In this example, Tank's Animal Hospital has sold 21,892 tablets of trazodone 100 mg in a 12-month period. This practice is open six days a week (312 days open total in a year) and places their order once per week. The lead time for trazodone 100 mg is nine days and the desired safety stock is three days.

Variables needed for the time-frame ROP example.

- Annual sales: 21,892 tablets
- Time-frame: two-week supply

$$Two\text{-}Week\ Supply = \frac{annual\ usage}{26}$$
$$Two\text{-}Week\ Supply = 842\ tablets$$

Variables needed for lead time ROP example.

- Annual sales: 21,892
- Days open per year: 312
- Lead time: nine days
- Days of safety stock: three

- Step 1: calculate the average daily use.

$$Average\ daily\ use = \frac{annual\ usage}{number\ of\ days\ open\ per\ year}$$
$$Average\ daily\ use = \frac{21,892\ tablets}{312\ days}$$
$$Average\ daily\ use = 70.2\ tablets\ per\ day$$

- Step 2: calculate the ROP.

$$Reorder\ point = \left(average\ daily\ use \times lead\ time\right) + safety\ stock$$
$$Reorder\ point = \left(average\ daily\ use \times lead\ time\right) + \left(average\ daily\ use \times days\ of\ safety\ stock\right)$$
$$Reorder\ point = \left(70.2 \times 9\right) + \left(70.2 \times 3\right)$$
$$Reorder\ point = 631.8 + 210.6$$
$$Reorder\ point = 842.4 \approx 842$$

As you can see, the process for the lead time method is more involved but you can fine-tune any of the variables if needed. The time-frame method is a more brief calculation but is not as precise. At the end of both methods, the ROP is the same in this example. But if you order more than once per week or want to adjust your safety stock levels, the two ROP calculation methods will start to differ.

"Best Practice" Questions to Consider

- What method are you currently using to calculate your ROPs, if any?
- Is this system working? Why or why not?
- Is there another method you'd like to try for calculating your ROPs?

Next, I invite you to try experimenting with the different calculation methods to see the results and explore how ROPs might be integrated into your practice.

3.7   Reorder Point Exceptions

Implementing ROPs into your inventory can be a game-changer but there are several exceptions to keep in mind. Some products or categories of products might not remain consistent throughout the year and have changes in demand depending on the season or time of year. These will vary depending on your unique practice, but it's essential to keep in mind that **seasonal products should be calculated differently**.

Normally, ROPs are calculated based on annual usage. For seasonal ROPs, I like to calculate two different ROPs based on **peak and lull times**. The goal of calculating a separate peak and lull time ROP is to avoid overstocking when sales have decreased and not understocking when the product is flying off the shelf.

Some practice management software systems allow you to enter different ROPs depending on the time-frame. Others, unfortunately, do not. If your PiMS only allows for one order point to be entered, you can update your order points at the start of the peak or lull season. Alternatively, seasonal ROPs can be tracked manually by adding the different order points to reorder tags, minimum and maximum labels, or simply adding to a calendar or planner (Figure 3.3).

Let's examine a scenario: Vectra® 3D, a flea/tick prevention, is a seasonal product and the demand significantly increases as the weather gets warmer during the spring and summer months. After reviewing a report from the PiMS, the monthly sales information is as shown in Table 3.5.

After evaluating this dataset, it becomes clear that there are two "seasons" of demand for this product. The demand is significantly higher from April to July than for the rest of the year. Also, it's helpful to note that demand starts to ramp up in March and winds down in August. March would be a good time to start using the higher ROP; in August, it would be time to start using the lower ROP.

Now, let us calculate this peak and lull time ROP together. In this example, I'm going to show how to calculate them using the time-frame method using a two-week supply. The first step in this

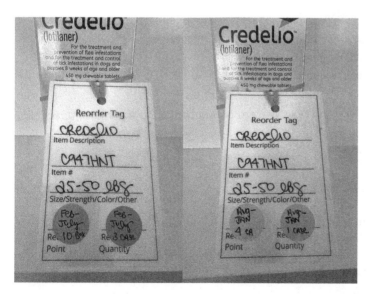

Figure 3.3 A method for displaying seasonal reorder points on reorder tags. In this example, colored dots were put on a laminated reorder tag. As the season and time of year change, the reorder point and reorder quantity can easily be adjusted and swapped with a different time-frame. Nicole Clausen.

Table 3.5 A data set of monthly usage for Vectra 3D, a seasonal product.

Month	Monthly usage (in units)
January	11
February	8
March	19
April	47
May	53
June	54
July	49
August	21
September	12
October	9
November	7
December	10
Total	300

process is to determine the peak and lull times. Then, calculate the number of months and two-week periods within the two different seasons. Once this information is outlined, the two-week supply order point can be calculated.

3.7.1 Calculating Seasonal Reorder Points

3.7.1.1 Peak Reorder Point Calculation

- Number of months during peak season: five
- Number of two-week periods during peak season: 11
- Total product usage during peak season: 222 units

$$Two\text{-}week\ supply = \frac{total\ peak\ usage}{number\ of\ two\text{-}week\ periods}$$

$$Two\text{-}week\ supply = \frac{222\ units}{11}$$

$$Two\text{-}week\ supply = 20.18 \approx 20\ units$$

During the peak season (from March to July), the ROP is 20 units. Once the stock level reaches that point, it's now considered low and should be ordered.

3.7.1.2 Lull Reorder Point Calculation

- Number of months during lull season: seven
- Number of two-week periods during lull season: 15
- Total product usage during lull season: 78 units

$$Two\text{-}week\ supply = \frac{total\ lull\ usage}{number\ of\ two\text{-}week\ periods}$$

$$Two\text{-}week\ supply = \frac{78\ units}{15}$$

$$Two\text{-}week\ supply = 5.2 \approx 5\ units$$

During the lull season (from August to February), the ROP is five units. Once the stock level reaches that point, it's now considered low and should be ordered.

Calculating the two different ROPs will help you stock seasonal items more accurately throughout the year.

Another instance of a potential ROP exception is **emergency drugs**. This may not be the case for larger practices, emergency, or specialty centers where emergencies happen more frequently and likely have a more consistent demand. But for smaller practices, these critical items should be handled differently.

ROPs work best for things with generally consistent demand. If injectables expire before they are even used, they should not have a ROP and should be ordered as needed. For items that aren't injectables, such as vitamin K tablets, a good starting point is to keep a minimum on hand for what you'd need to treat an average-to-large patient. Ultimately, I like to create a list of all emergency products and drugs (urgent supplies included!) and review these with the veterinarians at my practice to decipher the minimum amounts to keep on hand.

Special orders are another situation where ROPs aren't helpful. Special ordered products do not have a consistent demand, so they should be handled differently and with care. There are several options when it comes to these items. Ideally, if your practice offers it, clients can purchase exactly what they need through an online pharmacy. Typically, most online pharmacy platforms will allow you to submit or recommend a prescription directly to a client. This will send a notification right to their email, making the whole process easier and more streamlined for the client. Special orders can also be ordered on an as-needed basis. If this is the case, I always recommend clients pre-pay for the special order.

As you start to calculate and add ROPs to your inventory, you will likely discover practice-specific nuances as well. Do not forget this is an iterative process and is not going to be perfect from day one. Do not be afraid to be curious about what might work in your inventory, and try different strategies!

"Best Practice" Concept Quiz
1) In what circumstances do ROPs not work? Why not?

3.8 You've Calculated Your Order Points ... Now What?

Once you have done the incredible work of calculating your ROPs, what's next? What do you do with all the information? Here comes the fun part. With our ROPs, we have quantified what "low" means. Now, we do not have to guess or wonder if a particular product is low. We can always revisit or calculate that minimum order level.

So far, we've learned how to answer the first question of demand forecasting, which is "What does low mean?" Now, let us explore the second question of demand forecasting, "Once something is low, how will you know it's low and needs to be ordered?" Rather than relying on your team to tell you by writing in the "want book" or on a whiteboard, you can set up reorder flags that will help streamline the process. Let us explore what this can look like.

3.8.1 Reorder Flags

There are a number of different types of reorder flags, but I classify them into three major categories or "buckets." The first type of ROP is electronic. The second is a manual or visual ROP, and the third is a physical ROP. Different categories of items might work better with different types of reorder flags. For example, a reorder checklist might work better for the retail area or the dental cart than your pharmaceuticals. Additionally, a single item can have multiple types of ROPs and act as a double-check system.

Electronic ROPs are those that are entered in a PiMS, dispensing cabinet (such as Cubex or Omnicell), or other electronic software. These all function differently but generally, once ROPs are entered, the system will flag once an item either reaches or falls below the threshold. Most systems have a "reorder report" that shows all the items that need to be ordered and the quantity to reorder. This process significantly reduces the time spent compiling an order, which is great news for everyone, obviously.

Electronic ROPs work best for things that are already tracked in your PiMS and dispensed to clients. This includes vaccines, pharmaceuticals, injections, diets, supplements, and retail items. They do not work as well for things not tracked well in the software system or not sold to clients, like hospital supplies, white goods, needles, syringes, large bottles of liquid, etc.

Remember that while using electronic ROPs, on-hand counts must be maintained and reasonably accurate in the software system. If on-hand counts aren't accurate, ROPs will not flag at the appropriate time and you risk stockouts or forgetting to order something. If your counts are often inaccurate, consider what needs to shift. With that being said, one of the benefits of regular inventory counts and keeping your inventory counts accurate is that you'll have the opportunity to utilize your reorder report.

Entering ROPs into a dispensing cabinet system works similarly. In the setup of each item, a minimum and maximum quantity order can be entered. Then, whenever the on-hand quantity reaches the minimum level, it will be flagged on a purchase order or reorder report. Depending on the system and how it's set up, purchase orders can be sent directly to distributors or vendors automatically.

Manual or visual ROPs include tools like the "want book," visually inspecting what's low, and checklists. For example, a checklist for the vaccine refrigerator lists the vaccines that should be stocked, the minimum to be kept on hand, and the quantity to order when it reaches the minimum threshold. Then, whenever it's time to place the weekly order, the checklist is reviewed to see if anything needs to be ordered. This is also helpful for a dental cart and surgery suite. Using this method, other team members can assist in the ordering process, or if your practice has department leaders, they can be in charge of their "zones."

Other examples of checklists include a **VIP products list** – a list of things your practice never wants to be without, such as euthanasia solution, rabies vaccines, in-house laboratory rotors, anesthetics, etc. That list can act as a double-check system so that even if you have reorder flags set up elsewhere or you are in a hurry, you can use the VIP products list to verify you are not running low on any critical items.

Other helpful product lists could be for a traveling specialist who needs specific items or medications, a controlled substance checklist, an emergency or crash cart checklist, or any other zone or situation where it would be helpful to have a double-check system in place.

Visual or manual ROPs include the "want book" which can be another helpful double-check aid or act as a list for special orders. Just remember that each team member will have a different viewpoint of what is "low" so the want book should not be used exclusively as an ordering strategy.

The **physical ROPs** category includes such tools as reorder tags, reorder bins, minimum and maximum labels, and anything that serves as a physical "flag" for when an item is running low. Physical ROPs work for all items but they work best with hospital supplies, white goods, and other items that aren't dispensed in your PiMS. Physical ROPs provide an indicator of when something is running low without having an accurate on-hand count in the PiMS. Because they aren't connected to your software, you can use physical ROPs to order anything in your practice: Office and janitorial supplies, hospital supplies, break room candy, you name it.

Reorder tags are a simple yet effective tool in your inventory management toolkit. A reorder tag is filled out with identifying information, as well as the ROP and the reorder quantity. Then, the reorder tag is attached to the ROP; this can be achieved with a rubber band, tape, zipper resealable bag, etc. (Figure 3.4). Once the on-hand amount reaches the ROP and a team member uses or opens the unit with the reorder tag attached, the reorder tag is then put in a bin. Then, when you are placing an order, you can grab all the reorder tags from the bin and add them to your order.

Let's use boxes of syringes as an example. Based on your purchase history, you calculate your ROP to be two boxes of syringes. If there are two boxes of syringes on the shelf, you are "low" and need to order more. The reorder tag (listing the ROP) will be attached with either tape or a rubber band to the second to last box. As soon as a team member grabs the second to last box, the reorder tag should be removed and placed in a bin. When it's time to place your order, you gather up the syringe reorder tag and add that to your order. Then, as soon as the syringes arrive in the practice, the reorder tag will be affixed to the second to last box and the process starts all over again.

Although reorder tags are a very "low-tech" tool, they are very helpful for things that are not tracked well in your PiMS. They can be used for anything, though! If prescription labels tend to be forgotten, use a reorder tag on them. Forget to order paper towels? Tape a reorder tag to the "ROP." They can also be used for primary IV lines, soda lime, laundry detergent, gauze squares, cast padding, povidone scrub brushes, and most things in your practice.

As helpful as they are, reorder tags do come with limitations and downsides. They are not as helpful for tablets, capsules, and other items that are tracked by unit. For example, let's say your

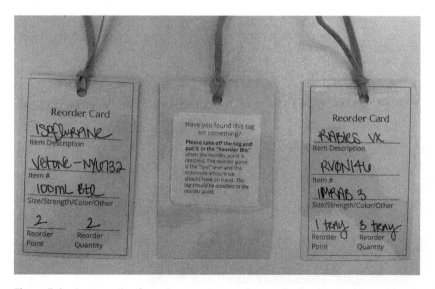

Figure 3.4 An example of reorder tags that can be attached to items with a rubber band. In the isoflurane example on the left, the tag would be rubber banded to the second to last bottle. Then, when someone takes that bottle, they would remove the tag and put it in a "to be ordered" bin. Nicole Clausen.

ROP for gabapentin is 187 capsules. It might be challenging for another team member to know exactly when you hit 187 capsules in a 500-count bottle. It also creates an additional step for other team members to remember when filling a prescription. For pharmaceuticals that are tracked per unit, typically ROPs in the PiMS work best.

An exception to this general rule is injectables or other liquids in clear or amber bottles. Reorder tags can be used with injectables or other liquids by drawing a line on the bottle, signaling where the order point is. Then, a reorder tag can be affixed with a rubber band. Once the liquid level reaches the line, the reorder tag can be removed and placed in a bin to reorder (Figures 3.5 and 3.6).

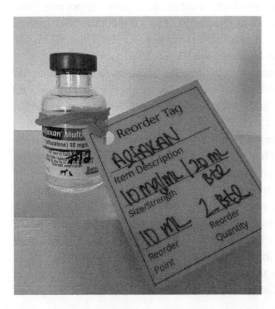

Figure 3.5 How to use a reorder tag with a bottle of liquid. Once the permanent marker line has been reached, Alfaxan® is now "low." The reorder tag should be put in the "to be ordered" bin. Nicole Clausen.

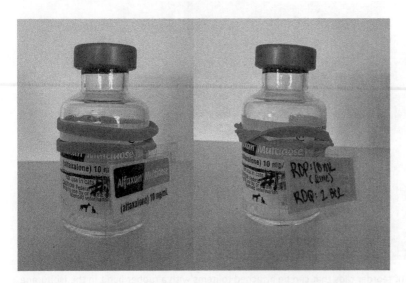

Figure 3.6 How to create a reorder tag from the item's packaging. This is helpful for products with a small bottle size or where a normal tag might be too cumbersome. Nicole Clausen.

In addition, reorder tags are only helpful if the tags get put in a bin or are otherwise given to the inventory manager. So if they end up in the trash or someone's smock, or just stuck on a shelf, that's not helpful. Therefore, I highly recommend getting your team on board and excited about the possibilities when using reorder tags. Some helpful ways to do this are to share your vision and the possibility of not running out of things with reorder tags, get them involved in what items to place reorder tags on, or decide where to put the "to be ordered bins." I also recommend putting "to be ordered" bins throughout your practice and not just having one (Figures 3.7 and 3.8). The goal is to remove as much friction as possible!

Figure 3.7 An example of a "to be ordered" bin. Use as many bins throughout your practice as you need to make it as easy as possible for your team. Nicole Clausen.

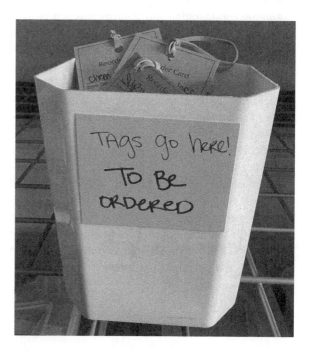

Figure 3.8 An example of an "ordered" bin. The purpose of this bin to keep track of what products have been ordered and provide a convenient spot until the items arrive. Nicole Clausen.

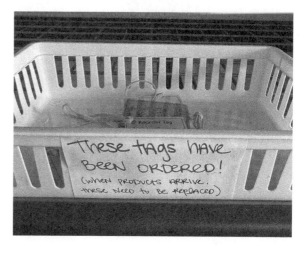

"Best Practice" Tips

- Use Command® strips to place bins in the central storage area or wherever there is a high concentration of reorder tags on products.
- Use bright-colored tags so they stick out.
- Kelly K, a fantastic inventory manager in Indiana, occasionally puts a piece of candy in the reorder bin so anyone who puts a reorder tag in the bin finds a sweet treat!
- Once your tags are finalized, laminate them so they last longer and seem more important than a scrap of paper.

Tip: reorder tags can also be color-coded by category (i.e., controlled substances, hospital supplies, or office supplies) or by the vendor.

Another consideration with reorder tags is how to attach them to the physical ROP. Depending on the item, different methods can be used. Rubber bands, tape, and zipper reusable bags are some of my favorites. Rubber bands can be used to attach the reorder tag to almost anything (Figure 3.9). Not only can they be attached to a box, but they can also be helpful in segmenting out the ROP. For example, a small animal practice might have a ROP of three 60 cc Luer-Lock syringes. Those three syringes can be rubber banded together with the reorder tag so that when all the other syringes in the box are used and a team member needs to grab one from the bundle, the reorder tag then gets removed and put in a bin.

Zipper resealable plastic bags can also be used creatively. These can be helpful when there are a lot of very small items, typically within a much larger container (Figure 3.10). For example, mini StatSpin® urine separator tubes, micro blood sample tubes, or male adapter catheter caps. Let's say that for one practice, the ROP for EDTA purple-top microtubes is 21. Twenty-one tubes are then put in a plastic bag, along with the reorder tag, and placed in the main 100-count container. Throughout the normal course of patient care, all the other 79 tubes in the container are used. Then, when someone needs to reach into the plastic bag to remove a tube, they also remove the reorder tag and put it in the order bin.

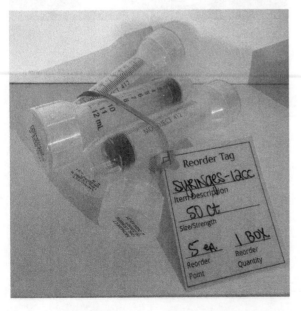

Figure 3.9 How to use a reorder tag and a rubber band attachment for white goods or hospital supplies that are used infrequently and have a low reorder point. Nicole Clausen.

Figure 3.10 How to use a reorder tag with smaller items. In this example, a reorder tag was placed in a plastic, reclosable bag with 22 gauge, 1 ½″ needles. The team would use the other needles outside the bag. Once the remaining needles were gone and they grabbed a needle from inside the bag, they would also pull out the reorder tag and put it in the "to be ordered" bin. Nicole Clausen.

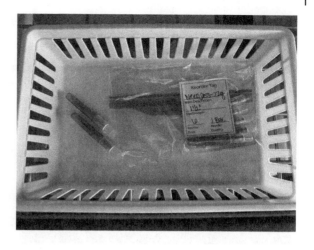

Reorder tags can also be helpful for those items that are infrequently used, but when you need them, you really need them. This can help avoid the situation of someone forgetting to write it down or to tell you that it was used. Although simple and "low tech," ROPs have a lot of helpful applications for many inventory items!

Reorder bins are another very helpful physical reorder tag. As with reorder tags, reorder bins are very helpful for hospital supplies and other things not tracked well in the PiMS. There are two main ways to utilize reorder bins. The first is to separate one bin with a divider. The divider serves as the ROP. Everything in front of the divider is used and as soon as something is grabbed from behind the divider, that signals it's time to reorder that product (Figure 3.11).

With this system, the key to successfully implementing it into your practice is that each and every team member must clearly understand how the reorder bins work and should "respect the divider" and first grab from in front of the divider. This system also pairs well with using double-sided labels that say "in stock" and "restock needed." It can also be used in conjunction with

Figure 3.11 An example of indicator reorder bins. In this example, the team would grab syringes from the first section. Once all the syringes are gone from the first section, then someone must grab from the second section. Once the divider has been "breached," it means this item is now "low" and should be ordered. Additionally, the bin can be turned around so the second section is now facing out. This is a great way to view at a glance which products need to be replenished. Nicole Clausen.

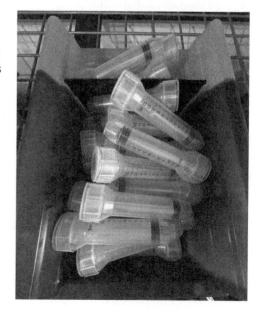

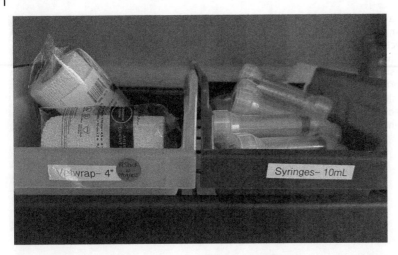

Figure 3.12 Indicator reorder bins in use. On the left, this bin has been flipped around, signaling the vet wrap is "low," and units from the first section are gone and need to be restocked. There is also a dot added that says "restock in progress." On the right, the first section facing outward is a visual cue that there are plenty of 10 mL syringes in stock. Nicole Clausen.

reorder cards so that when the reorder level is reached, the team member puts the card in a "to be reordered" bin (Figure 3.12).

Tip: create a standard operating procedure (SOP) (with visuals) on exactly how to use the reorder bins and reorder tags in addition to hosting a training session. This SOP should be posted in the central storage area or wherever the practice has reorder bins.

The two-bin system works similarly but is best with items where a larger quantity is used and kept on hand. With the two-bin system, there are two bins on the shelf, with one placed in front of the other, and they are filled with one item (for example, primary IV lines or CoFlex rolls). The two-bin step-by-step process is as follows.

1) Add inventory to both bins.
2) Use the inventory from the front bin first.
3) Once the first bin is empty, that's a signal that it's time to reorder.
4) Once it's noted that the product will be (or has been) ordered, move the full second bin to the front (the empty bin should now be behind the full bin).
5) Once the order comes in, restock the bins and the process repeats.
6) Note: It can also be helpful to have labels on the front of the bin that can be flipped to signal that the product is currently on order (Figure 3.13).

Another helpful physical ROP is **min/max labels on inventory items**. These labels can be added to any item and, at the very least, specify what the item is, the minimum that should be kept on hand (typically your ROP, including any safety stock), and the maximum quantity (typically your ROP plus the reorder quantity; we'll explore this concept later in this chapter). These labels can be helpful when someone is visually inspecting the inventory on hand and can use the labels to identify if something is low and should be ordered immediately (Figure 3.14). Min/max labels are helpful because everyone on your team can use them and feel empowered to know when something is running low.

There are a number of different types of reorder flags, but I've found they work best together as a symphony of flags to know when everything is low. Two or more types of ROPs can be used on a single product. For example, bottles of ear cleanser could have ROPs set up in the PiMS, a reorder

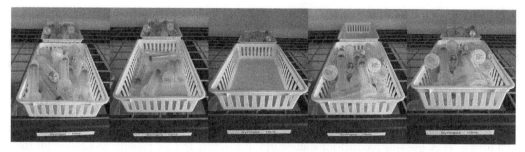

Figure 3.13 The two-bin system workflow (from left to right). Two bins are filled with inventory and put on the shelf, one in front of the other. Inventory is grabbed, as needed, from the front bin first. Once the front bin is empty, this item is low and it's time to reorder. Once it's been ordered or a restock is in progress, move the empty bin behind the full bin. Once the item arrives, restock the empty bin. Then, the process repeats. Nicole Clausen.

Figure 3.14 An example of a min/max label for carprofen 100 mg. Once there is only 0.25 of a bottle left, this item is considered "low" and should be replenished. In this example, one bottle should be ordered to bring this product back up to the maximum level. Nicole Clausen.

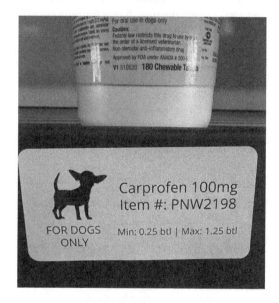

tag rubber banded to the ROP, and a min/max label affixed to the shelf. The various ROPs work together as a double-check system so that there are multiple reminders for when something is running low, significantly decreasing the chance an item will not get ordered or will be forgotten about.

Finally, different ROPs will have various levels of success at different practices, so it's essential to be curious and experiment to find what works best for your unique practice.

"Best Practice" Considerations
- Which of the methods in this section do you feel most drawn to?
- Which feels most chaotic?
- If you were combining a few methods to solve your current inventory woes, which ones do you want to implement and why?

3.8.2 Reorder Point Examples

In this section, we'll cover common products that practices run out of and how ROPs can help. First and foremost, you can make inventory less manual and automate the process by leaning on the three different categories of reorder flags: visual or manual, electronic, and physical ROPs. This will help you shift away from relying on the "want book" and visually inspecting every item in the practice to know what's going on.

For pharmaceuticals, tablets, pills, and liquids (think: gabapentin, amoxicillin, vitamin B injectable, or joint supplements), these items can all be tracked in your PiMS so that they could be set up with an electronic ROP in the PiMS. You could also use a reorder tag, in addition to the PiMS, as a "just in case" safety measure. In addition, if any of these items are critical to the function of your practice or to a patient's care, they can be added to a "VIP product list" as an additional double-check.

Let's go back to Tank's Animal Hospital. They use a lot of Cerenia® injectable and they have run out before. They use this product for some surgical patients and for patients as needed for their treatment plan. Additionally, they had a veterinarian join the practice six months ago. Their practice is new to using ROPs. After reviewing their sales history, they discovered they had used 217 ml in the past three months.

For this practice, because they are new to ROPs and have had a change in veterinarians, calculating a ROP using the time-frame formula over the last three months would be my recommendation.

3.8.2.1 Example Reorder Point Calculation: Cerenia Injectable
Variables required.

- Three-month sales = 217 ml
- Number of two-week periods in the time period = 6.5

$$Two\text{-}week\ supply = \frac{units\ sold\ in\ time\ period}{number\ of\ two\text{-}week\ periods}$$

$$Two\text{-}week\ supply = \frac{217}{6.5}$$

$$Two\text{-}week\ supply = 33.4$$

After calculating the ROP, they discover that approximately 33 ml is "low" and the minimum level they should have on hand.

After discussion, they decide to set up an electronic ROP in their PiMS and have a reorder tag set up as a "just in case" double-check.

For refrigerated items: for refrigerated items, you could have a "fridge stocklist" and every time you place your order, you could use that as a guide. It could list all the items in the fridge, the minimum level to have on hand, and the reorder quantity. This could include any vaccinations, in-house lab testing supplies, and medications stored in the refrigerator. For any of the items that are tracked in the PiMS, you can set up an electronic order point. You can also set up a physical ROP and use tags on vaccine trays.

For IV lines or other hospital supplies (think: kennel food, cast padding, CoFlex, extension sets, t-ports, isoflurane, etc.): for things that are not in your software, manual and physical reorder tags work best. You could set up reorder tags or reorder bins for your IV lines, white goods, and any product that is consumed and used rather than sold. For your kennel food, you could have a reorder tag set up. Or you could create a kennel "stock list" and delegate your kennel team to check this list on a daily, weekly, etc. basis.

For 3 ml syringes and needles: for syringes, you can set up reorder tags to flag when boxes are running low. You could also set up a "central storage" (or "syringe and needle storage") stock checklist to review prior to each order. A note on syringes and needles: Generally, I do not recommend keeping track of each individual needle and syringe. It's typically not worth your time, and there is little return on investment for the time spent. I recommend keeping track of unopened boxes instead.

Pro-Pectalin™ tabs, probiotics, other over-the-counter supplements, and prescription diets: these inventory items can be tracked in your PiMS, so I would start with an electronic ROP. In addition, you could also add a reorder tag or a "diarrhea-related (or other ailment) product" checklist to review each time you place an order.

These are just a few examples of how ROPs can be utilized in your practice so that you can start relying less on the "want book" and create more strategic systems.

3.9 Calculating Reorder Quantity – How Much to Order?

Now that we have answered the first two questions of demand forecasting, we understand what "low" means for a particular product, and there are systems in place to indicate when something is running low and must be ordered. The final question of demand forecasting is, once we have determined there is a need and an item should be ordered, how much will we order? This question can be answered utilizing **reorder quantity** (ROQ).

Like peanut butter and jelly, the reorder quantity is the second key piece of ROPs. They are used in conjunction and are often entered into the same area of the practice management software system or listed together on reorder tags or reorder bins. Just as with ROPs, this important piece of information is calculated using the usage or purchase history of a practice. Keep in mind that for things tracked or dispensed in the PiMS, the sales history should be used. For things that are not, the purchase history should be used.

Calculating the reorder quantity also requires understanding the turnover goal of the practice. An easy rule to remember: *the ultimate ordering goal is to use or sell it before you have to pay for it.* How much you purchase at a time will likely differ for various items. For lower-cost items (like tongue depressors or cotton balls), you might order less frequently but more at a time. For high-cost, high-turnover items, you might order more frequently but less at a time.

Overall, for practices that are on statement billing, this means that an item should come in and leave the practice within 25–30 days. For high-cost, high-turnover items, you might consider purchasing what you would sell in two weeks. If you only have to pay for an item once per month, it may not make sense to order that item four or five times throughout the month, thus increasing your labor costs.

I like to use the example of grocery shopping. If you know that your family goes through a bag of oranges every single week, would you go to the store every day for one orange or would you buy a bag of oranges at the beginning of the week?

Additionally, some practices can get very creative with billing term timing and using credit cards for extra time. Some practices, especially large animal and equine practices, will purchase in bulk at the beginning of their peak season. So, it's important to keep your unique practice in mind as you go through these calculations. In my experience, I would say that when setting reorder quantities, the majority of practices want to order anywhere between a two-week supply and a 30-day supply.

Bulk and promotional purchases should be calculated differently. You'll review that in the following chapter.

Helpful Definitions
- **Inventory turnover**: a measure of how quickly an item(s) comes in and leaves a business; this is a great measure of inventory efficiency. A high turnover means items are not just sitting on the shelf. A low turnover means they are on the shelf for long periods before being used or sold.

For a practice that is on statement billing, a good overall turnover goal is 12–14 times per year. This means that an inventory manager should order (at most) what will be used within 25–30 days. Order any more than that and your holding costs will increase. Plus, that is capital tied up on the shelf, not selling. Ordering less, though, will increase labor costs. There is always a balance between having too much on hand and not enough, where you are either running out or ordering a particular item all the time. Finding the balance for your unique practice is key.

There are some exceptions to this rule. Because prescription diets take up so much storage space, a turnover goal of 24 times per year is ideal. This means that ordering what will be used within two weeks works well for prescription diets. If there are any products that take up a lot of space, maintaining a healthy turnover will be especially important. For things that take a long time to arrive (think Class II controlled substances, ordered on a DEA Form 222), ordering slightly more might be beneficial.

To calculate the reorder quantity, use the following formula if you want to purchase a 30-day supply.

$$Reorder\ quantity = \frac{units\ sold\ or\ purchased\ in\ time\ period}{number\ of\ months\ in\ time\ period}$$

Use the following formula if you want to calculate a two-week supply.

$$Reorder\ quantity = \frac{units\ sold\ or\ purchased\ in\ time\ period}{number\ of\ two\text{-}week\ periods\ in\ time\ period}$$

To calculate the reorder quantity, use the following formula if you know how many days worth of stock you want to purchase.

$$Reorder\ quantity = average\ daily\ use \times number\ of\ days\ worth\ of\ stock$$

where

$$Average\ daily\ use = \frac{annual\ usage}{number\ of\ days\ per\ year}$$

3.9.1 Examples

3.9.1.1 Reorder Quantity Calculation Example

In this example, Tank's Animal Hospital has a turnover goal of 12 times per year, so they want to purchase 30 days of stock at a time. After reviewing a usage report from their software, it's determined that Product A sold 8,673.0 units in the last 12 months.

Variables required.

- Annual usage = 8,673.0
- Turnover goal = 12

$$Reorder\ quantity = \frac{annual\ usage}{number\ of\ months\ in\ time\ period}$$

$$Reorder\ quantity = \frac{8,673.0}{12}$$

$$Reorder\ quantity = 722.75 \approx 723\ units$$

In this example, once it's determined that Product A is low and should be reordered, 722 (or the nearest package quantity) should be ordered.

3.9.1.2 Calculating Reorder Points and Reorder Quantity Together

In this example, Tank's Animal Hospital will calculate both a ROP and reorder quantity for gabapentin 100 mg. This medication has an annual usage of 3,925. Tank's Animal Hospital is new to calculating ROPs and will use the time-frame method to calculate a two-week supply. They also have a turnover goal of 12 times per year and want to purchase a 30-day supply.

ROP calculation.

$$Reorder\ quantity = \frac{annual\ usage}{number\ of\ months\ in\ time\ period}$$

$$Reorder\ quantity = \frac{3,925.0}{12}$$

$$Reorder\ quantity = 327.08 \approx 327\ units$$

In this example, gabapentin 100 mg has a ROP of 151. When the on-hand level reaches that threshold, it is now considered low and should be ordered.

Reorder quantity calculation.

$$Reorder\ quantity = \frac{annual\ usage}{number\ of\ months\ in\ time\ period}$$

$$Reorder\ quantity = \frac{3,925.0}{12}$$

$$Reorder\ quantity = 327.08 \approx 327\ units$$

In this example, once the ROP of 151 units is reached, 327 units (or whatever is the closest package quantity) should be ordered. Because it is fairly inexpensive and a large patient can be prescribed a significant number of capsules at once, they decide to round up and purchase a 500-count bottle rather than three 100-count bottles. In addition, they'll set this ROP and order quantity up in their PiMS, as well as create an order tag as a backup (Figure 3.15).

I have always found calculating and implementing ROPs to be empowering and confidence boosting in the inventory! It's the bridge between shaking bottles and wandering around the pharmacy, wondering what is low, to feeling confident and in control of exactly what needs to be ordered and how much.

3.9.2 Inventory Manager Spotlight

Meet Shanise Burney-Farr, purchasing manager!

"I have been the inventory/purchasing manager for Bay Animal Hospital for 17 years. I started out as a tech and was given the ordering duties early on. Initially, I just shook bottles and really just ordered what looked low or what was written on the want list. We ran out of stuff all the time! I started to stash backup items in different places in the hospital as I learned what we ran out of the most. I got pretty good at hiding stuff!

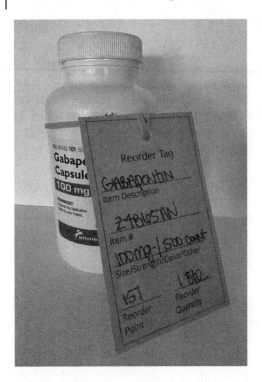

Figure 3.15 An example reorder tag for the gabapentin reorder point calculation. Nicole Clausen.

As the years progressed and I took inventory classes and learned on the job, I learned about ROPs, cycle counts, seasonal use, etc. Now, the system that works for us is delegated department management, reorder tags, and ROPs. So we have a designated staff member inventory their assigned area weekly, biweekly, or monthly, depending on the area. We have someone assigned to the treatment area/exam room supplies, surgical supplies, hospital-use injectables, refrigerated and lab supplies, pharmacy items, office supplies, pet food and OTC items, and janitorial and grooming supplies.

Each team member completes a form indicating what they have and what they need me to order. And I use these lists to build my purchase orders. I also have reorder tags on the items in my central storage area and a backup refrigerator. The reorder tags are basically aligned to the ROPs in our veterinary software. We also have a sign-out sheet for items removed from central storage. Daily, I remove the reorder tags that have been placed in the order bin and the sign-out list and use them both to build on my order (Figures 3.16 and 3.17).

I also generate a want list through our veterinary software and cross-reference that list with the sign-out sheet, reorder tags, and the lists from the different departments. It sounds like a lot but it's pretty routine, and I've been out on injury for three months and have still managed to keep the boat afloat by working remotely and just having the lists emailed to me!"

3.10 Calculating the Minimum and Maximum Level

Slightly different from the reorder quantity is the **maximum level**. This is the maximum level of the inventory you should have on hand. This can also be referred to as the overstock point because anything above the maximum level would be considered overstock. Some PiMSs will have

Figure 3.16 Shanise's reorder checklist for grooming and cleaning supplies.
Source: Courtesy of Shanise Burney-Farr.

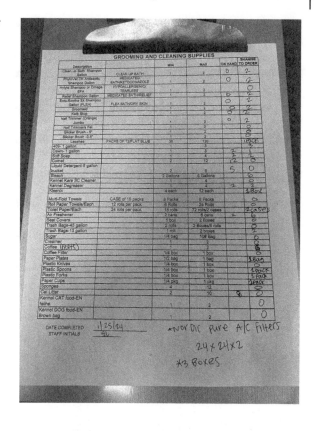

Figure 3.17 Shanise's reorder tags. *Source:* Courtesy of Shanise Burney-Farr.

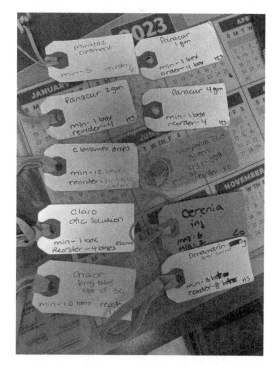

a minimum and a maximum inventory level rather than a ROP and a reorder quantity. Let's talk about the differences.

The minimum level in your inventory is the same as your ROP. Once you reach your minimum level or your ROP, you'll "order up" to the max. For example, let's say your maximum inventory level for gauze squares is 22 sleeves. As you place your order, you find that you have seven sleeves of gauze left and want to reorder. You'll "order up" to the max and purchase 15 sleeves to bring you back up to the maximum level of 22 sleeves.

Your reorder quantity and the maximum level are not the same. There are many different ways to calculate the maximum level for a product. But, in the spirit of not overcomplicating, my favorite way to calculate the max level is to add the ROP and reorder quantity together.

$$Maximum\ Level = Reorder\ Point + Reorder\ Quantity$$

Back to Tank's Animal Hospital. Dr Tank calculated that they purchased 103 boxes of 6 cc syringes in the last 12 months. They use the time-frame ROP calculation method and decide that when they have two weeks' worth of stock left, they'll order an additional 30 days' worth.

The first step is to find the ROP or the minimum level. In this case, the ROP is a two-week supply.

$$Reorder\ point = \frac{annual\ purchases}{26}$$
$$Reorder\ point = \frac{103}{26}$$
$$Reorder\ point = 3.96 \approx 4\ boxes$$

The next step is to calculate and find the reorder quantity. In this example, Tank's Animal Hospital purchases a 30-day supply at a time.

$$Reorder\ quantity = \frac{annual\ purchases}{12}$$
$$Reorder\ quantity = \frac{103}{12}$$
$$Reorder\ quantity = 8.58 \approx 9\ boxes$$

Now that both the ROP and reorder quantity have been calculated, the maximum quantity can be found.

$$Maximum\ Quantity = Reorder\ Point + Reorder\ Quantity$$
$$Maximum\ Quantity = 4\ Boxes + 9\ Boxes$$
$$Maximum\ Quantity = 13\ Boxes$$

In this example, their maximum level is 13 boxes of 6 cc syringes. When ordering, if there are five boxes on the shelf, they would order up to max and purchase eight boxes of syringes. If there were three boxes left, they would order up to max by purchasing 10 boxes.

Although slightly different from the reorder quantity, the maximum level allows for a bit more flexibility when ordering if you are under or over the ROP or minimum level. It's also helpful to know the maximum level to investigate if you are overstocked on a particular item and have too much on hand.

As an example, let's say that you suspect that you have too many bags of one particular type of food. You could calculate the maximum quantity and see if you were above that level. To take it one step further, you could compare how many bags you have with your 30-day supply to see how many months' worth of stock you have on hand. We'll review this concept in more depth later in the book.

"Best Practice" Questions to Consider

- Does your PiMS use the maximum level or the reorder quantity level? Or both?
- Are there any products that you suspect might be overstocked for which you could calculate the maximum level and verify?
- How might you integrate the maximum level into your practice to help find the balance between too much and not enough?

3.11 Calculating the Economic Order Quantity

The economic order quantity (EOQ) is another method for calculating how much to order (Heinke 2014, p. 334). The formula finds the order quantity that will meet your demand but also minimize your holding and labor costs. It essentially helps to find the "sweet spot" for a particular item and the balance between too much and not enough.

Using this formula will determine the best quantity of a specific item to order each time an order is placed.

$$Economic\ order\ quantity = \sqrt{\frac{2 \times A \times F}{H \times UC}}$$

where

- A = annual demand in units
- F = fixed ordering costs incurred per order
- H = holding costs expressed on an annual basis as a percentage of unit cost
- UC = unit cost to purchase from vendor or supplier

Let's review an example together.
Variables required.

- Annual demand in units (A) = 15,983
- Fixed ordering costs per order (F) = \$35.00
- Holding costs = 25%
- Unit cost = \$0.37

$$Economic\ Order\ Quantity = \sqrt{\frac{2 \times A \times F}{H \times UC}}$$

$$Economic\ Order\ Quantity = \sqrt{\frac{2 \times 15,983 \times \$35.00}{25\% \times \$0.37}}$$

$$Economic\ Order\ Quantity = \sqrt{\frac{1,118,810}{0.0925}}$$

$$Economic\ Order\ Quantity = \sqrt{12,095,243.24}$$
$$Economic\ Order\ Quantity = 3,477.82 \approx 3,478$$

In this example, the best or most economical amount to order for this product would be 3,478 units.

The main downside of using this model is that it's fairly complex in comparison to other methods for determining how much to order. Not only that, but it has other limitations. First and foremost, it assumes a fairly constant demand for a particular product so it might not be helpful for seasonal products or if your practice is growing or has a change in demand related to new or changing veterinarians. Additionally, as you can see from the example above, it does not take into account the storage space that's available.

Other limitations include the following.

- The EOQ model assumes fairly steady labor and holding costs. Your practice's labor costs may change due to raises, a changing team, etc. Holding costs can also change due to inflation, changes in rent, storage costs, etc.
- The EOQ only really considers qualitative factors and does not take into account product expiry, storage space, and other considerations that might be unique to your practice.

Although it can be helpful to know the EOQ and quantify the "sweet spot" for ordering a particular item, there are some downsides to consider, including whether this model would be in alignment with your unique practice and your inventory.

3.12 Putting It all Together

We have explored demand forecasting and how to answer the three quintessential questions to know what to order and when.

- What does "low" mean?
- Once something is low, how will you know when it's reached the "low" threshold and should be ordered?
- Once you know that something is low and should be ordered, how much will you order?

Let's review how you can put together your ROPs, reorder quantities, and reorder flags to maintain the "flow" of inventory in your practice. Here are some examples of products, ROP calculations, and types of ROPs to use as inspiration for using ROPs in your inventory.

3.12.1 Product A

Product A is a shampoo mousse. According to the sales report from the PiMS, 43 were sold in the last six months.

Variables required.

- Number of two-week periods = 13
- Sales in the time period (six months) = 43

- Step 1: calculate the ROP using the time-frame method.

$$Reorder\ point = \frac{sales\ in\ time\ period}{number\ of\ two\text{-}week\ periods\ in\ time\ period}$$

Figure 3.18 An example reorder tag for the mousse reorder point calculation. Nicole Clausen.

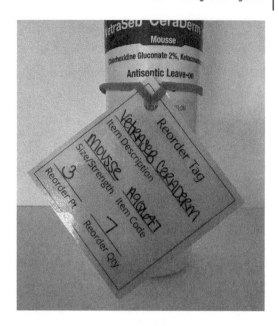

$$Reorder\ point = \frac{43}{13}$$
$$Reorder\ point = 3.3 \approx 3\ bottles$$

- Step 2: calculate the reorder quantity.

$$Reorder\ quantity = \frac{sales\ in\ time\ period}{number\ of\ months\ in\ time\ period}$$
$$Reorder\ quantity = \frac{43}{6}$$
$$Reorder\ quantity = 7.2 \approx 7\ bottles$$

In this example, when you have three bottles of mousse left on the shelf, you are "low" and need to reorder. Three is the ROP for this product. When this product is "low," you will order seven bottles of mousse.

For this product, because it is sold in the PiMS, ROPs could be added to your software, a reorder tag could be used, or you could create a "bathing/grooming" product checklist (Figure 3.18).

3.12.2 Product B

Product B, amoxicillin 500 mg, an antibiotic, comes in bottles of 100 or 500. According to the sales report from the PiMS, 5,104 were sold in the last year. In this example, when your practice has a two-week supply on hand, you'd like to order another two weeks' worth of stock.

- Step 1: calculate the ROP using the time-frame method.

$$Reorder\ point = \frac{annual\ usage}{26}$$

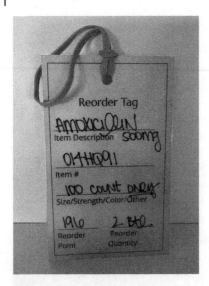

$$Reorder\ point = \frac{5,104}{26}$$
$$Reorder\ point = 196.3 \approx 196\ capsules$$

- Step 2: calculate the reorder quantity.

$$Reorder\ quantity = \frac{annual\ usage}{26}$$

$$Reorder\ quantity = \frac{5,104}{26}$$

$$Reorder\ quantity = 196.3 \approx 196\ capsules$$

In this example, when you have 196 on hand, you are "low" and need to order. When you are low, you will order two bottles of 100 (Figure 3.19).

I would add ROPs to the PiMS for this product.

One of the challenges of using reorder tags for pharmaceuticals is that it's hard to use them for open containers. For example, if you have a 500-count bottle of gabapentin,

Figure 3.19 An example reorder tag for the amoxicillin reorder point calculation. Nicole Clausen.

your team might not recognize when the ROP of 338 has been reached. In this case, the ROP of 196 is very close to two 100-count bottles, so a reorder tag could be used in this situation.

3.12.3 Product C

Product C is primary IV lines. According to your purchase history, 152 IV lines were purchased in the last three months. In this example, when your practice has a two-week supply left, you want to order a 30-day supply.

- Step 1: calculate the ROP using the time-frame method.

$$Reorder\ point = \frac{purchases\ in\ time\ period}{number\ of\ two\text{-}week\ periods\ in\ time\ period}$$

$$Reorder\ point = \frac{152}{6.5}$$

$$Reorder\ point = 23.4 \approx 23$$

- Step 2: calculate the reorder quantity.

$$Reorder\ quantity = \frac{purchases\ in\ time\ period}{number\ of\ months\ in\ time\ period}$$

$$Reorder\ quantity = \frac{152}{3}$$

$$Reorder\ quantity = 50.6 \approx 51$$

In this example, when you have 23 IV lines on hand, you are "low" and need to order. Then, when you are low, you will order 51 (or round down to 50).

For this product, use a reorder tag, the two-bin system, or a bin with a shelf label listing the ROP and reorder quantity for this item (Figures 3.20 and 3.21).

Below is an example ROP strategy for your entire inventory.

- Electronic ROPs in the PiMS for things that are sold/dispensed in the software.
- Shelf labels listing the ROPs on each item in central storage.
- Order checklists for the dental cart and surgery suite "zones."
- Reorder tags for cabinets/storage areas that aren't seen often (red rubber catheters, etc.).
- Draw a Sharpie® line and use reorder tags for liquids and injectables.
- Order checklists for prescription diets and the reception retail area.
- Finally, place an Amazon Echo device in the treatment area so team members can "speak" to Alexa and add products to the "want list."

A note on injectables or bottles of liquid (or the big tubs of Panacur® granules): Once the ROP has been calculated, you could draw a Sharpie line around the bottle to indicate the reorder level. Once the reorder level has been reached, a team member would pull off the tag and put it in the "to be ordered" bin.

3.13 A Quick Story from the Author

When I was just getting started with ROPs and demand forecasting, I remember feeling the biggest wave of relief as I started calculating and setting up order points for various items. For most items, when I had a two-week supply on the shelf, I would order an additional 30-day supply. We were a growing practice, and a 30-day supply gave enough of a "buffer" for those extra busy weeks and months. No longer did I have to carry this mental load of "Should I order this?," "I wonder if this is low?" or "Why did someone not tell me we were low until after we were out?"

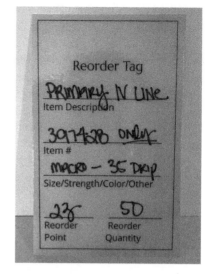

Figure 3.20 An example reorder tag for the primary IV line reorder point calculation. Nicole Clausen.

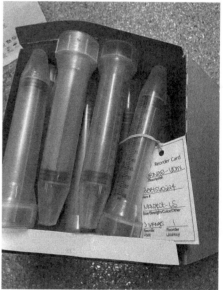

Figure 3.21 An example of using reorder tags with 60 ml syringes and a low reorder point. Nicole Clausen.

It was such a breath of fresh air and gave me a much-needed "I can do this" confidence boost.

Each time I would place an order, I would go through and calculate ROPs for each item I was purchasing. I used my emotional support calculator, and I would add them to my PiMS. It was a little bit of a transition process and trial and error. Sometimes, it led me down a rabbit hole of needing to reset codes and restructure how procedure and inventory codes were linked. Other times, after trying out the order point for a cycle or two, I would need to readjust.

It worked well for my brain (and the time I had available to me) to enter them as I ordered them. But I've coached other folks who prefer to enter order points into each product A–Z, or they'd go from category to category. One thing I've noticed is that for 90% of your items, ROPs will be fairly straightforward. For the remaining 10%, you might have to get creative and add your own flavor of razzle-dazzle. For example, this could be having two types of reorder flags set up for one item. It might look like for long-term, chronic medication refills (like thyrosyn), rounding up your ROP to an average script size. This might take a round or two of adjustments and/or problem solving.

It probably will not be perfect the first time. But your practice could not run without your knack for puzzling through inventory issues, setting up systems, and getting your team what they need. You can do this!

4

Efficient Ordering and Replenishment

4.1 The Ordering Process

Ordering is the pinnacle and peak of all our hard work and effort in demand forecasting and determining precisely what to order. I've noticed that ordering is sometimes the only aspect of inventory management that our team recognizes because this process is more visible. I've certainly felt like I was seen as just the "order girl" before. What's not seen is all the work that goes into managing inventory to help get us there.

Ordering can sometimes feel chaotic. You're scrambling to place an order in between appointments. Or it's your day off and you're trying to place a super-quick "emergency" order. Or maybe it feels uncomfortable because you do not know exactly what to order. My goal for you in this chapter (combined with the previous chapter on demand forecasting) is for you to feel confident each week when it's time to place your order. Throughout this chapter, I'll outline strategies for ordering in a way that best supports your practice's goals.

When it comes to ordering, it's not just about physically placing the order. It's also about evaluating where you are ordering from, how often you are ordering, who is ordering, and being mindful of any order fees or minimums. Throughout this chapter, you'll be reviewing each of these important aspects. As with all the processes and workflows you create, it's helpful to document them and create standard operating procedures (SOPs).

Whenever thinking about how much to order and just ordering in general, always use the lens of "we want to sell or use an item before we have to pay for it." All my ordering decisions are filtered through this lens. This is an important goal, whether you are ordering a bulk purchase, a normal order, or anything in between.

This means that, with statement billing and strategic timing, once you order an item, you generally have 25–30 days before paying for that item/invoice (depending on the billing terms of your vendor). So, in this case, unless it's a special circumstance, you would not want to order more than what you would use in 30 days. Of course, sometimes that is just not possible with the manufacturer's packaging size but it's something you want to strive for!

If your vendor has billing terms of 14 or 60 days, ideally, you'll purchase what you would use in 14 or 60 days, respectively. In addition, I know of some practice managers who get extra creative with their timing and use a credit card for payment, increasing the amount of time.

It's important to remember that there are more costs involved with ordering than just the product cost. There are also two main indirect costs: labor and holding costs. **Labor costs** include the inventory team's time to place, receive, enter, and manage orders. **Holding (or carrying) costs**

Inventory Management for Veterinary Professionals, First Edition. Nicole I. Clausen.
© 2024 John Wiley & Sons, Inc. Published 2024 by John Wiley & Sons, Inc.
Companion website: www.wiley.com/go/clausen/inventory

include rent, opportunity costs, insurance, temperature controls, and insurance, among others, to keep that inventory item safe and protected until it's sold. A primary goal with ordering is to (i) understand these indirect costs and how they affect your practice and (ii) create your systems to balance the two indirect costs.

Let's explore different strategies for ordering, replenishment techniques, and other best practices to consider.

Helpful Definition
- **Replenishment**: adding or ordering more stock to replace what has been used or sold.

4.2 Replenishment Techniques

There are a number of different replenishment or ordering techniques that you can use in your practice to help manage inventory more smoothly. Do not feel overwhelmed or discouraged by the terms or the jargon that's used (be a detective!). What's helpful here is not necessarily the exact term but the concept. Depending on your practice and your goals, different techniques might work better than others for you. I will typically use and recommend a combination of the various strategies. The goal is to craft an ordering and replenishment strategy that works with you rather than against you!

Here are some common inventory replenishment strategies.

- **Reorder point (ROP)**: this method involves calculating ROPs based on lead time, demand, and ideal levels. Then, a minimum ROP level is determined. Once that ROP has been reached, that item should be reordered. (See Chapter 3 for more information about calculating and implementing reorder points.)
- **Just-in-time (JIT)**: this replenishment technique is a "lean management" tool where inventory is ordered and replenished JIT to be used or sold again. This method can help reduce holding costs and prevent overstocking, but you must pay close attention to your inventory levels. You can also run the risk of being "too lean" if you have any sudden significant increases in demand.
- **Minimum and maximum levels**: using this method, there are precalculated minimum and maximum levels. Once the minimum is reached or the quantity on hand falls below the minimum level, an order is placed to bring it back up to the maximum level. Some practice management systems use the min/max level method rather than ROPs. They might seem similar but they are different! (See Chapter 3 for more information.)
- **Periodic replenishment**: instead of monitoring inventory levels to see what's low, orders are placed at specific time intervals, such as weekly, monthly, or seasonally. The order quantity is determined based on demand forecasting and how much will be used or sold during the replenishment time period. This method is not used as often in veterinary practices. An example of this might be purchasing in bulk before the busy season for an equine practice or purchasing heartworm prevention in bulk prior to the spring. (See "Special Purchasing Considerations" later in this chapter for more information.)
- **Economic order quantity (EOQ)**: this is a formula-based approach for determining how much to order that minimizes total inventory costs, such as ordering and holding costs. This method is infrequently used. (See Chapter 3 for more information.)
- **Kanban system**: this method is popular in manufacturing but can also be helpful in veterinary medicine and healthcare. The Kanban method is a "lean management" technique that uses visual

cues or cards to signal that something is running low. I find this works exceptionally well for hospital supplies and other consumables. (See "Two Bin System" in Chapter 3 for more information.)

Helpful Definitions
- **Lean management**: this is like the business version of minimalism! It's about minimizing waste – whether it's time, resources, or extra steps in a process – to make everything work smoothly and save money.
- **Holding (carrying) cost**: the cost of keeping an item on the shelf.
- **Demand shift**: a change in what products are needed. This can be due to changes in medication preference, seasonality, changes in the care team, an increase or decrease in overall patient visits, or a change in a specific kind of case (for example, if you see eight cases of pancreatitis in one week whereas you usually see two a month), among other factors.

I invite you to be curious about what replenishment strategies might work best for your practice. Similar to the different types of ROPs, different tactics work better for particular categories or items. For example, the Kanban system might work best for hospital supplies in your central storage area, whereas periodic replenishment might work best for bulk flea, tick, and heartworm prevention. Ultimately, you might discover that for 95% of your inventory, it works best with ROPs.

"Best Practice" Questions to Consider
- What methods of replenishment are you currently using? You might already be using one primary method without realizing its technical term.
- Do you think adding other techniques for other types of items would be beneficial?
- Are there any tactics you want to try out or add to your inventory?

4.3   Creating an Order Schedule

4.3.1   Author's Story/Note

When I think about water, I cannot help but think of this story. I remember when I took Tank camping for the first time. I had snagged a campground spot right on the lake. It was the clearest, most beautiful blue and green water I had ever seen. Tank had never really been a fan of swimming but would occasionally splash and run around. He had an independent streak a mile wide due to his livestock guardian dog roots. He had to be on a long line. On this particular trip, though, I brought him down to the water, and he was immediately enamored.

He started running up and down the edge of the water, splashing the cold water everywhere, and his long legs almost did not keep up with his excitement. The "zoomies" were in full effect. The edge of the lake was pretty shallow, and he eventually went deeper into the water and started swimming and, for lack of a better word, frolicking in the water. He was filled with so much joy and excitement. We played in the water for a long time! It's a memory that I hold so near and dear to my heart. He was normally a fairly reserved, stoic dog, especially as he got older, so it was so precious to see him so full of joy.

When you think about the flow of inventory in your practice, creating an ordering schedule can help regulate the cycles and create consistency. It's also helpful to have a schedule and a routine to follow each week. Not only that but when planning orders, you can also plan your other corresponding tasks. When I follow this process, I'll know (generally, as long as there aren't delays) when

Table 4.1 An example ordering schedule.

Sunday	Monday	Tuesday	Wednesday	Thursday	Friday	Saturday
	Herbal order (every other week)	Main order (cutoff is 2 PM)		Unpack and receive the main order	Order food vendor #1 (cutoff is 12 PM)	
			Unpack and receive food order			

my orders will arrive and when they need to be unpacked and received. If I know that, I can plan to receive orders on specific days and/or make a plan for orders with controlled substances or temperature-controlled items.

To create an ordering schedule, list the vendors you normally order from or the types of orders (for example, Food Vendor #1, Main Weekly Order, etc.). Then, determine when and how often you'll order. I'm a visual person so I like to add it to a calendar so I can see exactly what I need to be doing on a particular day. This can also be helpful when you want to create pockets of uninterrupted inventory time throughout the week.

An example of this schedule is shown in Table 4.1.

Mapping out your order schedule can give you insight into when you'll need to do certain inventory tasks and can help make an alternative plan when you are on vacation or get limited "inventory time" due to being short-handed.

4.4 Ordering Workflow

Setting up a workflow for your ordering days can help you get into a routine and a rhythm. It can also help ensure that nothing gets forgotten! This workflow will likely depend on a number of different factors: How often you place an order, what other roles you have outside of inventory, and what vendor you are purchasing from, among other factors.

My ordering flow looked very different when I first started compared to when I had gotten some experience and confidence under my belt! When I first started, I would walk around the hospital, shaking bottles, rummaging through cabinets, checking the want list, and seeing what was running low that day. Then I'd order it. During my first week on the job, I remember my team members calling items into the distributor throughout the day to be ordered. I often forgot to check things (hello, neurodivergence!). If they were out of sight, they were sometimes out of mind. At this point, I was probably ordering every day. It's a bit wild (and embarrassing) to think about where I started. I try to give myself grace, remembering that I had no training and I was just trying to do the best I could with what I had at the time.

As I got more experience and became comfortable with inventory management, I was able to set up my ROPs and flags so that I wasn't critically low on items all the time. I also had a much better indicator that something was low, rather than relying on the "want book" or the whiteboard. I settled on ordering twice weekly for most things and once weekly for herbals and diets. I would print the "Reorder Report" from AVImark®, check the want list, and do a walkthrough of all my items. Eventually, I learned about reorder tags and added additional "flags" for hospital supplies and white goods, so I did not have to dig through cabinets any more.

Each morning of ordering day, I would pull all my different flags together (the report from my software, tags for some items, etc.), and then I would quickly verify that nothing else needed to be changed or added. Each of my reorder flags also listed the quantity to order, so I always knew how much I needed to reorder. Then, I would log in to the ordering website and place my order.

"Best Practice" Creating an Ordering Workflow

The first step in creating an ordering workflow that works for you is to think about the following.

- What is your ordering cadence? How often will you be ordering and what vendors will you need to purchase from? Will some vendors be on a consistent ordering schedule, and others might be as needed?
  - For example, if you are an equine practice that places a large bulk order at the end of the year during American Association of Equine Practitioners (AAEP) promotions, your ordering workflow for that extra large bulk order will likely be different than a normal weekly order.
- What order flags do you have set up? Do you use your practice management system or other inventory software? Do you have reorder tags? Is part of the order delegated to another team member?
- Are there any other considerations that you'll need to keep in mind?

Then, start to outline your workflow. It might make sense to have a different ordering workflow depending on the type of order. As an example, listing out the steps for a big yearly bulk purchase can help make sure nothing is forgotten!

Let's explore a few examples together.

Georgia, the lead inventory manager at Tank's Animal Hospital, is rethinking her ordering workflow after adding different kinds of reorder tags. Here's what she came up with.

1) Each Tuesday and Thursday morning, review the "Reorder Report," grab the reorder tags from the "to be ordered" basket, and give Amelia the dental cart reorder checklist and Dr Tank the controlled substance reorder checklist.
2) Once the reorder checklists are back from Amelia and Dr Tank, quickly review all the items that need to be ordered.
3) Then, check the appointment calendar for the upcoming week to see if any patients or cases need specific inventory items or special ordered items, or if any appointments will significantly alter normal demand (like an appointment with two litters of Great Pyrenees puppies for vaccines!).
4) Finally, do a quick once-over to make sure nothing was missed.
5) Then, add the items to reorder and their corresponding quantities to the shopping cart.

Tank's Animal Hospital places a yearly bulk purchase of heartworm prevention to take advantage of the savings. Here's the workflow that Georgia outlined.

1) Learn more about the promotion: what are the terms, what products are included, and what limitations or specifics are there?
2) After learning the special financing terms, pull the date range from the same time period from last year to see how much was sold for that time-frame (as an example, if the promotion outlines 90-day special financing and you are purchasing for February–April, run a report for that same time period in a previous year). for more information and best practices for bulk or promotional purchases, see the "Special Purchasing Considerations" section of this chapter.
3) After calculating how much to order, confirm with Dr Tank and order through the preferred rep to take advantage of split billing.

Creating and outlining an ordering workflow can help ensure that no items are forgotten and that each section or task is completed before ordering.

4.4.1   Example Preorder Checklist

- Find and determine what's low and needs to be ordered.
  - Gather the reorder tags from the "to be ordered" bin.
  - Run a reorder report from your practice management system or other inventory software to see if anything is flagged as low.
  - Review the "want list" or special order list.
  - Check to see if any specific products need to be ordered for any upcoming special procedures.
  - Double-check your "VIP products."
  - Do a quick "once over" and see if anything was missed.
- Determine how much to order for each item that is running low (your reorder quantity). Ideally, your reorder quantity should already be calculated and documented somewhere.
- Start adding your low items and their reorder quantities to the cart in your ordering platform.

4.4.2   Placing Your Order

Once you know what you need to order, the next step is to place the order! I often recommend placing an order using the vendor's, distributor's, or manufacturer's website, or another online ordering platform. I'm dating myself slightly but I remember watching my first practice manager fax her order in. In all seriousness, I prefer to use an online ordering platform of some kind over calling, faxing, or texting your order because you have more control over exactly what item you'd like to purchase and can see pricing information.

One of the mishaps that can happen is ordering the wrong quantity of something. When I was an inventory manager, I once ordered just one catheter instead of a whole box. There were quite a few times when I only received one of something, thinking I had ordered a whole case. It can also go the other way! Inventory managers have told me they thought they were ordering a box of 12 bags of fluids but instead received 12 boxes of 12 bags. This can happen because there are times when the units that you are purchasing aren't exactly clear. "Am I ordering one unit, or am I ordering one case of 10?" for example. Before placing your order, I recommend verifying the quantity and the cost for each item. Does it seem to align? Or am I purchasing $20,000 in fluids?

Another thing that I've found helpful is to create "shopping lists" in your ordering platform. This is helpful because you essentially create a list of items and then it's much easier to add an item to the cart without having to search for it. For example, you might create a shopping list for all your vaccines. Then, when you need to order, you can go to the shopping list, enter the quantity, and add it to the cart.

Utilizing the list can eliminate having to search for the item and potentially accidentally ordering the wrong one. Another instance where a shopping list might be helpful is with preferred hospital supplies and white goods. If your team is particular about a specific brand or type of supply, you can use the list to make sure you are always purchasing the correct one. Alternatively, if shopping lists aren't available to you, you can add the item identification code to your reorder list, tags, etc., so you can quickly find the exact item.

Once your order has been placed, I invite you to give yourself a big pat on the back and celebrate somehow. Maybe take a few minutes to walk outside and get some sun on your face, make a cup of your favorite tea, or just take a moment to drink some water or nourish your body. What you do matters. Just because you might not have your hands on a patient during these moments does not make your role and your work any less important. So take a breath. Remember, you are a human being doing a job. Take care of your human beingness throughout the day.

4.5 Strategies for Navigating Backorders

Hands down, I think one of the most frustrating parts about managing inventory is navigating backorders and supply chain issues. When a backorder happens, you often do not control when you will start receiving the product again. Not only that but you often do not get a heads-up that something will no longer be available! Then, to top it all off, sometimes your team does not understand why something is unavailable and what that really means.

In this section, you'll review strategies for navigating backorders and how to make it easier on yourself and your team.

Helpful Definitions
- **Backorder**: a product that is not available for purchase for a variety of reasons. Sometimes, you can place an order to go on a "backorder list" and as soon as it's in stock, the order will be shipped out to you.
- **Supply chain**: the journey a product takes from individual raw components to a final finished product in your practice. Disruptions can happen anywhere along the supply chain, impacting the availability of a product.
- **Allocation**: when a product has limited availability, the vendor or company limits how much can be purchased at a time to avoid it being completely out of stock. It helps manage limited stock and ensures the product is distributed fairly.

There are four main issues to consider when trying to navigate backorders.

1) Communicating with your team.
2) Researching and discovering backorders.
3) Identifying alternatives.
4) Navigating current backorders.

4.5.1 Communicating with Your Team

There is no doubt about it – backorders are incredibly frustrating for you and your team. One of the most useful things you can do is create a communication strategy and action plan so that your team is aware of things on backorder. This helps to ensure that they aren't trying to prescribe backordered products while seeing patients. Or getting irritated at you (or the inventory manager), assuming that the product was simply not ordered.

I personally prefer to have a multi-pronged approach so communication is covered from different angles. Here are some of my favorite methods.

- **Add a "marker" to the label or spot on the shelf**: this can serve as a visual cue or reminder that the item is on backorder and it's not just out. Plus, if it has information about an alternative product listed, it helps our team not feel so "stuck" and powerless about the backorder. For example, you could use a bright, specific-colored garage sale sticker dot with "B.O." written on it to denote it's on backorder. You could also have a brightly colored "On Backorder" sticker.

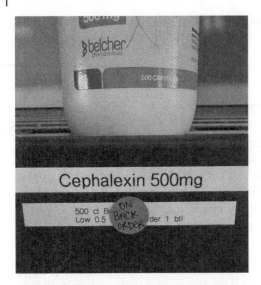

Figure 4.1 An example of a marker that can be added to backordered products. Nicole Clausen.

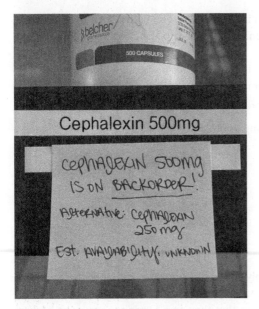

Figure 4.2 Another flag that can be added to backordered products. Nicole Clausen.

Or you could use a sticky note and list information on the backorder and any available alternative product (Figures 4.1 and 4.2).

- **Create an alert in your practice management system**: some practice management systems allow you to create an alert from an individual product. When the product is ordered on a patient's medical record, the alert will pop up. If a product is on backorder, an alert could be added with any backorder information, alternative products, estimated arrival details, or other helpful information.

- **Create a backorder communication system**: in addition to adding labels to the shelf and creating an alert in your practice management system, it's also helpful to create a backorder "master list" or a system for giving your team updates all in one location. This can be done with a Slack channel with your entire team as members. A Slack channel is also a great hospital-wide communication method for any updates, not just inventory. This can also be created with a Google Sheets document or a physical whiteboard.

It can be helpful to list the date an item went on backorder, product information, any alternative products, and the date of expected arrival (if known).

4.5.2 Researching and Discovering Backorders

Depending on whether you are being proactive and trying to identify any upcoming backorders or you have already discovered a product is on backorder and you are trying to navigate the situation, there are a number of helpful strategies.

Some of these methods might not work for everyone but the key is to be curious! Ask yourself what might work and see what might be helpful for you.

- **Build a relationship with your distributor or manufacturer representatives**: your distributor and manufacturer reps can be an invaluable resource (and not just for backorders!). Your reps often will have information about what might be going on backorder or allocation. They might already release information or resources regularly about any upcoming availability issues.

When I was an inventory manager, my inside sales representative at my main distributor was always incredibly helpful. She would try to find items in an alternative warehouse, add me to a backorder list to receive them as soon as they were available, and give me allocation and availability updates.

Tip: If the online ordering website you are using shows that an item is out of stock, call your inside sales rep (ISR)! The website will only show availability for your specific warehouse, so it may be in stock in another location. Your ISR may be able to order some through another warehouse. Keep in mind that items that ship from an alternative warehouse might take longer to arrive.

- **Have accounts with a mix of smaller and larger distributors**: when products are hard to find, it's beneficial to have accounts with as many vendors and distributors as possible. You'll have access to more opportunities to find that particular product.
  Tip: I find it helpful to have a mix of smaller and larger distributors because smaller companies might have different availability than larger companies. Also, some suppliers or vendors might have a particular "specialty" where certain products are more often available.
- **Set up daily alerts with the FDA drug shortage database**: the FDA maintains a drug shortage list (for human medications) that lists drugs or ingredients that are currently in shortage or have been resolved. Although it does not typically include veterinary-specific drugs, if something is used in both human and animal medicine, it might be helpful. On this site, you can set up daily email alerts for any new or updated drug shortages.

4.5.3 Navigating Current Backorders

If you find that a particular item is on backorder, I recommend first communicating with your team. Is this a critically important item (like something related to anesthesia or euthanasia solution), or is it more of a "nice to have"? Knowing this information can help determine your path forward. Does an alternative need to be discussed or will you just need to wait until it comes off backorder? For example, if opioids go on backorder, it's important to make an alternative plan for anesthetics and surgical procedures.

Here are some tips for when a product is currently on backorder.

- **See if it's available compounded**: if an item is on backorder and has no estimated date of return, see if the product is available to be compounded. Compounding pharmacies often offer alternatives for some products. For example, pimobendan can be compounded for those times when Vetmedin® is unavailable. Other products may not be available (for example, if there is a raw material shortage) but it's always worth checking!

"Best Practice" Tip
Kelly K, a wonderful member of the Veterinary Inventory Strategy Network, creates a shopping list with all the current pertinent backorders to view them all in one place. That way, she does not have to search for each item she's tracking.

- **Create an action plan with your team**: after discussing the products that are on backorder, create an action plan with the next steps. You might consider the following.
  - What tasks need to be completed? Do alternatives need to be researched? Does a medication backup plan need to be crafted (if opioids or euthanasia solution go on backorder, for example)?
  - Who will be in charge of each task? Does anything need to be delegated?

- Set goals or a goal timeline for completing the action plan.
- What follow-up communication (if any) will be necessary with your team?
- What resources or other tools do you have available that would be helpful? Would your ISR be helpful? Would another vendor or compounding pharmacy be beneficial?

It can be beneficial to set up a "Backorder Standard Operating Procedure" or have a documented process that lists the steps that you'll follow if a backorder does happen. That way, the disruption will be communicated to your team, you can identify any alternatives, and no part of the process gets missed.

4.5.4 Example Backorder Process

When you notice an item is no longer available or out of stock:

1) check to see if it's available through a different vendor, manufacturer, or distributor
2) if not, call the ISR at your main distributor and see if there is any in a different warehouse. Check to see if they have any availability updates or if you can be added to a backorder list
3) communicate the backorder to your team. This might involve posting in a practice communication channel, sending a group email, or posting it on a communication board or backorder list
4) add an alert to the product in your practice management system (if possible) and add some kind of note/marker to the item's location on the shelf
5) discuss with the management team or medical team to determine if an alternative product or increase in another product is necessary
6) research different alternative options and present them to the team for review and approval.

4.6 Utilizing Purchase Orders in Your Practice Management System

Once you have placed your order, creating a purchase order in your software system can make receiving much easier. The term "purchase order" might vary depending on the PiMS or other inventory software you are using. Essentially, you want to create a list of the items that you purchased with the corresponding quantities so that when the shipment arrives, it's really easy to update the software with how much was received.

Rather than manually updating the quantity on hand for all the items purchased, you can quickly update the quantity on hand, cost, and any other pertinent information with the receiving function. In Chapter 5, you'll cover in more detail how to use your software system to make receiving easier.

4.7 Special Purchasing Considerations

In the previous chapter, you reviewed how to calculate ROPs for your items and use data and your consumption patterns to estimate future demand. The premise of these calculations was to maintain a healthy turnover and not keep too much on the shelf. However, there are times when it might make financial sense to purchase on promotion or in large quantities, which can offer significant savings, rebates, or other financial incentives. But in order to capitalize on any bulk purchasing benefits, it's important to order strategically.

I have seen quite a few instances where purchasing in bulk has gone sideways. Most often, the purchaser ordered too much and at the end of the billing period, a huge payment was due but barely any of the product had sold. In quite a few of those instances, it had significantly impacted cash flow and the practice was in danger of not being able to afford payroll. Other times, a large order was purchased and the practice still had some on the shelf a year later, and quite a bit of it expired.

By remembering your demand forecasting principles, you can more effectively order for bulk or promotional purchases and eliminate those scary situations above. It's also important to remember that just because something is on sale or promotion does not necessarily mean it makes sense to buy it.

4.7.1 Are Bulk Purchases Worth It?

Bulk purchases have often been calculated by applying a certain growth percentage to what was purchased the previous year. But that does not take into account how much was actually sold. Did any of the products purchased expire? Did ordering that much product negatively impact the practice's cash flow? Did the product just sit on the shelf collecting dust? To help avoid these instances and keep our bulk purchases from negatively impacting the practice, it's important to purchase according to what has sold, not based on purchase history.

When considering purchasing larger quantities, it's essential to understand the billing terms. Often, vendors or manufacturers will have promotions at different times of the year with special financing terms or significant discounts. The terms will vary depending on the specific promotion, the vendor, and often the "tiers" or categories of products that are purchased.

Your distributor representative sometimes has the flexibility to work with you on creative billing terms, like split billing (payments are split up evenly over X number of months) or delayed billing (for example, you might have 90 days to pay rather than the regular 25 days). So, if you are considering purchasing larger than normal quantities, check with your distributor representative first.

After understanding the specific billing terms for the larger order, the next step is to calculate the amount to order based on your practice's sales or usage for that product. Generally, when making bulk purchases, only order what you will use or sell within the special financing period. For example, if a distributor offers you 90 days delayed billing, only order what would be used within the 90-day time period.

Use the following formula for calculating bulk orders.

$$Bulk\ Order\ Quantity = Average\ Daily\ Use \times Billing\ Terms\ \left(in\ Days\right)$$

where

$$Average\ Daily\ Use = \frac{Annual\ Usage}{Number\ of\ Days\ Open\ per\ Year}$$

Let's explore two examples together. Tank's Animal Hospital wants to purchase Product A from Distributor C and has agreed a 90-day delayed billing period. They have an annual usage for this particular product of 3,819 units. In addition, the hospital is open five days a week.

Variables required.

- Annual usage = 3,819 units
- Number of days open per year = 260 days
- Billing terms = 90 days

The first step is to find the average daily use for Product A.

$$Average\ Daily\ Use = \frac{Annual\ Usage}{Number\ of\ Days\ Open\ per\ Year}$$

$$Average\ Daily\ Use = \frac{3,819\ Units}{260\ Days}$$

$$Average\ Daily\ Use = 14.69 \approx 15\ Units$$

Once the average daily usage has been calculated, the next step is to calculate the bulk quantity to order.

$$Bulk\ Order\ Quantity = Average\ Daily\ Use \times Billing\ Terms\ \left(in\ Days\right)$$

$$Bulk\ Order\ Quantity = 15\ Units \times 90\ Days$$

$$Bulk\ Order\ Quantity = 1,350\ Units$$

In this example, Tank's Animal Hospital's suggested purchase is 1,350 units of Product A. If they decide to purchase this amount, they would likely sell what was purchased before the bill for Distributor C becomes due.

In another example for Tank's Animal Hospital, the item they are interested in purchasing in bulk is a seasonal product (Product B). They would also get 90 days of delayed billing for this product. In that case, if an item is seasonal and has very different average sales during the peak time versus the slower season, I like to calculate how much to purchase a little differently.

Let's explore an example of calculating the amount to bulk purchase for a seasonal product. There are two ways Dr Tank and Georgia (his lead inventory manager) could go about this. Using the first method, they could review a sales report for the same time period last year. They would still want to purchase what they would use or sell in the special financing time period but rather than calculating the average, they would look to see what sold last year.

They are planning on purchasing Interceptor® Plus to arrive at the practice at the beginning of March. As a reminder, they have negotiated 90 days of special financing so Dr Tank and Georgia want to see how much Interceptor Plus was sold starting in March for 90 days of the previous year. Table 4.2 shows the sales report data.

Table 4.2 An example sales report for Interceptor Plus.

Month	Amount sold
February	28 boxes
March	87 boxes
April	123 boxes
May	94 boxes
June	41 boxes

To purchase what's anticipated to sell within the special delayed billing financing terms (starting in March), Georgia would add together the amounts sold in March, April, and May from the previous year.

$$Bulk\ Order\ Quantity = Amount\ Sold\ During\ the\ Same\ Period\ of\ The\ Previous\ Year$$

$$Bulk\ Order\ Quantity = March + April + May$$

$$Bulk\ Order\ Quantity = 87 + 123 + 94$$

$$Bulk\ Order\ Quantity = 304\ Boxes$$

In this example, Tank's Animal Hospital would purchase 304 boxes (rounded to the nearest case, if applicable) of Interceptor Plus.

The decision whether or not to purchase in bulk or with a promotion is a business decision unique to your practice and should be taken strategically with your practice's specific goals and financial health in mind.

4.7.2 What about Promotional Purchases?

Throughout your inventory adventures, another purchasing consideration you might come across is whether or not to purchase an item on promotion. This is not as cut and dried as purchasing in bulk and will come down to whether or not it makes sense for your unique practice. First and foremost, it's key to understand the terms. Is it a 5% discount across the board? Or do you save 15% if you purchase $10,000 worth or more and have 90 days of delayed billing? The terms of the promotion can vary wildly, so it's crucial to understand what that looks like.

Then, it's important to understand how much you use or sell in the context of the promotion.

- If it has delayed billing or special financing terms, how much do you normally use or sell within that time period? Is it significantly different from the promotional order requirements?
- Is this an "A" or top-selling item? Alternatively, does it only sell occasionally? I invite you to reflect and consider if you are purchasing it because it's on sale or if it will help your practice financially.
- If there aren't any special billing terms, can you talk to your distributor rep to negotiate any?

It's also helpful to think about other logistical components.

- Do you have enough storage space for the item?
- Is there a high risk of shrinkage such as theft, loss, product expiry, or other reasons for loss if you purchase more than normal?
- How will this purchase affect cash flow? Will spending money at the end of the year decrease taxable profits and be beneficial in that sense?

If you decide that the promotion is worth buying the extra product, determining how much you'll need is key to taking advantage of the discount. If there are special financing terms and delayed billing, I recommend purchasing what you'll use in that timeframe. If there is no delayed or split billing, I recommend reviewing the previous demand for the item, your storage space, determining what would be "too much" to purchase, and considering any other factors that may impact your practice.

Let's explore two different examples and how you might decide to move forward and take advantage of the promotion or not.

Example 4.1

Recently, Dr Tank went to a large veterinary conference and found quite a few enticing promotions. First, there is Cerenia® injectable. This is a top-selling product at Tank's Animal Hospital, and it's one of the top 10 items sold. If he purchases $5,000 worth of products, he will receive a 10% rebate.

To start, Dr Tank calculates the average daily use of the item. His practice is open six days a week, for a total of 312 days per year. After pulling a sales report, Dr Tank identifies that the practice sold 2981 ml in the last 12 months.

Variables required.

- Annual usage = 2,981 ml
- Number of days open per year = 312 days

$$Average\ Daily\ Use = \frac{Annual\ Usage}{Number\ of\ Days\ Open\ per\ Year}$$

$$Average\ Daily\ Use = \frac{2,981\ ml}{312\ Days}$$

$$Average\ Daily\ Use = 9.55 \approx 10\ ml$$

On average, Tank's Animal Hospital uses 10 ml per day. Each bottle of Injectable A contains 20 ml and costs $265.00. Knowing this information, Dr Tank can do some additional calculations.

The promotion requires a purchase of $5,000, which is equivalent to roughly 19 bottles (approximately 380 ml). After calculating the average daily use, the next step is to find out how long roughly 380 ml will last.

$$Days\ of\ Stock = \frac{Total\ Number\ of\ Units}{Average\ Daily\ Use}$$

$$Days\ of\ Stock = \frac{380\ ml}{10\ ml}$$

$$Days\ of\ Stock = 38$$

In this example, Dr Tank calculated that $5,000 of Injectable A would last approximately 38 days. In this case, the practice had the storage capacity and there wasn't a high risk of theft. Due to the consumption pattern, Dr Tank felt comfortable purchasing the product on promotion.

Let's take it one step further and say that Dr Tank was able to negotiate delayed billing of 60 days, so he wants to purchase what the practice would use in 60 days. He uses the bulk order formula from above to calculate this.

$$Bulk\ Order\ Quantity = Average\ Daily\ Use \times Billing\ Terms\ (in\ Days)$$

$$Bulk\ Order\ Quantity = 10\ ml \times 60\ Days$$

$$Bulk\ Order\ Quantity = 600\ ml$$

then

$$ml\ to\ Bottle\ Conversion = \frac{600\ ml}{20\ ml\ per\ Bottle}$$

$$ml\ to\ Bottle\ Conversion = 30\ Bottles$$

In this example, Tank's Animal Hospital's suggested purchase is 30 bottles of Injectable A for a total cost of $7,950. If they decide to purchase this amount, they would likely sell what was purchased before the bill comes due. Additionally, Dr Tank would receive a rebate of $795.

Example 4.2

In the next example, Dr Tank learned of another promotion for a bathing product, Shampoo A. If the practice buys 10 bottles, they'll get two free. This item does not sell very frequently, so he's unsure if purchasing this product on promotion would make sense. Let's explore this example together.

To start, Dr Tank calculates the average daily use of the item. His practice is open six days a week for a total of 312 days per year. After pulling a sales report, Dr Tank identified that the practice sold 14 bottles in the last 12 months.

Variables required.

- Annual usage = 14 bottles
- Number of days open per year = 312 days

$$Average\ Daily\ Use = \frac{Annual\ Usage}{Number\ of\ Days\ Open\ per\ Year}$$

$$Average\ Daily\ Use = \frac{14\ Bottles}{312\ Days}$$

$$Average\ Daily\ Use = 0.04\ Bottles\ per\ day$$

Next, he calculated how many days 10 bottles would last.

$$Days\ of\ Stock = \frac{Total\ Quantity}{Average\ Daily\ Use}$$

$$Days\ of\ Stock = \frac{10\ Bottles}{0.04\ Bottles\ per\ day}$$

$$Days\ of\ Stock = 250\ Days$$

In this example, if Tank's Animal Hospital purchased the 10 bottles of Shampoo A on promotion, it would last on the shelf for approximately 250 days before selling. Dr Tank decided not to take advantage of the promotion due to the minimal benefit and low turnover.

Whether to purchase an item on promotion will depend heavily on the item, its consumption pattern, and if it makes financial sense for your practice. The key is to weigh the variables to see if the benefit outweighs the cost or whether the product would just sit on the shelf.

4.8 It's More than Just the Cost of an Item

Often when thinking about inventory costs, people just think about the direct costs of an item: how much the practice paid to purchase an inventory item, piece of equipment, supply, or anything else. But that's not the whole picture. There are other costs associated with inventory that are also important to keep in mind. These **indirect costs** can quickly add up if you are not careful.

Let's say that you are in the market for a new vacuum cleaner and you spend hours researching different brands, reading reviews, watching testimonial videos, and trying to figure out which vacuum would be the best fit. You finally find the perfect one and purchase it. In addition to the direct cost of the vacuum, there is the indirect cost of all those hours spent researching.

Let's explore another situation. You are working on placing your order for the week. You realize that you can purchase a bottle of gabapentin for $1.00 less from another supplier, but you do not need to purchase anything else from that supplier. So, you might save $1.00 upfront but now you have another shipment to unpack, an additional invoice to receive into your software, and additional work for your book keeper. So, it can be helpful to determine if you are really saving money on the item or if you are only saving on the direct costs while increasing your indirect costs.

There are two main categories of indirect costs: labor and holding costs. **Labor costs** include the inventory team's time to place, receive, enter, and manage the order. **Holding costs** are those associated with keeping it on the shelf and include costs such as rent, opportunity cost, insurance, and temperature controls, among others, to keep that inventory item safe and protected until it's sold. It's important to understand how indirect costs might affect your practice and try to find the balance between labor and holding costs.

When you purchase *more of something less frequently, it means higher holding costs but lower labor costs.* When you purchase *less of something more frequently, it means lower holding costs but higher labor costs.*

4.8.1 Indirect Costs: Holding and Labor Costs

Holding costs include costs associated with "holding" or keeping that item on the shelf. Depending on the practice, these costs could consist of the utility and facility costs of protecting that inventory item from heat, cold, and humidity, insurance premium costs, any pharmacy licensing fees or regulatory costs, any loss due to expiry or shrinkage (for example, theft, missed charges, etc.), taxes paid on the value of the inventory, and any facility costs to store that inventory item, among other factors. Generally, the holding costs for a veterinary practice range between 8% and 15% (Heinke 2014) of the total unit cost. The longer the product is "held" and kept on the shelf, the higher the holding costs will be.

Labor costs include any costs related to your (or another team member's) time to manage the flow of inventory in the practice and complete the five R's of inventory replenishment: recognize, react, reorder, receive, and restock. Your time to determine what needs to be ordered, compile an order, place the order, unpack, receive, and restock the order. The idea is that the more orders that are placed throughout the week and the longer an order takes to be placed, the higher the labor costs will be. Generally, labor costs account for 15–20% of the total unit cost (Heinke 2014).

What does this mean for you, and how does it affect your practice?

Let us explore a scenario. Say that in an effort to reduce inventory costs and keep your orders on the smaller side, you only buy a little bit at a time for each inventory item, no matter how quickly it sells. For a particular flea/tick prevention that often flies off the shelf, it seems like you have to constantly order a sleeve or two every other day. Although you might keep your average purchase amount per order on the lower side, you are purchasing that item 6–10 times a month but only paying for it once for statement billing. Think about all the extra indirect labor costs associated with ordering, unpacking, receiving, stocking, and book keeping an item so frequently.

Calculating and leveraging your ROPs can be a great way to find the balance between your labor and holding indirect costs!

4.9   Choosing and Evaluating Vendors

In vet med, there are a number of different options for vendors and distributors, both small and larger companies. Before you dive into strategies for evaluating different vendors, let's review some terms together.

Helpful Definitions
- **Distributor**: a distributor is an intermediary between the producer or manufacturer of a product and a veterinary practice (examples include MWI Animal Health, Covetrus, Patterson Veterinary, and Midwest Veterinary Supply). They are essentially like Dunder Mifflin in vet med.
- **Manufacturer**: a company that makes goods for sale (examples: Nutramax Laboratories Inc., Zoetis, Elanco Animal Health, Boehringer Ingelheim Vetmedica, Ceva Animal Health, Hill's Pet Nutrition).

With ever-present supply chain disruptions and frequent backorders, I like to have a mix of accounts open with small and larger distributors. This allows the opportunity to check availability across multiple companies and not be as limited.

Think of it like grocery stores. I have quite a few in my area that I could go to if something is out of stock, but I have a main grocery store that I usually frequent; they have a great selection of produce and great pricing, and the staff are always kind and friendly.

"Best Practice" SOP
When selecting a vendor, manufacturer, or distributor, here are some aspects to consider.

- **Product selection**: what is their range of products? Do they have any specialty items or a line of generic products or supplies? Evaluate the range of products to see if they align with your practice.
- **Support services**: in addition to the products they sell, what other services do they offer to help your practice? Would you have a territory manager who can assist you? Do they have equipment maintenance services? Evaluate to see what is available to you and who might be working with you at this company.
  - Having relationships with your distributor's territory manager and ISR can benefit your practice greatly, so it's helpful if you enjoy working with them!
- **Pricing**: what is their product pricing like? Is it in alignment with other distributors that you currently use? Is there room for any negotiations? Do they work with any group purchasing organizations (GPOs) that you are part of? Keep in mind that for some items, you'll pay the exact same no matter which distributor you use. Other items have a variable cost and will be different from distributor to distributor.
- **Sustainability and environmental impact**: what does the company do to minimize its environmental impact, and what are its efforts toward sustainability? What is its packaging like? What efforts does it make to minimize waste and excessive packaging?
- **Shipping and delivery times**: what are their shipping and delivery times? When should you expect the shipment to arrive after placing your order? What are their cutoff times, and do they offer weekend delivery? Explore their shipping and delivery times to see if they align with your practice.
- **Ordering platform and website**: is their ordering website easy to navigate and purchase from? Is their website accessible or are there challenges? Does the ordering platform offer any helpful features for ordering? How much of a priority for you is an easy-to-use and accessible ordering website?

- **Shipping charges or ordering minimums**: explore what their shipping costs are and if there are any order minimums. Are there additional shipping charges if you do not meet the order minimums? Is there room for negotiation on any of the shipping charges or minimums?
- **Rebates, discounts, or other incentives**: what loyalty programs, rebates, discounts, or other incentives do they offer? How will you be notified of new promotions or rebate programs? Explore what this looks like and how you might benefit.
- **Returns, recall, and backorder/allocation policies**: what are their policies on product returns? What is the process if you need to return something, and do you get a credit? What are their policies if there is a recall or supply chain disruption? How does that get handled, and how will you be impacted or involved?

Evaluating your vendors to make sure they are the best fit for your practice is so important!

4.10 Creating and Using a Budget

Inventory budgets are hard in vet med. There are a few reasons for this, but part of the reason is that the cost of goods sold (COGS) as a category is a challenge to define. Veterinary medicine is a service-based industry, so there is inventory sold and inventory consumed. To add another layer to the complexity, there are also costs included in COGS (like reference laboratory costs), and the total expenses are unknown until the statement arrives, and you cannot limit them as the month goes on.

For example, you would never say to Mrs Jones "I'm so sorry that we cannot run Fifi's lab tests because we are over budget on our reference lab expenses this month." You certainly would never tell someone "I'm so sorry, we cannot cremate Buddy after his euthanasia because we are over budget on our cremation expenses this month." In-house and reference lab expenses are considered part of the COGS but you do not know the grand total until the statement comes in after the billing cycle. Especially if you are a practice that's very diagnostic forward, this can be a significant portion of your COGS.

When it comes to budgeting, it's important to understand that there are two types of expenses included in COGS. First, items that are purchased. With these items, you have more control over the total amount spent. With the second type, nonpurchase costs (i.e., cremation services and laboratory costs), you do not have visibility (or much control) over the grand total until the statement arrives.

When trying to lower inventory costs or add a budget, some use a "top-down" approach by assigning a budget of a certain percentage to last week's revenue (for example, your budget is 15% of last week's revenue). They then expect the inventory manager to shoehorn all their expenses into this amount. This approach does not work because it is a reactive way to fix the problem, and the problem persists. The purchaser then needs to make a judgment call on what's "important enough" to reorder. But if we have sold the item, that means it needs to be purchased again in order to provide patient care and sustain revenue creation.

Ideally, if you are trying to reduce your inventory costs, you should use a "bottom-up" approach by first optimizing your inventory by removing unnecessary and redundant products, increasing turnover by reviewing and recalculating reorder levels, and evaluating your inventory overall. Then, once you streamline your inventory, you can overlay a budget for "guard rails." But if you try to assign a budget first without evaluating or optimizing your inventory, it will often be significantly more challenging (and frustrating!) for the inventory manager.

Inventory managers are often put in the middle between the care team (which expects to have everything they need for patient care in stock at all times) and the leadership (which assigns the budget). Let's set the inventory team up for success as much as possible.

So, how can you craft a budget that works with you rather than against you? There are several different methods for creating a budget and a few tactics for keeping track of your progress throughout the month, and how well one method or tactic works for you depends mostly on your practice. Be curious about what would work well, and keep in mind that it's probably not going to be perfect from the start.

"Best Practice" Concept Check
- Why are budgets hard in vet med?
- Have you ever had a budget that felt impossible to meet? How did you navigate the situation?
- Before implementing a budget (using the bottom-up approach), what should you do first?

4.10.1 Three-year Average Method

In this method, you'll first estimate the practice's future revenue based on the average revenue growth over the last three years. This method is helpful if your growth has been relatively stable or if your practice stays reasonably consistent, revenue- or growth-wise. The next step is to project and estimate your COGS based on the last three years of information as well.

If you break your costs into subcategories, you can create smaller, more specific expense categories. For example, within the overall COGS, you might have subcategories like pharmacy or dietary product costs. By dividing costs into subcategories, you can create individual budgets for each category. For instance, you might have a budget specifically for purchases (like vaccination or injection costs) and another budget for overall COGS, which includes all costs related to patient care. It's beneficial to categorize expenses for clearer budgeting and analysis, allowing your practice to understand its spending patterns.

The American Animal Hospital Association (AAHA) Chart of Accounts is a great resource for categorizing your chart of accounts into different categories and subcategories, including all of your COGS expenses.

Helpful Definitions
- **Chart of accounts**: in accounting, a chart of accounts is like a map that organizes all the financial transactions of a practice. It's a list of all the different types of accounts where the money, assets, debts, and expenses are recorded. Each account has a specific code or number (specifically called a general ledger code) that helps keep everything organized and easy to find. Think of it as a directory that helps accountants track and manage the practice's finances effectively.

"Best Practice" Calculate a Budget using the Three-year Average Method
- Step 1: project annual and monthly revenues.
- Step 2: determine the average cost of goods as a percent of revenue. Estimate expected COGS annually and monthly.
- Step 3: determine if the projected COGS is aligned with your practice's COGS goals.
  - If not, how can you optimize your inventory and work on reducing your COGS so that you can take a "bottom-up" approach?
- Step 4: establish subcategories for your hospital and project expenses for each of these subcategories.
  - For example, you might want to have a separate subcategory for items that are purchased versus not.
- Step 5: track spending by category using whichever method is most convenient. This might include using general ledger codes, Excel, or another purchasing budgeting tool or software.
- Step 6: the budget progress should be reviewed on a regular basis.

If it's consistently hard to reach budgeted spending goals, it's important not just to try to "spend less" but also to optimize your inventory. Chapter 9 has strategies on how to optimize your inventory, and Chapter 10 includes tactics and strategies for evaluating your inventory.

Tip: If you are new to budgeting, it's okay! It can feel overwhelming, so do not be afraid to either start small and simple or go step by step. You can do this!

4.10.1.1 Annual Revenue Projections

Start by determining your annual revenue for the last three years. This information can typically be found in your profit and loss statement from your accountant. Then, calculate the change in revenue (by percentage) from year to year. Once you have determined the percentage change in revenue, the next step is to find the average change in revenue. Then, multiply last year's revenue by your average change in revenue to project next year's revenue.

In this example, we'll be creating a budget for Tank's Animal Hospital. Georgia has put a lot of effort into optimizing and streamlining their inventory. Now, Dr Tank and Georgia will sit down together and walk through the process of calculating their budget for the upcoming year.

First, they'll find the revenue for the last three years (Table 4.3).

Then, they'll calculate the difference between the revenue of that year versus the previous year (Table 4.4). For example, Dr Tank will calculate the difference in revenue from three years ago to two years ago.

Then, they'll find the percent difference from year to year. To find the percent difference, use the formula below.

$$Percent\ Difference = \frac{Revenue\ Change\ in\ \$}{Annual\ Revenue} \times 100$$

As an example, Georgia uses the formula to calculate the percentage change in the practice's revenue from two years ago.

$$Percent\ Difference = \frac{Revenue\ Change\ in\ \$}{Annual\ Revenue} \times 100$$

$$Percent\ Difference = \frac{\$\ 300,000}{\$\ 3,100,000} \times 100$$

Table 4.3 Revenue for the last three years for Tank's Animal Hospital.

	Three years ago	Two years ago	Last year
Revenue	$2,800,000	$3,100,000	$3,300,000

Table 4.4 Revenue and the change in revenue for the last three years for Tank's Animal Hospital.

	Three years ago	Two years ago	Last year
Revenue ($)	2,800,000	3,100,000	3,300,000
Revenue change ($)	↑ 89,000	↑ 300,000	↑ 200,000

Table 4.5 Revenue, change in revenue (in dollars), and the percentage change in revenue for the last three years for Tank's Animal Hospital.

	Three years ago	Two years ago	Last year
Revenue ($)	2,800,000	3,100,000	3,300,000
Revenue change ($)	↑ 89,000	↑ 300,000	↑ 200,000
Revenue change (%)	3.2	9.7	6.1

Percent Difference = 0.0967 × 100

Percent Difference = 9.7%

They'll continue to find the percentage change between each of the years (Table 4.5).

Once the revenue change percentage has been found for each year, the next step is to find the average percentage of revenue change (Table 4.6).

Once the average percentage change in revenue is calculated, then multiply the average change by last year's revenue to calculate the projected annual revenue for this year (Table 4.7).

Dr Tank and Georgia have now projected their revenue for next year!

You might be thinking to yourself at this point, "Nicole, that seems like way too much work. I'm not sure I can do this." I can certainly understand! Keep in mind that you only have to do it once per year. If you'd rather start small, that's okay too! Check to see if your accounting program has the option to walk you through creating a budget or work with your accountant to help you with this process.

Table 4.6 Revenue, change in revenue (in dollars), and the percentage change in revenue for the last three years for Tank's Animal Hospital. It also demonstrates the estimated growth in revenue for the upcoming year.

	Three years ago	Two years ago	Last year	This year's projection
Revenue ($)	2,800,000	3,100,000	3,300,000	
Revenue change ($)	↑ 89,000	↑ 300,000	↑ 200,000	
Revenue change (%)	3.2	9.7	6.1	**6.3%**

Table 4.7 Revenue, change in revenue (in dollars), and the percentage change in revenue for the last three years for Tank's Animal Hospital. It also demonstrates the estimated growth in revenue and the projected revenue for the upcoming year.

	Three years ago	Two years ago	Last year	This year's projection
Revenue ($)	2,800,000	3,100,000	3,300,000	**3,507,900**
Revenue change ($)	↑ 89,000	↑ 300,000	↑ 200,000	
Revenue change (%)	3.2	9.7	6.1	6.3

4.10.1.2 Monthly Revenue Projections

The next step in this process is to estimate the monthly revenue. This can be done one of two ways.

- Divide the projected annual revenue by 12 months. However, all months are not created equal, so I prefer to project my monthly revenue a little differently.
- An alternative is to apply the average growth percentage to the same month last year (i.e., for March 2025, apply the growth percentage to March 2024).
  - In the example above, let us say revenue for March 2024 was $159,000. Multiply the growth percentage Dr Tank found above (6.3%) by $159,000 to get the projected March 2025 revenue ($169,017) (Table 4.8).

4.10.1.3 Annual COGS Projections

Similarly to determining the annual revenue projections, Dr Tank's next step will be to determine the annual COGS projections. This information can be found in the profit and loss statement from the accounting software.

Tip: If you have questions at any time, check with your accountant!

First, find the COGS for the last three years. It's usually helpful to find the costs of any subcategories as well. In Table 4.9, I've included a simple "inventory purchases" row to separate inventory that was purchased versus the entire COGS category.

Once Dr Tank has found the COGS and inventory cost information for the last three years, the next step is to find the average for each row to calculate this year's projections (Table 4.10). They'll find the average in this step rather than applying a growth percentage like in the revenue projections because the COGS should not increase the same way the revenue does!

Table 4.8 Projected revenue for March 2025, based on the revenue from March 2024 and the calculated estimated growth percentage for Tank's Animal Hospital.

Revenue from March 2024	**$159,000**
Growth percentage	6.3%
Projected revenue for March 2025	$169,017

Table 4.9 The COGS as a percentage of revenue, the COGS amount spent, the inventory purchases as a percentage of revenue, and the inventory purchases dollar amount spent for the last three years for Tank's Animal Hospital.

	Three years ago	Two years ago	Last year	Current year projection
COGS as a % of revenue	23.6%	24.8%	27.1%	
COGS $ spent	$660,800	$768,800	$894,300	
Inventory purchases as a % of revenue	18.1%	16.7%	21.2%	
Inventory purchases $ spent	$506,800	$517,700	$699,600	

Table 4.10 COGS as a percentage of revenue, the COGS amount spent, the inventory purchases as a percentage of revenue, and the inventory purchases dollar amount spent for the last three years for Tank's Animal Hospital. It also demonstrates the estimated inventory expenses for the upcoming year.

	Three years ago	Two years ago	Last year	Current year projection (average)
COGS as a % of revenue	23.6%	24.8%	27.1%	**25.2%**
COGS $ spent	$660,800	$768,800	$894,300	$774,633
Inventory purchases as a % of revenue	18.1%	16.7%	21.2%	18.6%
Inventory purchases $ spent	$506,800	$517,700	$699,600	$574,700

Table 4.11 Tank's Animal Hospital's monthly COGS projection in table form.

Budget for:	March 2025	
Projected monthly revenue	$169,017	Actual monthly revenue
Projected total COGS	$42,592	Actual total COGS
Projected inventory purchases	$31,437	Actual inventory purchases
Projected subcategory 1 purchases	$12,100	Actual subcategory 1 purchases

4.10.1.4 Putting It All Together

Now that Dr Tank and Georgia have estimated the monthly projected revenue ($169,017) from the previous step, as well as a COGS projection (25.2%), the COGS and inventory purchase budget for March can be calculated. The COGS budget for March 2025 is $42,592 and the inventory purchases budget is $31,437.

If it's helpful, subcategories can be broken out further or divided into weekly sections (Table 4.11).

Dr Tank and Georgia have now walked through the entire process for projecting and estimating their budget for the next year. As you go through this process for your practice, keep in mind that if you are not in a stable growth era and your revenue keeps increasing significantly year over year, the three-year average projections might be too conservative for you. In that case, explore projecting the average growth percentage over the last two years or whatever method for estimating growth seems most accurate for your practice.

If that feels too overwhelming, here are some other methods to try.

- **Using your accounting software**: the accounting software you use might have a budget feature where you can enter your projected growth percentage, and it will create a monthly budget based on your previous year's revenue and your specified growth percentage. You can use the growth percentage you calculated above or a growth percentage from your finance team, and it will save time not to calculate much of the information above by hand.
- **Using the previous week's revenue**: another method of budgeting is using your previous week's revenue and setting your budget to be XX%, a percentage, of that revenue. I've found this number can range anywhere from 13% to 18% (but can also be higher or lower). That means that if your goal percentage was 15% and the previous week's revenue was $68,000, your budget for

this week would be $10,200. As I mentioned earlier, this method of calculating the budget is very reactive and can put a lot of unnecessary pressure on the purchaser.

If you want to use the previous week's revenue budget method, or really any budgeting method, it's important first to optimize your inventory!

"Best Practice" Questions to Consider

- Is your practice currently using a budget? Does it seem to work well or is it a constant challenge to stay under budget?
- Is there another type of budgeting that you'd like to try that might be more effective?
- If you have a hard time consistently staying under budget, how could you optimize your inventory to make it easier?

5

Receiving and Restocking Your Inventory

5.1 Author Note

Managing inventory, planning, and organization just makes my brain happy.

As a child, I had a few different ideas for what I wanted to be when I grew up. First, I wanted to be a marine biologist working with whales. (Well, I actually still want to do that but I think everyone probably does.) I also wanted to be a business owner and an entrepreneur, even though I wasn't sure exactly what that meant or looked like.

I remember visiting my grandparents' home in Maple Valley, Washington. My cousin and I huddled around my notebook in the living room, drafting pet store plans at the tender age of seven. We thought of everything. We planned what we wanted to carry and even drew plans for the layout of the store.

Fast forward a few years, I wanted to open an ice cream stand in our driveway on a rural dead-end street. Despite the obvious (but overlooked) location problems, I got to work outlining what treats my sister and I would carry, how we would spread the word, and how we would price our inventory.

Sometime later, I started a mock newsletter all about different shells and shellfish species. I spent hours writing the newsletter, creating the layout, and putting it all together. It did not stop there. When I was 15, my dad started a custom concrete countertop business. I designed all of the marketing materials including the logo, custom letterheads, brochures, you name it.

When I got to college, no major ever felt right. I went from nursing to general studies to business management to animal science. Over the years, I started to fall in love with operations and inventory. It was always in the back of my mind that I wanted to be a business owner, but I just wasn't sure what that would look like or how that would come into play. Today, I love drafting plans and envisioning adventures as much as I did back then. Looking back now, it's so interesting to realize that the games we used to play had such a direct correlation to the work I do.

After years and years of being an inventory manager and helping other practices with their inventory, I know two things to be true: (i) breaking down boxes is cathartic and relaxing, and (ii) facing a shelf is an automatic habit. Whenever I walk into a store and there are messy shelves, there's an immediate urge to start straightening and tidying the shelf. Making the products look presentable and "fluffed up." Often I'll have to physically stop myself from doing it!

This chapter is all about exploring systems and best practices for receiving and restocking your inventory.

Inventory Management for Veterinary Professionals, First Edition. Nicole I. Clausen.
© 2024 John Wiley & Sons, Inc. Published 2024 by John Wiley & Sons, Inc.
Companion website: www.wiley.com/go/clausen/inventory

5.2 Receiving Inventory

Once you have recognized what's low, compiled a list of what's needed, and placed your order, the next step is receiving that order into your practice and restocking what was low. Although the process for receiving your inventory is fairly straightforward, that does not mean it's not important to review. Receiving is the "gateway" of inventory into your practice and the first line of defense against expired or otherwise substandard items.

I've noticed that receiving is often one of the most delegated aspects of inventory. If you are short on time or wear a bazillion "hats" in your practice, it can be a huge time saver to create a stream-lined and efficient process that your team can carry out. This is also an excellent junction at which to set up systems to prevent theft and diversion.

Think about it: What if someone puts items away and a team member cannot find the proper medication during an emergency because it wasn't in the correct spot? What if someone put away syringes in the wrong place, and then you ordered more because you thought the syringes were out of stock? What if someone did not follow the proper procedures for controlled substances and compliance with the Drug Enforcement Administration (DEA) wasn't maintained? Establishing reasonable procedures for receiving and restocking inventory keeps our practice organized, reduces costs (including labor costs), and supports compliance with regulatory bodies.

There are two main components to receiving and restocking your inventory. The first is to replenish the physical inventory; the second is to receive and update your practice management system (PiMS) (or inventory software) with the new order. The goal of restocking the physical inventory is to ensure everything that was ordered arrives correctly, appropriately store all the items that arrive, and prepare the new arrivals to either sell or use.

The goal of receiving the new order into the PiMS is to update the quantity on hand (QOH) (and any shipment information like the current costs, etc.) to reflect what is in stock accurately. This is the first step in keeping your PiMS accurate! Throughout this process, most PiMSs will allow you to update costs, expiry dates, or lot numbers and increase prices all at once with specific functions. Throughout this text, I'll refer to the amount the practice pays for an item as the cost and the amount the client pays as the price. Most PiMSs use similar terms, and it's best not to use these terms interchangeably. Inventory can get complicated, after all.

5.3 Guidelines for Receiving and Restocking

When an order arrives in the practice, it's helpful to follow the same workflow every time so that no part of the process gets missed. It's most beneficial that all involved team members are fully trained and comfortable with the entire process at every stage. Although receiving inventory might seem like an insignificant piece of the inventory management system, this is where items come into your practice, and prices increase as costs increase and many important processes happen. This is the time when items get organized and restocked, reorder tags get readded, controlled substances start their journey, and items are replenished.

When I perform an inventory audit and analysis for a client, it's common to find items priced lower than an item's cost because they slipped through the cracks of the receiving process. This is also a key time for ensuring compliance with controlled substances for the DEA. Plus, inventory receiving is the "safety net" or checks and balances system for ensuring that our patients get the best (for example, not expired, short-dated, damaged, etc.) products possible.

It works well to train your entire team to recognize when a new shipment comes in. The goal is that someone can immediately identify if there is a cooler with temperature-controlled items that should be unpacked immediately. This will be especially important in the summer when the ice packs aren't as cold for as long. Many distributors and vendors will have stickers on the outside of the box identifying that it's a refrigerated or frozen product. These boxes should have priority and be unpacked and received as soon as possible.

Even if not everyone in the team unpacks boxes, it's helpful for everyone to be on the lookout for when they arrive. Personally, I love unpacking boxes and organizing the order as I put it all away, but it is something that is often delegated. There are two considerations here.

First, from a theft prevention perspective, it's important that the person who receives the inventory is different from the person who orders it. Consider this situation. Let's say the inventory manager orders and receives all the orders. Let's say that they ordered an extra bottle of gabapentin to take home. When the boxes arrive, they quietly put the bottle in their backpack. Then, they enter one less bottle into inventory. The stolen bottle will not raise any red flags because it was never entered into the system and accounted for.

Second, I like to create an "inventory team" of several helpers who are fully trained in the receiving process. That way, more than one person understands the process, multiple people are properly trained, and it does not turn into an unpacking "free for all." It's vital to include team members who aren't seeing exam rooms all day and have some "flex time" in the treatment area. It's also helpful if someone is out sick or out of the office on vacation.

Now, of course, you know what's best for your practice, but splitting the ordering and receiving duties can add a safety measure to your inventory.

Shipments that aren't temperature sensitive can be unpacked and put away whenever is convenient for the practice during the day. However, it's preferable to receive (unpack) any shipments on the same day they arrive. If items aren't stocked promptly, there is a higher risk of running out and a team member reordering (or suggesting it's out) when in reality it's already in the building. My preference is to strategically plan my order days around when the shipment will arrive to ensure the practice will be properly staffed and available to receive as needed. This is especially important for orders containing controlled substances as these items will have more requirements and steps for receiving.

"Best Practice" Tip
Try to strategically plan your order days around when the shipment will arrive to ensure the practice will be properly staffed and available to receive as needed.

5.3.1 Receiving Workflow

Receiving is a process that will flow differently depending on the practice. If you are instituting these guidelines in your practice, remember to be curious. Consider what might work best for you and try different things to eventually reach the "best fit" for your unique practice and team culture. Here are some elements and an example workflow that can be adjusted to fit your needs.

1) As soon as a shipment arrives in the practice, the inventory team is notified and any temperature-controlled boxes are identified. Alternatively, if it's a larger practice, the shipments are delivered directly to the pharmacy. If the inventory team is unavailable, another team member may unpack and put away refrigerated or frozen items, ensuring proper invoice processing procedures are followed.

2) The inventory team will gather all the boxes together for unpacking. If it's a large shipment with multiple vendors, group the packages together by each vendor or distributor.

3) Open each box and locate the packing slip or invoice.

4) Once the packing slip or invoice has been located, start unpacking the items from each box. Check to see if any products are damaged, short-dated, expired, or otherwise not in good condition.

5) At this point, the process may vary. Some people like to unpack everything from the box and put it on a treatment table. Others prefer to put it away as they go. Either route is perfectly acceptable!

6) As items are unpacked, check off on the invoice that the product arrived with the correct quantity. If any items are missing, short-dated, expired, damaged, etc., highlight these items on the packing list or invoice. Once the particular shipment has been received fully, the vendor or distributor is called and alerted to the "problem" items.

7) If any controlled substances are in this shipment, these items are addressed first. Keep in mind that controlled substances will often be included with other items in a box, but they will likely have a separate controlled substance-only invoice. First, controlled substances are inspected to see if they are short-dated. Then, they are assigned a unique bottle number and logged into the unopened container log of your controlled substance log.

8) The substance is then checked off on the packing slip or invoice, and the proper quantity received is verified. Once that has been completed, it is dated, signed, or initialed by the person unpacking and a witness. Keep in mind that anything involving controlled substances should have a witness to protect everyone involved. If any of the substances are Class II, the DEA Form 222 Purchaser's Copy should be noted with the number of packages received and the date received. In addition, once the invoice has been checked off, a copy should be made. The original should be retained in a controlled substance invoice file, and the copy should be used for accounting purposes.

9) Once all items have been unpacked and checked off on the invoice, they are put away where the products belong. Place the new arrivals behind any currently stocked items. More specifically, the items that expire first are toward the front, and bottles with the furthest expiry date are last. That way, the products that will expire first will be used first.

10) If your practice utilizes reorder tags or reorder bins, the reorder tags are put back on the items and reorder bins are adjusted accordingly.

11) Once all the items have been put away and the invoices settled, call any vendors or distributors to report anything that's amiss.

12) Once these steps have been completed, the invoices are set aside to receive into the PiMS, and garbage and recycling are taken out.

Throughout this process, it's really important that each item gets put away in its proper place and not just shoved somewhere that has an empty spot on the shelf. This includes pharmaceuticals and hospital supplies or white goods. Each item in the practice should have a designed "home" and defined backstock location (with labels!) so that each team member knows where to find something every time. It's also useful to avoid "layering" on the central storage room shelves so that items aren't stacked on top of each other; each item should have its own lane.

Once items are received physically and put away in the proper location, the next step is to receive those items in the PiMS. The goal of receiving items into your PiMS is to update the QOH, cost, expiration dates, and lot numbers. Depending on your system, if you have a markup percentage entered, your software will automatically recalculate the price as your cost increases.

As I mentioned before, receiving into your PiMS is the first step in keeping the inventory accurate in your software! QOH must be accurate so that reorder points will be flagged at the appropriate time. Having an accurate QOH also helps for reporting purposes and monitoring the value of inventory on hand. Additionally, accurate reports allow you to track key performance indicators and troubleshoot any particular areas of your inventory. Some PiMSs do not track expiry dates or lot numbers well, so depending on your system, this may not apply to you.

Expiry and lot number side note: Sometimes, a PiMS will try to keep track of expiry dates and lot numbers and will assume which bottle is being used to dispense a prescription. Unfortunately, this assumption is often incorrect and it creates a snowball of inaccurate information that can take an incredibly long time to correct. If you are not currently using your PiMS to track lot numbers or expiry dates and would like to do so, start slow with vaccines or a small number of items and test how the system works and responds before diving in completely. Alternatively, some PiMSs will keep track of just one expiry date, and is unable to keep track of multiple expiry dates. I've found that most practices will just track expiry dates and/or lot numbers for vaccines or other items where that information is essential.

5.3.2 Receiving Inventory into Your Software

The most efficient way to receive invoices and packing slips into your PiMS is through a purchase order (PO) or receipt (different PiMS call these different things) function. Most software systems have a function where you can receive a list of items rather than individually updating each one. With that being said, the traditional use of POs is creating one and emailing or faxing it to the distributor, which I do not recommend. Instead, I recommend using POs as an internal document or tool to help with receiving.

Typically, most practices have more time when placing orders than receiving them. Often, adequate time is scheduled or given to order but receiving is done "on the fly" and ends up being rushed. As a result, if a PO is created when the order is placed, it can make the receiving process much more efficient. Another benefit to this is you'll see exactly what strength and quantity of each specific medication you ordered, so if the wrong concentration or strength were sent, it would be immediately identified. If the invoice is not reconciled with what was actually ordered, there is a possibility of stocking out of a particular item if the wrong strength or quantity was sent.

A PO or receipt in your PiMS is essentially a list of all the things ordered from a particular supplier with the quantity ordered and the cost of an item +/− additional information like expiry date, lot number, etc. When a PO is received, it will automatically update the on-hand amount and the cost of that particular item. I've worked with many practices that will go in and manually update the QOH for each individual item rather than receiving it on a PO. Using a PO saves a significant amount of time!

"Best Practice" Tip
Some PiMSs will put all the items that are flagged low on the reorder list together on a PO, reducing the amount of time spent creating the PO.

The exact process for receiving a PO will depend on your specific software system, but the general process should be fairly consistent. I recommend receiving any invoice or packing slip within 24 hours so that any cost increases can be passed on to the client immediately. A PO should be created before, during, or after the order is placed (remember, this is just an internal document or tool), listing each item and the quantity ordered from each vendor.

Once this is put together, there is typically some way to "release" the PO, signaling that everything listed is on order. Some PiMSs even have a flag, icon, or other marker signaling that it's on order for the rest of the team. At this point, I also like to post the order confirmation or display it so the rest of the team knows what's on order and what should arrive shortly at the practice. My stance is the more communication, the better!

Once the order has arrived, been physically checked off, and received, open up the previously created PO, switch to receiving mode if necessary, and start to verify that the quantity and items ordered are correct and update any costs. Once the entire invoice or packing slip has been received, verify that the total cost matches the total on the invoice. If the cost does not match, this is a great indication that there is likely an error somewhere. When the PiMS PO's total matches, the receipt can be finalized. Depending on the PiMS, if a cost has increased and markup percentages are utilized in the system, it will ask to verify the new prices.

"Best Practice" Tip

I highly recommend utilizing the markup percentage function in your PiMS to ensure that prices are appropriately increased as costs increase. I've caught too many items that are priced lower than the cost of the item!

Receiving inventory in the PiMS is helpful for a number of reasons. First and foremost, it provides a much more efficient way to update the QOH for a particular item and update or increase any prices as necessary. Second, keeping your on-hand count accurate opens up the possibility to track your inventory. This helps to utilize reorder points in the software, recognize waste and overstock, and use the data to troubleshoot high inventory costs, missed charges and excessive discounting, and make more data-informed decisions.

Ultimately, your PiMS is an expensive software and can be a treasure trove of tools to help make managing inventory that much easier (Table 5.1).

5.3.3 Reconciling Errors

One of the most challenging aspects of managing inventory in the PiMS is the level of effort required to maintain the proper inventory on hand. Sometimes, it feels like there are "gremlins" in the software changing the numbers because no other explanation makes sense. When the on-hand

Table 5.1 Examples of what should and should not be received into the practice management system.

Include in your PiMS	Do not include in your PiMS

• Anything that is related to patient care or that's sold to a client
• Examples:
  – Hospital supplies (gauze, syringes, needles, IV catheters)
  – Medications (gabapentin, dasuquin, injectable oxytocin)
  – Retail items (toothbrushes, pet odor candles, etc.)
  – Food (prescription diets, treats, canned food)
  – Liquids related to patient care (chlorhexidine solution, alcohol, hydrogen peroxide, Diff-Quik® stain)
  – In-house laboratory items (in-house lab machine rotors, blood tubes, in-house lab machine maintenance supplies)
	• Things not related to patient care or things not sold to a client
	• Examples:
	  – Office supplies (paper, stamps, envelopes)
	  – Janitorial supplies (toilet paper, paper towels, bleach, etc.)
	  – Office equipment

count is inaccurate, all the benefits of managing inventory in the PiMS go right out the window. With that being said, there are common errors within these systems that I find often and a trouble-shooting process that I follow. Later in this book, you'll review strategies for keeping inventory accurate in your software.

When the QOH is incorrect regularly in the PiMS, it can often be traced back to an item that was set up incorrectly or an error during the receiving process. In my experience, one of the most common culprits is not correctly setting up the units or package quantities correctly. In AVImark®, this is called the package quantity. In Cornerstone, it's called the buy/sell ratio. Other software systems call them different things. The idea is that this number or ratio tells the system how to interpret when something is sold and received.

Let's look at some examples of items and various pitfalls.

Example A: In AVImark, amoxicillin is set up with a package quantity of one. AVImark reads this as one unit (or capsule) per bottle. As a result, when receiving this item, it's really important to put the number of capsules received (i.e., 500 capsules). Let's say that during the receiving process, a team member did not realize they needed to put the total units and just entered a quantity of one (for one bottle). Now, AVImark will think the practice received one bottle containing one capsule. That means that the amount on hand will be inaccurate but, more importantly, it lists the cost per capsule as the cost of one bottle. That's when your pricing and your on-hand quantities get off track.

Example B: In Cornerstone, prednisone is set up with a buy/sell ratio of one bottle equal to 1000 tablets. Cornerstone reads this as each time one bottle is received, 1000 tablets were received in that bottle. But let's say that the usage of prednisone has decreased and you now purchase the 100-count bottle. The buy/sell ratio has not been updated to reflect that so, rather than updating the QOH by 100 for each bottle purchased, Cornerstone adds 1000 per bottle. As a result, the on-hand count shows significantly more on hand than what's true.

Let's look at how this affects the price of the item.

- Old buy/sell ratio: one bottle = 1000 tablets, so $137.92 per bottle = $0.14 per tablet.
- Incorrect buy/sell ratio: one bottle = 1000 tablets (correct amount = 100 tablets) so $15.98 per bottle = $0.02 per tablet.
- Correct buy/sell ratio: one bottle = 100 tablets so $15.98 per bottle = $0.16 per tablet

From the example above, having incorrect cost information for the product could lead to under-charging the client. Alternatively, the value of inventory on hand could appear much lower or higher than it actually is.

Setting up the package quantity or buy/sell ratio in your software incorrectly can have a negative impact on your prices and on-hand quantities. I know what a long process it can be to get everything set up correctly, but the time you put in now will pay dividends down the road! Keep going, it's worth the effort.

"Best Practice" Tip

When receiving in your software, make sure the total on the invoice you are receiving matches the PO or receipt in the PiMS. If they do not match exactly, that's often an indication that a product is not set up appropriately or there is an error. When I was an inventory manager and was in the "messy middle" of getting all the items in my software updated, I would always check that the two totals matched. More often than not, if they did not match, it meant an item wasn't set up correctly and had the wrong units, or I had forgotten an item or quantity.

5.4 Setting up Your Software to Optimize this Process

If POs have not been received before into the PiMS, you might have to do some initial software cleanup to make the process go smoothly. The quantities on hand for items might be way off; there may be duplicates, items that have not sold in a long time, or products that have not been updated in years. If you want to utilize your software for inventory and receiving, taking the time to ensure each item is properly set up can significantly impact this process. This is the first step in making sure your QOH is accurate!

Considering this, if the on-hand values in your PiMS are inaccurate (i.e. −3895 units), I recommend doing a full physical count and updating the counts prior to starting to receive POs. By doing this, you'll start with a clean slate. Then, once POs start to be received, the on-hand counts will be more accurate, and you can investigate counts that are incorrect to find out where they went. This might include missed charges, setup errors in the software system, theft, and more. For example:

- if your on-hand count in the software is −4815, we know that's not possible and the number is not real
- alternatively, if you have 430 tablets on the shelf and your software says there are 370 on hand, that difference can be realistically investigated and adjusted.

If you have not received invoices or POs into your PiMS before and do not use the price markup feature in the system, it's helpful to enter markup percentages. Once the markup percentages are entered and the POs start to be received, most PiMSs will recalculate the price (if the cost has increased) based on the new data and the markup. This process will catch up with any outdated prices and help ensure that your prices are appropriate. Some PiMS systems also have the ability to set up markup break pricing. For example, one dose could be set up with a markup of 150%, while six doses could be set up with a markup of 100%. This feature is helpful for setting up quantity discounts.

So, to help leverage your PiMS as much as possible, I recommend:

- starting with accurate physical counts. This might mean doing a full physical count or spot-checking and updating your counts as needed
- setting up each item with the correct package quantity or buy/sell ratio, as well as the markup percentage for each item.

Although not required, taking these steps will make the most of all the time and effort you are putting into receiving! Think of this like pumping your healthy inventory ecosystem full of nutrients to make sure the structural foundations are strong and keep any parasites from entering the environment.

5.5 Training Your Team

One of the most commonly delegated responsibilities of inventory management is unpacking and receiving boxes. This can be a great way to involve your team while freeing up time to attend to other inventory or management tasks. When delegating, unpacking boxes, or receiving inventory, the best practice is to train specific people so that you can check in with them, provide feedback, and track who is doing what.

The first step is to choose the right person (or people) for the task. When it comes to unpacking and receiving, whoever is doing this is responsible for ensuring that all pharmaceuticals, medications, biologics, etc. arrive correctly. They are the first line of quality control and need to understand the importance of their role in the inventory ecosystem. They aren't just putting things on shelves to get them out of the way but need to take pride in the organization and functionality of the stock systems. They utilize their proactive attitude and strong attention to detail to check for refrigerated items, identify errors, and alert the inventory manager to anything that's amiss in a timely manner.

After you have identified the best team member(s) for unpacking and receiving, it's important to set them up for success by thoroughly explaining and training them on the process. They should know clearly what steps to follow, what is expected of them, what to look out for, and what to do if something goes wrong. When delegating this role, you are also delegating responsibility and authority to this person (or people) to make empowered decisions. Someone who is drawn to special projects, organizing, and attention to detail, and who enjoys taking ownership of new tasks may be a great fit for this role.

"Best Practice" Tip
It's ideal for the receiving inventory team member to have dedicated time each week (depending on how many orders are placed) for unpacking boxes, checking in shipments, and any other related tasks. It's very difficult to avoid small mistakes that make a big difference while multitasking. Although to other team members, it might seem like spending time managing inventory is not valuable in comparison to caring for patients, that is certainly not the case. Without inventory, we simply cannot care for our patients.

"Best Practice" Tip
Only someone who has excellent attention to detail and is fully trained and comfortable with inventory should receive invoices or packing slips into the PiMS.

5.5.1 An Example Receiving Checklist

Below is an example receiving checklist to assist your team in receiving inventory.

- If it is a large shipment, group all the same distributor boxes together.
- Open each box, find the packing slip, and unpack the contents.
- Examine each item.
  - Check for short-dated expiries.
  - Check to make sure all items are there.
  - Ensure there are no damaged/opened items.
  - If you are tracking expiry dates or lot numbers, write them down for each item in the margin of the packing slip or invoice.
  - Highlight any missing, broken, or short-dated items, and call the manufacturer or distributor.
  - Check off any item that has arrived correctly.
- For controlled substances, assign a unique bottle number and log each bottle into the unopened container log.
- Once the packing slip has been reconciled, put each item away in its designated spot. Write the date the box was unpacked, and initial whoever unpacked it on the packing slip.
  - Note: Items with the furthest expiry date should be put in the "last" spot.
- Receive the packing slip, invoice, or PO into the PiMS within 24 hours.

- File the packing slip to be reconciled with the statement at the end of the billing period.
- If the shipment contains a controlled substance, the invoice gets initialed by the receiver and a witness and dated, and each item that arrived is checked off. The invoice is copied and the original is kept on file.
- If a shipment contains a Class II controlled substance, the DEA Form 222 gets annotated with the number of containers received and the date of receipt.

5.6 Invoice and Statement Processing

Once an invoice is entered into the PiMS and all the inventory has been put away, collect and organize the invoices until the statement is reconciled. If the unpacking is delegated to another team member, it should have the initials of whoever unpacked it, the date, and checkmarks next to each item received on every invoice. Then, once that invoice or packing slip has been entered into the PiMS, it should be annotated. Personally, I always put "Entered ⊠ NC" (my initials) in the top right-hand corner so that I know the invoice has been entered and does not accidentally get received twice.

Invoices that list a controlled substance should be treated differently. The DEA requires that invoices for controlled substances are kept on file and readily available for two years. Keep in mind that some states require them to be kept for longer, so check your state regulations as well!

Just like a regular invoice, whenever a controlled substance packing slip or invoice arrives, it's essential to verify that the substance and the correct quantity listed were indeed shipped and accounted for appropriately. Then, the invoice needs to be signed, witnessed, dated, and checked off for each item. Then, a photocopy should be made. The original should be placed into a controlled substance invoice binder; a separate binder should be created for Class II and Class III–V drug invoices. Invoices for Class II and Class III–V need to be kept separate (21 CFR 1304.04 – Maintenance of Records and Inventories., 2024). The photocopy should be put with the other invoices or packing slips for book-keeping purposes.

For more information on controlled substances, see Chapter 12.

There are many ways to organize invoices but the most important thing will be to find a system that works well for you and your practice. Some practices only keep controlled substances hardcopy invoices and then scan the remaining invoices into QuickBooks™. Other practices keep all invoices and organize them by vendor and month. Other practices scan all invoices and keep no hard copies. If you do not have a system yet, start by researching your specific state and federal regulations for keeping invoices. Then, once the appropriate, legal way has been determined, consider what organization and storage method might work best for you.

"Best Practice" Tip

Check with your accountant on the best way to handle sales tax on your inventory items. Tax requirements vary from state to state and can change, so it's important to keep up to date.

5.6.1 Reconciling Invoices and Statements

Reconciling the invoices and statements together is an important part of financial management in inventory. Invoice and statement reconciliation is a process of comparing the monthly statement to the original invoices that were received throughout the month. It serves a number of different purposes. First and foremost, it is a double-check to ensure the amount listed to be paid on the statement is accurate and correct. Second, it's a great time to:

- ensure any appropriate returns and credits were issued
- ensure there are no duplicate invoices
- make sure all the invoices have been received into the PiMS and any accounting software
- double-check that all controlled substance invoices have been filed in the correct spot.

When I reconciled the statements each month, I started with the statement and then I'd grab the stack of invoices for that particular month. With my filing system, everything was already in chronological order and separated by vendor and manufacturer. I went down the statement and checked off each invoice that was present and accurate. I also checked to make sure everything had been received into the PiMS. After all the invoices I had were checked off, I looked to see if any invoices were missing. If so, I would get those from the vendor and determine why it was originally missing and if it had been received into the PiMS. After all the invoices were accounted for and accurate, I checked for any credits that had been issued. Once I had verified that everything was true and accurate, I attached all the invoices to the statement, and it would go to the practice owner for payment.

"Best Practice" Tip

When the statement from the reference laboratory arrives, that's a great time to ensure that all labs were charged to the client and that the prices are accurate in the practice management software. It's also helpful to check to see if any veterinarian or staff discounts were applied appropriately.

The ultimate goal for reconciling the invoices and statements each month is to ensure that the practice is being charged appropriately and not overcharged, that any credits and returns were applied correctly, and that all items charged for were received and acceptable to be sold.

5.6.2 Example Invoice Processing Workflow

When I was managing inventory while still working in a veterinary practice, this is the workflow that worked the best for me.

1) When a shipment arrived, I unpacked the boxes, put away the inventory items, and checked them off appropriately on the invoice or packing list. Then, I put the invoice or packing slip in a bin labeled "To Be Received in PiMS" once the physical receiving process was complete.
2) Either that same day or within 24 hours, I received the POs into the PiMS. Once each invoice or packing slip was received, I wrote "Entered ☒ Initials" in the top right-hand corner.
3) If it was a shipment that contained a controlled substance, I made a photocopy of the invoice and put the original in the CS Class II or Class III–V binder as necessary.
4) Once all the invoices or packing slips were received, I put them into file folders. Each file folder had the name of a distributor or vendor on it, and I placed the invoices in the corresponding folders in chronological order. Note: I would reuse the folder each month.
5) Throughout the month, I kept adding to each vendor's folder until the statement arrived. Once the statement arrived, I took the invoices out of the folder and reconciled them. Because they were in chronological order, it was an extremely quick process.
6) Once a statement was reconciled, I paperclipped all the invoices to the statement and delivered it to the practice owner.
7) From there, it was paid and put into a storage box in chronological and alphabetical order.

5.7 Putting It into Practice

With receiving, restocking, invoice, and statement management, the keys are systems, routines, and proper training. When starting to integrate some of these processes into your practice, consider the following.

- Who on the team would be the best fit for unpacking boxes and receiving? Will this person be you? Who on the team has attention to detail and initiative, or has already taken an interest in inventory?
- Will they need dedicated time to do the tasks assigned to them?
- How can you ensure they get the proper training before taking these tasks over?
- What authority do they have?
- Will a controlled substance standard operating procedure for managing the movement be created?
- Who will receive invoices and packing slips into the practice management system? Will dedicated time be needed for this? What is needed to ensure these are entered into the PiMS within 24 hours?
- What will the invoice and statement workflow look like? Who will need to be involved in this process?
- How can checks and balances be set up to ensure each aspect is functioning properly?

6

Organizing, Storing, and Protecting Your Inventory

6.1 Author's Note

When I was a freshman, I skipped the second half of ninth grade and the first half of tenth grade, but I still had to meet the required graduation credits. As a result, in my senior year, I took community college classes and classes at my high school and was enrolled in an occupational program to become a certified nursing assistant. On top of that, I had a job (at a local veterinary practice), and I tutored and babysat in my spare time.

Did I also mention I was undiagnosed ADHD?

Throughout my academic "career," up until this point, I had not learned good systems or study habits because I never really had to. I never used a planner, I was bad at keeping track of assignments and due dates, and to top it all off, I had never learned how to set boundaries or structures of care for myself. I was taught to "push through" and do what needed to be done. Keeping everything in my brain and my tendency to keep busy kept me bouncing along.

As you can imagine, midway through my senior year, it started to take a toll on me. I forgot about big projects at school, missed an important exam, and was often late for my college classes. Keeping everything "in my brain" became impossible. Everything seemed to come crashing down around me, and I really did not know what to do or how to handle it.

I wish I could say that I learned my lesson, and that's when I became organized and set up healthy systems and structures for myself, but I struggled through my twenties. Honestly, I'm always learning and improving on the systems that help me stay organized, but now, I have the foundational structures and routines dialed in to support me and my brain.

Can you think of a time in your life (or even in your practice!) when the roof came crashing down because there were not enough organizational or support structures?

6.2 Why a Tidy Inventory and Pharmacy Matters

Why do organization and support structures in your inventory matter? In addition to high school, I can certainly think of quite a few times when it felt like everything came crashing down because I did not have systems or structures in place.

An organized inventory is important to a thriving and healthy inventory ecosystem. The ultimate goal of organizing your inventory is so that you and your entire team know where everything is

Inventory Management for Veterinary Professionals, First Edition. Nicole I. Clausen.
© 2024 John Wiley & Sons, Inc. Published 2024 by John Wiley & Sons, Inc.
Companion website: www.wiley.com/go/clausen/inventory

and can efficiently locate everything in your practice. Consider an unorganized inventory; the "central storage" area is filled to the brim with unlabeled boxes of things, bags of random hospital supplies, equipment manuals dating back to the age of floppy disks, broken printers, and bins of cords that plug into stuff that does not even work any more. When things are unorganized, it adds more chaos and inefficiency to you and your team. (Plus, no one wants to go into that dusty room. They feel dirty even thinking about it.)

When inventory is unorganized, it impacts your practice on multiple levels. First and foremost, knowing and seeing exactly what you have on hand at any given time is challenging. It's hard to determine if you have five primary IV lines or if there is another box or bag hidden somewhere. As a result, items can be overordered because a team member thinks you are low or out, writes it on the list, and it gets ordered – meanwhile, there is a large box hidden from view. On the opposite end of the spectrum, an item could run out because your team might assume there is more stashed away somewhere. As a result, this could lead to increased inventory costs, increased stockouts, and increased team frustrations.

We've covered the primary reasons for not having an organized inventory before. I know, you get it. But if you are working at a practice that does not have good inventory systems in place yet, this is something we need to cover. This is one of the most likely scenarios you will proactively try to avoid with your processes and the one you'll most likely need to fix.

A disorganized and chaotic pharmacy can also lead to medication dispensing errors. If people are buzzing around in the pharmacy, music is playing, dogs are barking, and the front desk is paging back, how easily could a script of prednisolone accidentally be filled with prednisone? What about carprofen 75 mg instead of 25 mg? What if 0.8 ml of ketamine was drawn up instead of 0.08 ml?

In addition, when your pharmacy and inventory areas are unorganized, it can increase the amount of time spent by the care team looking for items rather than seeing patients. For example, let's say that, on average, a team member spends five minutes searching for a particular hospital supply. But, if that area were organized, it would only take an average of 30 seconds to find this same item. Now, let's say that, on average, the team searches for an item 35 times a week for 52 weeks. With a disorganized hospital supply area, that's an average of 151 hours a year trying to locate hospital supplies. But if improvements were made and items could now be found in 30 seconds, the team would spend 15 hours a year. That is a significant difference in labor hours just spent searching (Table 6.1).

"Best Practice" Improvements Check

Utilizing this same before-and-after organizational strategy is a great way to test and quantify any improvements that you have made. If you want to create a test in your practice, start with a list of 20 items and time how long it takes to find the list of items. Then, divide by 20 to find the average time across all items. Once you have organized the area, time how long it takes to find that exact list of items and note the difference between before and after.

Table 6.1 An example of the labor hours spent searching before and after organizing.

Before organization	After organization
5 minutes of searching	30 seconds of searching
35 times a week	35 times a week
175 minutes or 2.9 hours per week	17.5 minutes or 0.3 hours per week
9100 minutes or 151.7 hours per year	910 minutes or 15.2 hours per year

6.3   Organizing Your Pharmacy

Pharmacy areas can be organized in a number of ways but ultimately, they should be organized in a way that makes the most sense for your practice and your team. One of the key factors in organizing your inventory is consistency. There are a number of benefits when everything is consistent and processes are defined. For example, team members always know where to look for something; when a new item is ordered into the practice, it's immediately known where that item will be stored, and in emergency cases, no one is running around panicking trying to find a specific item. Consistency calms chaos; it sets the foundation for building efficient habits and practices, and that's no different when it comes to organization.

I find it most helpful to create "inventory zones" throughout your practice. An inventory zone is when all items of a similar category or purpose are grouped together. For example, the zones in a particular practice could be pharmacy, laboratory, dental, surgery, treatment, exam room, mobile vehicle, central storage, overstock/backstock, etc. Once these areas are defined, they can be broken down into further categories. For example, the pharmacy could have "subzone" areas such as injectables, NSAIDs, controlled substances, parasiticides, behavioral medications, etc. Within each defined zone and possibly subzone, different areas will be managed differently. The way that IV catheters are organized and managed is going to be different from how gabapentin will be dealt with.

Once the various zones and subcategories are defined and documented, organizing can get even more granular. Each item should have a designated primary and secondary overstock or backstock location. This is paramount because it will provide the consistency that is so important. When anyone in your practice is searching for an item, they'll immediately know where to look for it. Oftentimes, I find that practices will have a defined primary location for many injectables or pharmaceuticals, but for hospital supplies, dental, or surgical supplies, that might not be the case.

"Best Practice" Inventory Tip

Each item should have a defined primary and secondary (or overstock) location.

Let's imagine a couple of scenarios: A bottle of injectable carprofen is open and someone does not know where it normally goes on the shelf and puts it back in the wrong place. The next person who goes looking for the open carprofen cannot find it, panics, opens another bottle, and orders two more. Now, there are multiple open bottles and too much overstock on the way.

Now, let's imagine that Clavamox® drops are on the shelf, bearing in mind that they must be purchased in a 12-pack and only three boxes fit on the shelf in the primary location. Let's say that particular item does not have a defined overstock or secondary location, so it gets put on any shelf in central storage. Someone uses the last box on the primary location shelf and looks for more but cannot find them. You are on vacation, and you receive a panicked text that Clavamox drops have run out. Your vacation is interrupted, and you tell your team member to order more, even though there is plenty on the shelf. The additional stock comes in and now your practice is overstocked, and six bottles expire.

One of the most interesting (and frustrating) things about inventory is that when there is a lack of organization, the effects tend to snowball quickly and can affect multiple areas and functions of your practice.

6.3.1   "Nicole's Organizational Method"

As mentioned previously, several different methods of organizing within a particular zone can exist. The pharmacy shelves could be organized by disease process or major symptom, alphabetical order, or another way that makes the most sense to your practice. My preference is to have all tablets, pills, and liquids organized first by disease process/symptom and then by alphabetical order within that. For injectables, I prefer to organize everything in alphabetical order. For cabinets where hospital supplies and white goods are stored, it can be helpful to group similar items together: Syringes with other syringes, all in-house reference laboratory supplies in one location, and all catheters and other tubing together in one spot.

The key is to find an organizational flow that works with the day-to-day operations of your practice.

6.4   Creating a Central Storage or Hospital Supplies Storage Area

Creating a central storage area or dedicated hospital supplies area in your practice can be beneficial for a number of reasons. Centralizing your inventory allows you to create an organized area in your practice dedicated to storing overstock and supplies to restock the rest of the practice. With a central storage area, there is often more room to intentionally organize your stock rather than shoving things in cabinets, hoping it will fit everything. Think of central storage as the main "inventory hub" that provides stock for all the different zones of your practice.

Thinking about our coral reef metaphor, central storage is like the main area that the water and nutrients flow into before moving out to different parts of the reef to nourish the various coral, plants, fish, and other sea creature species.

If you do not currently have a designated central main storage location, you can create one by assigning a closet or other area of your facility to this area. There are several main components of this area, including shelving to house the items, labels to note which items go where, and organizational tools (like bins, clear boxes, etc.) to keep things neat and tidy. Remember that the ultimate goals are to create a space where the team can find items easily and quickly, you can visually see exactly what you have on hand, and there is a place to restock the rest of your practice from.

When creating your central storage area, keep in mind the following points.

- Place heavier items on the bottom to mid shelves for safety and ergonomic purposes. Avoid putting heavy items toward the top!
- Place the most used items at mid to eye level.
- Do not put things on the floor, especially boxes. Keeping things off the floor protects the items from spills and dust bunny damage. Plus, "stuff" tends to collect on top of boxes and it quickly becomes a "shove stuff station."
- Try to group similar items together. For example, keep all intravenous tubing and fluid administration supplies together.
- It's preferable to use adjustable wire shelving with bins for all items. It will likely be an investment upfront but will pay off significantly.
- Take pictures of the ideal cleanliness and layout of central storage to document a standard for this area. It's also helpful to post this (for example, on the back of the door) so it can be easily referenced.
- Labels should be affixed to bins and each item's location. The ultimate goal is for each team member to know exactly where each item "lives." There are a number of different options for labels, such as magnetic labels, plastic clip-on labels, and more.

Although investing in bins and other organization tools may seem like an unnecessary investment up front, there can be a significant return on investment due to limiting over- or underordering or reducing the time the team spends searching for items. As I mentioned earlier, it is incredibly helpful to group similar items together. You can also go one step further by color-coding the different items or groups of items within your storage. For example, a cadence of color coding could include the following.

- Yellow → Urinary items
- Brown → Gastrointestinal items
- Green → Wound care/bandaging supplies
- Red → Blood/IV/injection
- Blue → Respiratory
- Purple → Everyday items
- Orange → Specialty items

Color coding further decreases the amount of time searching for a specific item.

6.5 (Re)Organizing Areas of Your Practice

If various areas of your practice need help in the organizational department, there is a framework that you can use to get any space under control. It can be used for areas as small as a drawer or as big as a massive storage facility for a 50+ veterinarian specialty center. This process, called 5S, is part of a lean methodology toolkit. Lean methodologies or lean processes are "designed to increase quality and efficiency by eliminating wasted resources like time, money, and effort" (Simplilearn 2023). Lean processes, for inventory management in particular, are very helpful to reduce waste and streamline different areas of our practice.

6.5.1 The 5S Process

The 5S process is a five-step framework that originated in Japan for organizing a space. The Ss are Sort, Straighten and Set, Shine, Standardize, and Sustain (https://asq.org/quality-resources/lean/five-s-tutorial).

6.5.1.1 Sort

Start by determining what you have and need in the space but, more importantly, what you do not need. For example, if you are working on a drawer that includes bandage supplies, remove anything that is not related to what's being stored there. This might include lube, silver nitrate sticks, and whatever other random supplies have been shoved in the drawer over the years. Depending on the size of the area, it might be helpful to remove everything and sort it into two categories: needed and unnecessary. Items that should be included in the unnecessary category are things that should be stored elsewhere, are never or rarely used (should these items be discontinued?), or patient-specific or special order items.

The unnecessary category can be broken down into further categories.

- Expired items
- Does not belong
- To be returned to the supplier
- Overstock to be used
- Mystery items
- Obsolete items

Once items have been sorted and you have determined whether they are staying or going, it's time for the next step of the framework.

6.5.1.2 Straighten and Set

In this step, find or create a place for everything that's going to "live" and put each item away. A motto for this step is "a place for everything and everything in its place." Keep in mind that the goal for this step is not only to create a place for everything but also for your team to be able to find each item quickly. As you were performing the sort step, how many overstocked, extra, and lost treasures did you find? We want to prevent that from happening moving forward. Some tips for this step.

- Use bins, dividers, and other methods to contain and organize each item.
- Use a bin size that is relative to the maximum quantity as a way to control overstock.
- Utilize the two-bin system and other physical reorder points.
- Use labels (reorder points or min/max labels are very helpful) for each bin. Include pictures so that anyone on your team can restock and recognize where an item belongs.
- If an item is constantly getting put back in the wrong spot, determine whether the location of that item should be moved or relabeled.

6.5.1.3 Shine

Once the items have been sorted and set into place, the next step is to shine. The entire area is cleaned: The shelves and drawers are dusted, the floor is mopped, and anything else the area needs is done until the room shines. If there are spills and mystery liquids or stains, determine the root cause and set up protocols to mitigate the recurrence of spills. The area should be cleaned on a regular basis; include routine cleaning and area maintenance on any weekly or monthly task checklists.

6.5.1.4 Standardize

The goal of this step is to ensure that everyone on the team knows, understands, and follows the proper procedures for this area. It's important so that the area does not revert back and the new guidelines are followed. This could mean standardization through visual management (i.e., color-coded bins, pictures on each label/bin, a picture of how the closet, cabinet, etc., should look on the back of the door, etc.), keeping each area consistent (each drawer is organized similarly or the different exam room drawers match each other), or creating a standard operating procedure (SOP) with roles and responsibilities for different team members. Ultimately, it's important to remove any friction and make it easy for the team to maintain these standards.

6.5.1.5 Sustain

This step is the most challenging part of the framework! It's easy to fall back into bad habits, so it will be important to integrate processes and behavior changes so things do not revert. One of the most helpful things is to clearly assign who is responsible for sustaining the area and what that job entails. An audit form is a helpful tool which could contain a picture of what the area should be like, along with several questions, plus a spot for the date, time, and initials of the person completing the audit. Questions on the audit form could include the following.

- Pick five items: Are they in the correct location?
- Pick five items: Is the appropriate amount of stock present (no overstock or within the min/max parameters)?
- Is the area clear of dust, spills, and trash?
- Does the area match the picture listed?

This audit will help identify any areas that need improvement. Once the area has been sustained, continually look for ways to improve the area. Could storage be maximized? Would an item make sense in a different location? How could it be easier for the inventory manager to order or the team to find and stock different areas of the practice?

A similar process can be used for exam rooms. This can help cut down on the "brain calories" required to find items because it adds familiarity and predictability to where items are stored and kept. As an example, if all the exam rooms have the same layout (or at least similar organizational or storage components), then the drawers and cabinets can be organized and stocked in the exact same way in each room. For the team, it starts to become a "muscle memory," and they can focus on the patient in the room rather than searching for what they need.

Not only that, but if a central storage area was constructed or added, the exam rooms and treatment area could be easily stocked from this main storage area. The whole exam room storage becomes predictable and systematized.

Let's imagine that weekly on Friday afternoons is the time you have set aside to restock the treatment and exam rooms. Your team knows what you are doing because the communication is clear and your schedule is consistent. You grab the treatment area and exam room restock checklist and move through the rooms one by one. Your checklist includes each item that's in each exam room and the ideal quantity. You take the checklist to the exam rooms one by one and use the list to compare what each room should have versus what is actually there. You make notes as to what you need from central storage. You make a note that you need four sleeves of gauze, a box of 20 g needles, and two boxes of 3 cc syringes.

You then return to central storage to grab these items. After doing so, you notice that the 20 g needles have reached the reorder point, and you pull the tag off and put it in the bin to be reordered. After restocking the exam rooms, you remove the items from the inventory in your PiMS with an adjustment. In just a short amount of time, the exam rooms were properly stocked, an item was flagged for reorder, and hospital supplies were removed from the PiMS.

"Best Practice" Time Saver

A quick note on hospital supplies: It's generally not worth your time to keep track of each and every syringe, needle, and square of gauze in your practice. Typically, when a box is opened, the entire box should be adjusted out of your on-hand quantity. Generally speaking, the amount of time it takes to count and monitor these items individually does not provide a financial benefit. There are much better ways you could spend your time and effort!

"Best Practice" Questions to Consider
- What restocking and organizing workflows make the most sense in your practice?
- Is there a particular area of your practice that needs immediate organizing attention?
- Are there any team members who would enjoy and excel at the organization process?
- What systems or processes could be developed and implemented to maintain and sustain any areas that are reorganized?

6.6 Integrating Physical Reorder Points and Inventory Organization

Organized veterinary practices and physical reorder points go hand in hand. As a reminder, a reorder point is the point at which you reorder. A physical reorder point serves as a flag that something needs to be reordered. (You can revisit reorder points in Chapter 4.) This shifts from you examining each item in the practice or relying on the "want book" for ordering. Be curious and experiment with what works best for each particular item and your unique practice. Some methods will work better than others for different practices, but the key is to test and continuously improve.

Min/max labels are a great double-duty tool; not only are they a shelf label but they also serve as a physical reorder point (Figures 6.1, 6.2, and 6.3). Often, they list the product name, the minimum quantity to have on hand, and the maximum product level. Anything above and beyond the max level would be considered overstock. These labels can be placed on any item in your inventory, but they are especially beneficial for hospital supplies in the central storage area. In addition, information that the inventory manager, purchaser, and the team would find helpful can be included, such as:

- the item code
- what vendor it's purchased from (if there's always a specific vendor)
- a backstock or secondary location, if applicable
- if there are special shipping requirements or a longer lead time.

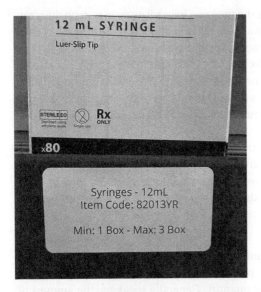

Figure 6.1 A min/max shelf label for syringes. Nicole Clausen.

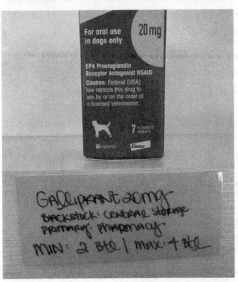

Figure 6.2 A min/max shelf label for Galliprant®. Nicole Clausen.

Figure 6.3 A min/max shelf label for Virbantel®.
Nicole Clausen.

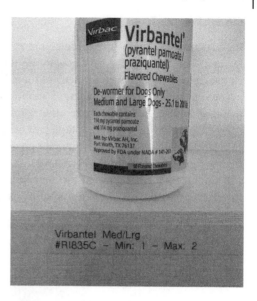

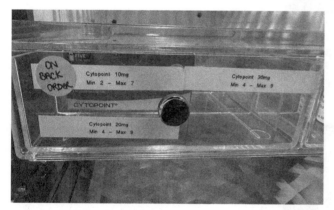

Figure 6.4 A min/max label for Cytopoint® with a sticker signaling that the product is on backorder.
Nicole Clausen.

These labels can be attached using plastic clip-ons, magnetic labels, or another type of adhesive that works well with your shelving.

"Best Practice" Shelf Label Tip
Highlight or put a sticker on backordered items so everyone in the practice can identify that it's on backorder rather than out of stock (Figure 6.4).

The most important aspect of these labels is to determine your minimum and maximum levels. The **minimum inventory level** is typically the reorder point for that item or the lowest inventory level you would want to have on hand. The **maximum inventory level** is different from the reorder quantity. It's the maximum amount you'd want on the shelf. A general rule for calculating the maximum level is the reorder point plus the reorder quantity. When using the min/max labels, you'll order the difference between what's on the shelf and the maximum quantity. The minimum level will serve as the signal that it's time to reorder. See Chapter 3 for information on how to calculate the minimum and maximum levels for items.

6.6.1 Reorder Tags

Reorder tags are one of the more common types of physical reorder points. In Chapter 4, you learned about reorder tags and how to use them in conjunction with your reorder points. In this chapter, you'll learn how to implement them into your practice.

These tags serve as a flag when an item reaches a "low" threshold. Let's examine an example together. For 3 cc syringes, the reorder point is two boxes and the reorder quantity is four boxes. A reorder tag is rubberbanded, taped, or otherwise affixed to the second to last box. When that second to last box is opened, the reorder tag should be pulled off and put in a bin, signaling that it's time to reorder (Figures 6.5, 6.6, and 6.7).

Reorder tags are exceptional for items that aren't tracked well in the PiMS, things that aren't invoiced easily or at all, like hospital supplies, large liquids (like fenbendazole granules or liquid),

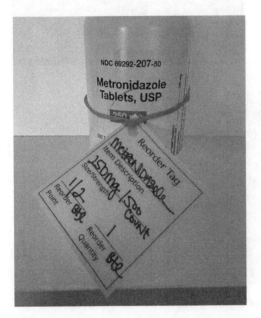

Figure 6.5 A reorder tag for metronidazole. Nicole Clausen.

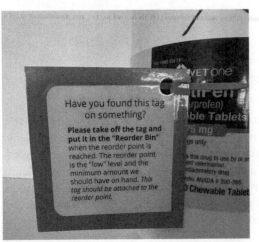

Figure 6.6 An example of instructions for team members that can be added to the back of tags. Nicole Clausen.

Figure 6.7 A reorder tag for Cytopoint. Nicole Clausen.

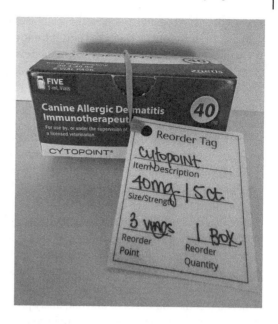

or even office and janitorial supplies. If there is a particular item that tends to run out or get forgotten, it's a great idea to add a reorder tag.

Although these tags can be very convenient and easy to use, they also have some challenges, including:

- team members forgetting to put them in the to-be-ordered bin (they can end up just being thrown on the shelf or in the trash)
- making sure the tag gets put back on the item correctly once it's been reordered
- the team grabbing every other box except for the one with the order tag.

There are several tips for ensuring reorder tags are implemented successfully.

- Laminate the tags and use rubber bands to help secure them.
- Place the to-be-ordered bins throughout the practice so that it's convenient for the team and reduces friction.
- Get buy-in from the team by involving and surveying them to find out what items work well for this system.
- Get creative and have a pizza party if no order tags are missed in 30 days (or something else your team would enjoy).
- Have a written SOP and designate a person (or team of people) for reattaching the reorder tags once the product has arrived in the practice.

6.6.2 Reorder Bins

Reorder bins are a great way to integrate physical reorder points into your central storage. There are a number of different options and directions you can take. For example, each bin can be divided into two different sections. A particular item (let's say primary IV lines) is placed in each section of the bin, but all of the product behind the divider, in a smaller section, is considered the reorder level. All the items in front of the divider are used (with care not to touch the product behind the divider). Once the items in the front section are gone, it's a signal that it's time to reorder.

The product is reordered and now the team uses the product behind the divider. Once it arrives in the practice, it should be restocked and the entire process should be repeated.

The process is similar in the **two-bin system**. Two bins are placed on a shelf, one behind the other. Both bins should be filled with the product. The team uses all the items in the front bin. When it's empty, it's the signal that it's time to reorder. Once the item has been reordered, the empty bin is moved to the back so that the full bin is now in front. Once the product arrives in the practice, it is restocked into the back bin first and the process starts all over again.

There are a number of different ways to utilize reorder bins in your practice, but keep in mind that the purpose is for the bins to serve as a physical flag that it's time to reorder.

Let's explore an example of how this could work.

Remember Georgia from Tank's Animal Hospital? Well, when she started at the hospital, things were a mess. The practice had been short-handed for a while and recently added two new veterinarians to their team, so inventory management took a back seat. Georgia's mission was to turn it all around. Let's set the scene and see how she cleaned up their inventory.

There were two smaller storage closets near the treatment room, and there was no rhyme or reason for how things were stored. In one of the storage closets were boxes full of a random assortment of white goods, gauze, and bandaging material. There were bottles of pharmaceuticals bunched together on the floor and old, dusty product brochures yellow with age on a shelf. The top shelves cradled random boxes of expired products and supplies, old broken equipment, and paperwork, including a staff birthday card for a team member who no longer worked for the practice. Next to that box was a broken printer that no one remembered putting there. The drawers and cabinets did not provide "homes" but halfway-there spaces, and whenever shipments of supplies came in, they were clearly dropped into whatever empty space could be found.

Georgia saw the proof of leaky profits immediately. How on earth did the team find what they needed in this mess? With some quick mental math, she knew that there were, at minimum, thousands of dollars of expired products in those boxes. She took a deep breath and mapped out the inventory "zones" by defining the different spaces and what should live there. She outlined which products would live in which cabinets going forward and mapped the changes. After her rough draft was done, she approached Dr Tank and the team and asked for feedback. With their opinions and ideas in mind, she finalized her zone plan.

Georgia walked through the **5S Process**. She pulled everything out of one area at a time (the west wall cabinet, the near-the-door drawer) and sorted everything into separate piles for what should be included, thrown away, moved, and decided on later. She added bins and labels for storage, pharmacy shelf dividers for backstock, and little drawer organizers to keep smaller items tidy. Finally, everything went into its new home and the area was cleaned.

Once everything shone, she documented it with pictures, a "planogram" (a diagram of where items should be placed in the zone), and written descriptions. Once she'd been through the 5S Process for each storage area in the practice and finished organizing each zone, she added labels and decided where they would use reorder flags. She added shelf labels to everything stored in cabinets or in central storage. Items that were stored in bins or little organizers were also given labels. In the pharmacy, shelf dividers were added. Georgia continued her documentation, took pictures of the new labels, and created a SOP. She also decided on the following.

- Reorder tags would be used for any supplies or items that were rarely used but very important to patient care. Tags would also be used for items that were stored only in drawers.
- Min/max labels would be used for any items that were stored in cabinets or in the central storage areas.

- The surgery, dentistry, and emergency carts would have a reorder checklist to help with ordering.
- For any remaining hospital supplies or white goods, reorder tags would be used.
- Georgia would use electronic reorder points for any pharmaceuticals and items that were tracked easily in their software.

After she had outlined exactly what reorder point flags she would like to use, the next step was to calculate the reorder points and create the flags.

Georgia started with the syringe cabinet to calculate the min/max levels for 1 ml tuberculin syringes. After checking with her ordering platform, she calculated that Tank's Animal Hospital purchased 117 boxes in the last 12 months. She decided it would be best for their hospital supplies that when they have a two-week supply on hand, they will order a 30-day supply.

First, to calculate the "minimum amount," Georgia calculated what a two-week supply would be for the 1 ml TB syringes. She divided the amount purchased in the last 12 months by the number of two-week periods in a year, 26.

$$Reorder\ Point\ or\ Minimum\ Amount = \frac{Annual\ Usage}{26}$$

$$ROP\ or\ Min = \frac{117\ Boxes}{26}$$

$$ROP\ or\ Min = 4.5 \approx 5\ Boxes$$

It was calculated that when Tank's Animal Hospital reaches five boxes of 1 cc TB syringes, they are considered low and need to be reordered. The next step was to calculate the reorder quantity (a 30-day supply).

$$Reorder\ Quantity = \frac{Annual\ Usage}{12}$$

$$ROQ = \frac{117\ Boxes}{12}$$

$$ROQ = 9.75 \approx 10\ Boxes$$

Now that both the minimum amount (the reorder point) and the reorder quantity were calculated, the last step was to calculate the maximum quantity.

$$Maximum\ Quantity = Minimum\ Quantity + Reorder\ Quantity$$

$$Maximum\ Quantity = 5\ Boxes + 10\ Boxes$$

$$Maximum\ Quantity = 15\ Boxes$$

For the 1 cc TB syringes, Georgia calculated that when they reach five boxes, they have reached the minimum quantity on hand and should reorder up to the maximum level of 15 boxes. So, if Tank's Animal Hospital were to have five boxes on the shelf, Georgia would "order up" to

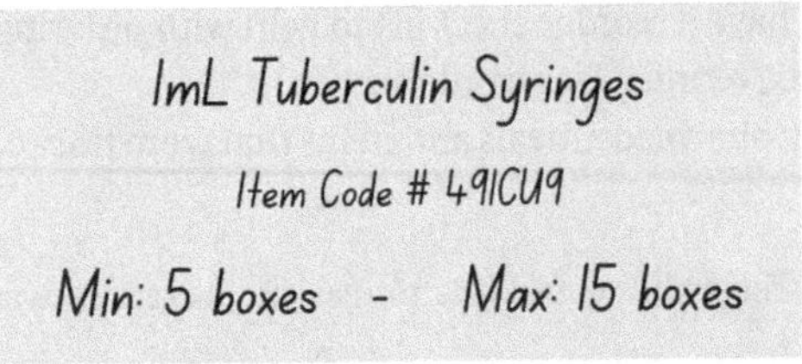

1mL Tuberculin Syringes

Item Code # 491CU9

Min: 5 boxes - Max: 15 boxes

Figure 6.8 The min/max label for the 1 ml tuberculin syringes calculation example. Nicole Clausen.

maximum by purchasing 10 boxes. If they had four boxes left on the shelf, she would "order up" to the maximum by purchasing 11 boxes.

Figure 6.8 shows the min/max label in action.

For the remaining products, Georgia calculated the reorder points and quantities and added the information to her tags, shelf labels, and bins. Success!

6.6.3 Inventory Manager Spotlight

Meet Tiffany McCumber, inventory coordinator extraordinaire! She was given the opportunity to take over the inventory at two of my hospitals in July 2006.

She says, "[Prior to that] I had *never* managed inventory before, so it was all new to me. I was given some training but learned a lot just by doing it. I am going on 18 years of doing inventory, and I could not be happier. I jokingly say that I am happier managing things on shelves rather than patients in cages!

My favorite part of inventory is making sure my team has all the things they need to perform their jobs to the best of their ability. I love it when they come to ask me if I have XYZ, and I can pinpoint exactly where that item they need is in my supply room. I am a quiet part of a well-oiled machine. I love it when I find a backorder that they need or find an alternative. I love offering ideas that they may not have heard before.

I am currently proud of the systems that I have in place for myself to make sure that I get all the things ordered and organized. I am very excited to work through my Certified Veterinary Inventory Professional course and fine-tune my systems and SOPs. I really want to grow within my company; I would like to help create a training program for future inventory coordinators in my company. I want to lower my COGS within my hospital, and hopefully teach others how to do it as well!"

Tiffany's supply room is lovingly called the "Chamber of Secrets" (Figures 6.9, 6.10, and 6.11). Her other storage room (shared with the laundry area) is called Narnia. She also has disco balls hanging from the ceiling. Who says inventory cannot be fun?

6.7 Protecting Your Inventory Investment

I wish I could say that theft or other misuse is not a possibility but unfortunately, it can and does happen. Whenever I speak at events on inventory, I hear stories of theft in attendee practices ranging from sneakily giving away services or inventory to a favorite client (without permission from management or the practice owner) to things as sinister as replacing the injectable controlled substances with water. I've heard some horrific stories and discovered a number of cases of theft of inventory in practices (some have even been over tens of thousands of dollars). A veterinarian once told me "It's not a matter of *if* you get stolen from; it's a matter of *when*."

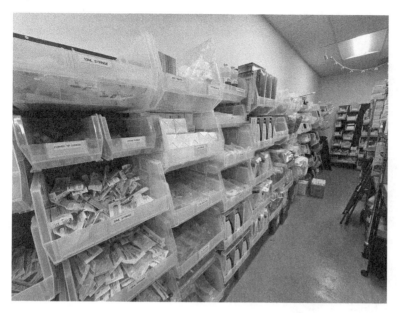

Figures 6.9 The supply room that Tiffany set up. Everything is labeled and grouped by category (syringes, surgery, bandaging, catheters, etc.). *Source:* Courtesy of Tiffany McCumber.

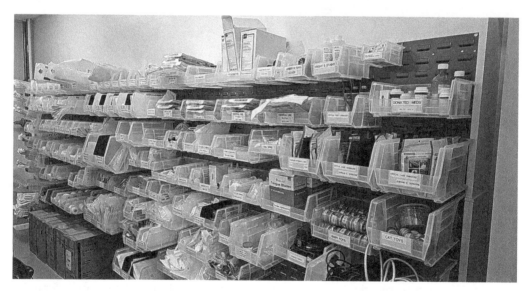

Figures 6.10 Another view of Tiffany's supply room. *Source:* Courtesy of Tiffany McCumber.

Knowing that theft and misuse are possibilities, protecting your inventory is an important aspect of managing inventory. One of the most helpful systems in preventing theft and diversion is checks and balances to ensure that more than one person knows the procedures for inventory so that not just one person is doing all of it alone. It's also important to implement a cycle counting schedule so that any off-counts and variances can be identified quickly.

Let's take gabapentin, for example. In many states (at the time of publication), it's not considered a controlled substance so it might not be monitored closely. If you were to count only once a year during

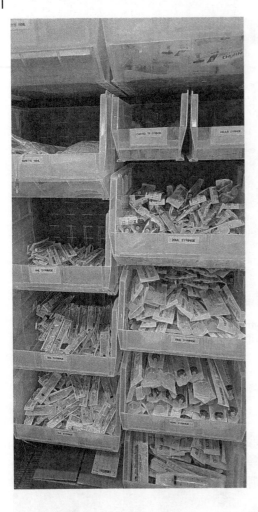

Figure 6.11 The bins and labels for syringes in the storage room. *Source:* Courtesy of Tiffany McCumber.

end-of-year counts, you might find you were missing 1763 capsules. How could you discover where they went? It would be extremely challenging (if not essentially impossible) to track down exactly where and how they went missing. But if you were to count more frequently, say biweekly or monthly, and you found you were missing 100, it would be easier and more efficient to track down where that 100 went.

6.7.1 What's Your "Win the Lottery" Policy?

Let's consider another scenario. An inventory manager was the sole person responsible for ordering and receiving. They ordered a product and before it was ever put on the shelf, they put it in their backpack. Then, when receiving the invoices into the PiMS, they did not "receive" that item (thus, the PiMS would not show any missing inventory). The invoice was then attached to the statement and paid. The item would not be flagged as missing on the shelf or on any reports! There would be no way to know that someone was stealing unless there were checks and balances in place. A great way to start is having a different person in charge of ordering versus receiving.

Having more than one person in charge of managing inventory is helpful for separating duties to safeguard your inventory. Not only that but if that inventory team member were to leave the practice, become ill, or win the lottery, other team members could step in and assist in the inventory process.

"Best Practice" Questions to Consider

- Have you had any instances of theft before? What was the result? What changed, or what processes were put in place as a result?
- Where could duties be separated to help prevent theft in your practice?
- Do you currently have a "win the lottery" policy in place so more than one person understands inventory?
- Who is considered "irreplaceable" on your team? What do you need to change so that their role can be filled if they leave?

One useful way to put this into practice is to have several people involved in the inventory management process, although one person could still be ultimately responsible. One person could be in charge of demand forecasting and ordering, while another is in charge of receiving (both physical receipt and receiving into the PiMS). A third person (like a book keeper) could be in charge of statement reconciliation. In addition, other (trained) team members could unpack and put away inventory when it arrives.

More oversight and additional protection measures should also be in place for ordering and receipt of controlled substances. In Chapter 12, we cover controlled substances in depth but here are a few ways to add protection for your controlled substances.

- The DEA registrant could review and "sign off" before any controlled substances are purchased.
- Only people who have been appropriately trained and verified to handle controlled substances should have access.
- Creating and regularly updating and maintaining controlled substance SOPs and processes.
- Anyone who is responsible for controlled substances (whether it's logging or another aspect of managing them) is required to take a controlled substance class prior to handling.

Over the years, I've heard of so many instances of controlled substance theft, from team members, to clients, and interview candidates. Do you think your theft control measures are enough? Where could you improve in this area?

6.7.2 An Example Workflow for Two to Three People

Let's explore an example workflow for two to three people involved in inventory management.

- Team member #1 could be in charge of demand forecasting and ordering. They would create a list of items that need to be ordered and place the order. Team member #2 should then review and sign off on all orders that were placed.
- Team member #2 could be in charge of unpacking boxes, receiving the inventory, and receipt into the practice management software. Team member #1 should review and sign off on all invoices or purchase orders received. It is important to note that only someone who is very well trained and has great attention to detail should receive packing slips or invoices into the software. This should not be a task for just anyone in the practice!
- Team member #3 (perhaps a book keeper) should reconcile invoices with statements. This individual could also receive inventory in the PiMS while team member #2 unpacked the boxes and physically received the inventory. If a third team member wasn't available for this role, the inventory manager could reconcile the monthly statements.

Segregating inventory management responsibilities helps create checks and balances and visibility to prevent theft and diversion. If you are thinking "Nicole, no way do we have time for this!," get curious about how the duties could be divided without taking a ton of extra time. For example, perhaps setting specific time aside once or twice a week for the second inventory team member to receive orders while scheduling the inventory manager frequent, dedicated time throughout the week.

"Best Practice" Considerations
- How could you implement more checks and balances in your practice?
- How could you ensure that not just one person knows and understands the inventory processes?

6.8 Strategies for Safeguarding Your Inventory

Protecting your inventory investment is key for expensive, valuable, or products prone to theft or diversion. This could include large bulk purchases, controlled substances, flea/tick/heartworm prevention, and a number of expensive items. Unfortunately, theft does occur in veterinary practices, either internally (from team members or others who have access to the pharmacy area) or externally (from clients or others with access to the building).

When it comes to safeguarding your inventory, as with most things in veterinary medicine and inventory management, what this looks like will depend on your practice and your unique situation. Below, I'll outline several ways and some inspiration to protect your expensive investments.

6.8.1 Add and Improve Visibility

One of the most helpful strategies for reducing theft in your practice is to make it clear that someone is paying attention and monitoring the inventory at any given time. If people know that inventory is watched, it makes it harder to steal. It would be quite easy to take something from central storage or backstock if it wasn't going to be counted, and no one would know it was missing.

6.8.1.1 Ways to Add and Improve Visibility

Cycle counting is one of the best things that can be implemented to reduce the possibility of theft. Cycle counting is when small amounts of inventory are counted frequently (focusing on and prioritizing valuable and frequently used items). See Chapter 9 for more information on cycle counts. With cycle counting, items are counted more often, which means (i) if theft did happen, it would be realized more quickly, and (ii) added visibility gives the team notice that inventory management is important and missing items will be found.

Create a process to regularly review purchase orders and invoices to ensure that what was ordered came in, was restocked appropriately, and was received into the PiMS. It would be very easy for someone to order something, not receive it into the software, and pocket the item. If there is no regular review process, this theft would likely go unnoticed. All invoices with controlled substances should be audited to ensure all proper processes are followed.

Another strategy would be to have two (or three) people involved in the ordering and receiving process to help separate duties (as exemplified above). For example, one person could order, another person could receive, and a third person could reconcile and review invoices and statements.

6.8.2 Limit Access to Inventory Overstock

In addition to adding and improving visibility, another tool in the "inventory protection toolbox" is to limit access to backstock or bulk purchases. Rather than allow the entire team access to all inventory, portions or sections would be locked to prevent theft. This strategy is particularly helpful for bulk purchases of valuable items like flea and tick or heartworm prevention, expensive large animal products, or larger orders of controlled substances. For example, the entire team might have access to a "working level" of stock (what the team will need for one or two weeks), and the remainder can only be accessed by the practice owner or practice manager.

6.8.2.1 Levels of Limited Access

(Mostly) unlimited access: almost all of the inventory is accessible to the entire team, except any bulk purchases or excessive levels of controlled substance backstock. The practice owner, practice manager, or member of the management team has access to the bulk product and distributes to the floor when necessary.

Example: Normally, you purchase fruit snacks from the regular grocery store. However, Costco was having a big sale, so you purchased two giant boxes from there. You would still give your team access to the regular-sized boxes of fruit snacks, but you lock up the Costco-size boxes and distribute them as needed.

Working stock access: the team only has access to the level of inventory necessary to treat patients for a week or two, and the remainder is locked away separately. This typically works best when only unopened containers are locked and open containers remain on the floor. It is helpful to purchase smaller quantity bottles (like 100-count containers of tramadol or gabapentin) rather than stocking the larger count bottles. This method can also limit the "multiple open bottles of the same product" scenario.

Example: You keep the fruit snacks you purchased under lock and key and will restock the snack drawer with how much your team will eat in a week or two. In this situation, it does not matter if the fruit snacks came from the regular grocery store or Costco.

Extremely limited access: with this access level, the entire team only has access to the level of inventory necessary to treat patients for a day or two, and the remainder is locked up. This method is extreme and should only be used in cases where internal theft is suspected and/or an internal investigation has been started. If there is no reason to use this level of restriction, it will likely be very cumbersome and inefficient. If this is necessary, only the practice owner and potentially the hospital administrator or practice management have access to the locked-up stock.

Example: You keep the fruit snacks you purchased under lock and key and will restock the snack drawer with how much your team will eat in a day or two.

Pharmacy-only access: with this method, the practice has an internal pharmacy and only pharmacy staff members have access to the entire inventory; team members order and request items from the pharmacy. Typically, the pharmacy team will fill all prescriptions as well and restock the practice as necessary. This method can be very beneficial, especially for larger practices with many team members. A "pharmacy-only access" type of setup can also be helpful for practices with many mobile or outcall vehicles. In order to restock their trucks, they must submit an order to the pharmacy. The pharmacy staff then makes sure the inventory is allocated to that specific truck or mobile vehicle. Setting up pharmacy-only access can also help with medication and dispensing errors.

Example: You keep the fruit snacks you purchased under lock and key in a "break room store," and the store clerk will only hand out the fruit snacks once someone has put in an order or otherwise requested them.

Examples of limiting access in your inventory include the following.

- Restricting access to the backstock safe of unopened controlled substances to only the DEA registrant and the hospital administrator.
- Restricting access to a large bulk purchase of flea, tick, or heartworm prevention to the practice owner, practice manager, and inventory manager and only putting two weeks' worth of working stock out on the floor.
- Restricting access to unopened injectables to prevent multiple open bottles.
- Not allowing employees to add items to their own accounts or dispense their own medications.
- Restricting access to the entire pharmacy to only the in-house pharmacy team who are responsible for dispensing and stocking all medications and supplies.
- Not allowing nonpharmacy staff in the pharmacy area to either fill medications or restock the treatment area.

6.8.3 Utilize Technology

Installing cameras throughout the practice is an excellent, cost-effective way to monitor and safeguard against theft. Even having a camera around the controlled substances is a great start! With the increase in popularity of home security, they are becoming more cost-effective.

There are many different ways to safeguard your inventory, so consider what will be beneficial to your unique practice and situation. Once you have established which methods to implement, document the process! Create SOPs and policies for the different processes and make it clear who has ownership of the different aspects. For example, what does the cycle counting process entail? Who is in charge of this process and who will they report to? What should be counted, and how should things be counted? If a discrepancy is found, what are the next steps?

Throughout this process, it's also important to review your practice employee manual and work with your lawyer or HR representative to see if anything related to theft should be added or changed.

7

Strategic Pricing for Your Inventory

7.1 How Your Practice's Values and Pricing Intersect

Pricing is a highly practice-specific decision. I often get asked about how to price something exactly. I do not believe there is an exact answer to what you should price something at, but there are some best practices and methodologies to consider.

"Best Practice" Rule for Pricing Your Inventory

Do not arbitrarily copy another veterinary practice's pricing. Pricing is specific to individual practices; you aren't saving yourself any time or benefiting your practice by mimicking someone else's decisions. You will set your practice up for success by intentionally pricing for your unique practice.

First and foremost, what are your practice's values? What does your clinic stand for? Let's explore an example of how this might come into play. Think about individual doses of heartworm prevention. Typically sold in a six-pack, your practice breaks up the packs to sell the single doses. Depending on your practice's values, you might consider two differing methods for pricing these.

- Because of the extra time and labor involved, the convenience to the client, and single doses being unavailable through online pharmacies, you decide to mark up single doses higher than the six-pack. In this example, 100% markup per single dose versus 60% markup for the whole box.
- You've found that the overwhelming majority of clients purchase single doses because they cannot afford to buy the entire box. So, rather than charge more to more economically challenged clients, you decide to have a consistent yet slightly higher markup of 65%, whether it's a single dose or a six-pack.

There is no right or wrong answer here. However, the decision to choose the first option rather than the second will depend heavily on your practice values. So, it's helpful to have clarity on where you stand prior to developing a pricing strategy.

Consider the "spectrum of care" with a range of options ranging from basic and lower-cost care to advanced, state-of-the-art, higher-cost care. Similarly, I like to think of the "spectrum of pricing." On one side, there could be low prices and lower margins (with a higher patient/client volume), whereas on the other side of the spectrum, there could be more boutique concierge pricing. This will look different for every practice. For example, a state-of-the-art metropolitan boutique specialty center will have different pricing from an extremely rural cattle practice.

Inventory Management for Veterinary Professionals, First Edition. Nicole I. Clausen.
© 2024 John Wiley & Sons, Inc. Published 2024 by John Wiley & Sons, Inc.
Companion website: www.wiley.com/go/clausen/inventory

There are a number of different ways to price your inventory. The most common is cost-based pricing which involves setting the price based on the cost of the item, plus any indirect costs, plus the desired level of profit. Value-based pricing involves setting the price of an item based on how much the perceived value is to clients. It's more about pricing the product based on its benefits and value to clients, not just the item's costs.

In this chapter, we'll be focusing on cost-based pricing strategies. But as I've mentioned, pricing is a highly practice-specific decision. You know your practice the best. You know your clients and the area the best. You can craft an intentional cost-based strategy that still considers your client demographics, desired compliance and purchasing behavior, and your practice's unique indirect costs. Plus, when your pricing strategy is intentionally crafted, it can be automated so no items or prices get left behind.

"Best Practice" Pricing Considerations

Whatever the nuances of your practice, there are some essential issues to consider.

- What are your practice's values? What does your clinic stand for?
- Where do you fall on the "spectrum of pricing"?
- Who do you serve? What are the demographics of your clientele?
- What are your indirect costs? Do you have high facility costs in an expensive neighborhood? What are your labor costs like for inventory management?
- What is your compliance rate with clients? Do you have a lot of competition from online pharmacies?
- Do your doctors work on production? Do their production percentages need to be taken into account?

At the end of the day, pricing your inventory is unique to your practice, but your profitability goals should be top of mind. Using your pricing strategy to support your practice's financial performance is important so that you can pay your team a living wage, invest in the growth of your practice, give back to the community, and ensure your practice is around for years to come.

Let's explore the nuances of pricing and how to develop a pricing strategy that aligns with your unique practice.

7.2 Introduction to Pricing Your Inventory

I like to approach pricing with strategy and sustainability in mind. How can you develop a pricing strategy that will not only serve your practice right now but also grow with it? Strategic pricing is more important now than ever before. With the increase in popularity of online pharmacies, our pricing strategy must balance profitability for our practice, build trust, and remain competitive for our clients.

Bottom line: Creating a pricing strategy can help practices maintain consistency and provide the ability to remain competitive yet profitable.

With the right policies in place, practices can plan for and maneuver cost increases appropriately and reduce the amount of unintentional chaos. The day-to-day activity in a veterinary practice is chaotic enough as it is: Someone came late for their appointment, another person brought two extra dogs, an emergency walked in, and a wellness exam unexpectedly turned into an urgent hospitalization appointment. If we can provide as much framework and structure as possible through standard processes (think: this is what to do, how to do it, and when), then we can eliminate some of the chaos that comes with not understanding what or how to do something.

Think about this situation: One of your team members excitedly tells a client about a product that just arrived today, and the owner wants to purchase it. The product has not been added or set up in the practice management system (PiMS) just yet. In an effort to sell the owner the product, you try to add and price the product really quickly. All of a sudden, you freeze up. How should I price this? What's our dispensing fee again? What does Chewy charge? What do other practices do? You check with a fellow team member to see if they remember. No luck. Now, you run upstairs to the practice manager's office but they are busy on a phone call. Your practice owner is in with a client and cannot be interrupted. This is all taking you away from other important tasks or projects, and the client is waiting.

That situation is what I consider unintentional chaos, the majority of which can be avoided with a clear standard operating procedure (SOP) for creating prices. With a documented pricing strategy, we are now able to price an item promptly and correctly without having to create extra stress or effort. Ideally, as soon as a new product is ordered, it is set up in the PiMS and priced appropriately. That way, when it arrives, it's ready to be sold. The ultimate goal with a pricing strategy is that products can be priced with confidence, that clients are charged appropriately, and that any cost increases can be properly adjusted and billed for.

There are two main pillars when creating your pricing strategy. The first is the pricing of the actual inventory item and the second is determining the fees added to the price of an item (such as a dispensing fee). In this text, **cost** refers to the amount the practice paid for an inventory, and **price** refers to the amount a client will be charged for that item. The additional fees, in addition to the price of the item, are often called **prescription fees**. These can include prescription dispensing fees, injection fees, handling fees, and controlled substance fees. A prescription fee can vary widely depending on the type and location of the practice.

"Best Practice" Highlight
There are two main pillars of your pricing strategy.

- Pricing the inventory item.
- Any additional fees, like a dispensing fee.

The purpose of the **markup** of an item (the difference between the cost of an item and its selling price) is important for a number of reasons. First, the markup of an item includes indirect costs such as holding and labor costs. **Holding costs**, as you remember from Chapter 4, include the cost of keeping an item on the shelf and can include such things as rent, insurance, etc. to house the item safely. **Labor costs** include an inventory manager or team member's time to purchase the item, receive it, and manage the movement of that particular item. It also includes any production pay or bonuses to the prescribing veterinarian or team member. The markup of an item is critical because if an item is priced too low, the costs of the practice may not be adequately covered.

The purpose of a **prescription fee** is different. A prescription fee covers the cost and expertise of the veterinarian to calculate the dose, determine the instructions, fill the prescription, review the medication with the owner, and the cost of the dram vial, among others. Similarly, the injection fee covers the time and expertise of the person administering the medication, etc.

A controlled substance fee can be added on top of the markup and other fees to offset the cost of regulatory compliance and controlled substance management tools such as log books or an electronic dispensing cabinet. Handling fees can also be added to cover any costs associated with storing, dispensing, or handling the item (Table 7.1).

Table 7.1 Differences in what's included for markup and any additional fees.

Item markup includes	Dispensing or injection fee includes
Indirect labor costs	Veterinarian and care team expertise
Indirect holding costs	Time to calculate dosage
Practice profit	Count prescription or prepare injectable syringe
	Cost of dram vial or needle and syringe
	Time and expertise to determine the instructions

7.3 Prescription and Dispensing Fees

In addition to creating a pricing strategy for your products, it's also essential to create a strategy for your prescription fees. Prescription fees can include prescription dispensing, handling, injection, or additional controlled substance or chemotherapy dispensing fees. Most practice management software systems have a way to include the additional fee into the price of an item so that it does not appear as two separate line items on a client's invoice.

For more information regarding using your PiMS to sell your inventory, see Chapter 8.

Helpful Definitions
- **Dispensing fee**: a service charge for filling the prescription. With this fee, the client is paying for the service and expertise that comes with filling the prescription.
- **Handling fee**: a service charge for extra care, expertise, and work involved in managing certain medications or products. This fee often covers additional effort, specialized storage, or any special precautions taken for that medication.
- **Injection fee**: a service charge for administering an injection. With this fee, the client is paying for the team's time, expertise, and equipment to administer the injection safely and properly.

Depending on your PiMS, your software might only have one fee type where the amount can be customized for each item. Alternatively, you might have different categories of fees (like prescription fees, handling fees, etc.) where the amount cannot be customized per item. Throughout this process, identify how your software system works for pricing, what the limitations are, and how you could translate your new pricing strategy into your software.

As with most things related to pricing your inventory, prescription dispensing or injection fees vary wildly depending on a number of factors, including your location, client demographics, practice type, and more. Prescription or dispensing fees are typically not included when utilizing the margin pricing method but can and typically are included when calculating pricing with the markup model, standard pricing formula, and the overhead cost pricing model. We'll cover all of those processes later in this chapter.

After working with hundreds of practices across the country, I've identified some common ranges and pricing patterns. Here's what I've found over the years (based on 2024 information).

- Prescription dispensing fees generally range from $8.00 to $25.00, but between $10.00 and $15.00 is most common.
- In some very rural and lower economic areas, it can be as low as $3.00 per prescription. Alternatively, some metropolitan areas or specialty centers can be above the high end of the range.

Table 7.2 Common ranges in practices across the United States.

Fee type	Fee range ($)
Prescription fee	8.00–25.00
Injection fee	15.00–45.00
Box, bottle, or noncounted prescription fee	3.00–10.00
Additional controlled substance fee	2.00–10.00

- Most injection fees are between $15.00 and $45.00. Many practices fall between $20.00 and $30.00.
- A lower "boxed" prescription fee for things that do not need to be counted can range from $3.00 to $10.00. Many practices typically range between not charging a fee for these items to $5.00.

"Best Practice" Tip

Controlled substances and chemotherapy can attract a higher prescription or injection fee because of the extra labor required for regulatory compliance and safety. This can vary depending on time, materials, and equipment required but most commonly, it is $2.00 to $10.00 per prescription or injection administration. While this practice is not the norm yet, adding an extra "surcharge" is becoming more common (Table 7.2).

7.3.1 Pricing Concept: Minimum Price

Some PiMSs allow you to set a minimum price. The goal here is to ensure that whatever is charged to the client covers, at least, the indirect and direct costs. If the price of an item plus the dispensing fee is less than the minimum price, the system will automatically charge the minimum price. If the dispensing fee plus the cost of an item is above the minimum price, nothing will happen. The minimum price is not in addition to the dispensing fee, and these two things aren't added together (unless your software does some very funky things!).

As an example, let's say that Tank's Animal Hospital has a minimum price set at $21.00. That means that no prescription will leave the practice for less than $21.00. So, if a script of 14 Thyrosyn is filled and the price is $11.10, the PiMS will automatically increase the price to $21.00.

This can be very helpful for inexpensive items. For example, if Tank's Animal Hospital has a minimum price of $25.00 but an injection fee of $20.00, rather than charging the client $20.02 for a vitamin B injection, the PiMS would automatically charge the client $25.00.

Typically, I recommend using both a minimum price and a dispensing fee. If just a minimum price is used, then any prescription over the minimum price will not have any additional fees to account for the team's time, expertise, and costs associated with filling that prescription or administering the injection. So when both the minimum price and the dispensing fee work together, any inexpensive medications below the minimum price threshold will be charged as whatever the minimum price is set for but any medications over the minimum price will have a dispensing or injection fee.

An example of this could look like:

- dispensing fee: $15.00
- minimum price: $20.00.

With that, no script will leave the practice for less than $20.00, but any script above the minimum price will be unaffected and still include a dispensing fee.

7.4 Pricing Models

7.4.1 Pricing Models at a Glance

- Markup model
- Total cost pricing model
- Margin Pricing model

The formulas in this chapter aren't new. They were discussed in *Practice Made Perfect* (Heinke 2014) and *Blackwell's Five-Minute Veterinary Practice Management Consult* (Ackerman 2020), and slight adaptations have been taught by different vet med educators for years. In this chapter, I want to outline and cover my considerations for adapting these to your practice, the different nuances, and what I've found works well (Table 7.3).

There are three main pricing models that can be used to price various inventory items and products. The first (and most popular) is using a **markup percentage** to increase the cost of an item. This is the most common method and what many veterinary professionals are used to. For example, gabapentin 100 mg has a markup of 200%.

The second and more precise method is to use a **total cost pricing formula** that takes into account indirect costs like labor and holding costs, veterinarian or care team production, and desired profit. The third is a **margin pricing** model, which adds a dollar amount to the cost rather than a percentage.

Each method has pros and cons and can be implemented differently in each practice. As with most things regarding inventory management, when creating a pricing strategy for your practice, what works best depends on your unique situation, culture, and business goals. I invite you to think about what method works best for you or if a mix of different methods is most helpful.

Imagine a pod of southern resident orca whales spending the warm summer months in the Salish Sea in Washington State. As a fun way to explore the nuances of the different pricing formulas, let us compare the pricing model concepts with how much each whale in the pod would eat.

Table 7.3 The three different pricing models reviewed in this chapter: markup model, pricing with formulas, and margin model pricing.

	Markup model	Total cost pricing model	Margin pricing model
Definition	The selling price is determined by adding a certain percentage to the cost of the product	The selling price is determined using a precise formula that includes cost factors specific to the individual practice	The selling price is determined by adding a certain dollar amount to the total cost of the product
Pros	Easy to set up, easy to maintain in the practice management system	Precise; includes specific cost information for the practice and can specify a desired profit margin	Especially for large patients, the selling price is often lower, making it more economical for clients
Cons	Only uses an overall percentage and does not include indirect costs or veterinarian production	Isn't easily maintained in the practice management system, and prices need to be manually recalculated as costs go up	For large patients, the profit per patient is lower than using the markup model and is not as profitable for the practice

Nova (J-51) is a happy male whale who, for the sake of learning the equation, is trying to figure out how much he and his sister, Crescent (J-58), need to eat. So he figures out his weight and Crescent's weight and does the math for each of them. Nova often explores with his family, so he likes simple equations.

He's 8200 lb and Crescent is 6900 lb. Nova knows that adult orca whales can eat up to 100–300 lb per day (https://whalemuseum.org/). Each whale in the pod would eat slightly different amounts of salmon depending on how large or small it is. Nova wants to make sure he and his pod members are eating appropriately but he would rather be doing whale things than math all day. But he knows different family members have more complexities. Tahlequah, he knows, is nursing her newborn calf. Would it work for her?

- *Markup percentage model considers body size and nutrition requirement.*
  Tahlequah (J-35) is a busy mom of two: Notch (J-47) and Phoenix (J-57). She noticed a very small school of her little ones' favorite meal and wanted to make sure each whale in the pod was able to have some of the highly prized squid. Tahlequah wants to determine how much to eat based on the margin formula for her and her calves; even with their different sizes, both whales would eat the same amount of salmon. To make sure everyone got a chance to eat, Tahlequah, her calf, and each member of the pod ate four squid.
- *Margin model = every whale, whatever their size, eats the same amount.*
  Kelp (K-42) is a big male orca who is always adventuring with his siblings. At the same time, he's also very conscientious and aware of the different needs of his family and the entire pod. Because of this, he wants to calculate exactly how much salmon each member of the pod would need to eat based on the water temperature, the activity level of each whale, their stage of life, and where they are in the reproductive cycle. In order to do this, he uses a formula but as time goes on, he realizes how much time it takes, and he constantly needs to recalculate how much salmon everyone should eat based on the changing environment.
- *Formula model considers water temperature, activity level, stage of life (pregnancy).*
  If you are just getting started developing your pricing strategy and you are learning, I invite you to start simple and start small. Pick one category and decide what type of pricing model you'd like to use and what that will look like for you. Sometimes, it can seem that because it's complicated or complex, it's automatically better. That is not the case! The key to remember is that your pricing strategy is intentional, and you are able to charge your clients accurately. Once you become more familiar with pricing and the different models, you can always change or improve them as you see fit.

7.4.2 Pricing Model: Markup Model

In the markup pricing model, a markup percentage is applied to a product cost to calculate the price. For example, gabapentin 100 mg costs $0.15 per capsule and has a markup of 200%. The selling price would be $0.45.

Revisiting our orca pod from earlier, Nova's method for calculating how much salmon to eat is similar to the markup formula. Because it's more percentage based, the whales would eat more appropriately for their body size. In your practice, the markup formula is helpful to make sure items are priced appropriately; it is easy to get started and easy to maintain, but might not take into consideration the different factors like Kelp's method of margin pricing.

The markup pricing model allows for consistency and makes pricing an item easy. Using the markup model is an excellent place to start, as it's fairly user-friendly and easily implemented.

Table 7.4 Common general ranges for markup percentages from across the USA. Markup can range from 15% to 400%+, so there is an extensive range to consider.

Category or practice type	Common markup percentage range (%)
Small animal general practice	100–300
Flea/tick and heartworm prevention	45–100
Over-the-counter or retail items	100
Prescription diets	45 or manufacturer's suggested retail price (MSRP)
Equine practice markup	75–150
Livestock and large animals	15–50

Table 7.5 The difference between the markup percentage for an item and the corresponding cost multiplier.

Cost multiplier	Markup percentage (%)
1.5×	50
2×	100
2.5×	150
3×	200
3.5×	250
4×	300

Each category can have its own markup percentage, and you can have various slide scale rules to allow for flexibility. For example, over-the-counter retail items might have a markup percentage of 100%, but prescription diets might have a 45% markup. Alternatively, very inexpensive items (example: <$0.05 per unit) might have a 500% markup, whereas very expensive items (example: >$1.50 per unit) might have a 75% markup.

The biggest benefit of using the markup method is that it's easy to implement and use with a PiMS, and it's easy to maintain when costs increase and you pass those increases along to clients.

Markups can vary greatly depending on what category you are marking up, where you are in the country, and your area demographics (Table 7.4).

There can be some confusion between what is called a cost multiplier and the markup of an item (Table 7.5). When your practice owner asks you to mark up the item 250%, your first instinct might be to multiply the cost of the item by 2.5. Seems reasonable, right? That might seem accurate, but the cost multiplier for an item does not equal the percentage increase. Occasionally, I'll hear these concepts used interchangeably but that is not accurate.

The cost multiplier and markup percentage are similar but they work in slightly different ways. The **markup percentage** calculates an amount that needs to be added to the cost of the item to find the selling price. Meanwhile, the **cost multiplier** takes the cost and multiplies it by the factor to arrive at the selling price.

Let's explore an example together.

In the markup percentage formula that you just learned, you find the percentage markup and then add it to the cost. The cost multiplier does that in one step.

250% markup example.

$$Price = \text{cost} + \left(markup \ \% \ \times \text{cost}\right)$$

$$Price = \$ \ 0.50 + \left(250\% \times \$ \ 0.50\right)$$

$$Price = \$0.50 + \$1.25$$

$$Price = \$1.75$$

3.5× multiplier example.

$$Price = \text{cost} \times multiplier$$

$$Price = \$0.50 \times 3.5$$

$$Price = \$ \ 1.75$$

The downside of using the markup model is that it does not take into account any indirect costs or production paid for the prescription or refill. So, if a particular item has high holding costs (it's expensive to store, sits on the shelf for a long time, or takes up significant storage space), the markup model will not take those into account and it may lower the overall profit margin. But, in some cases, the benefits outweigh any cons.

The majority of practice management software systems do not have a great tracking system for pricing increases unless a markup percentage is entered. Let's say a markup percentage is entered for a particular product and the cost increases happen. When receiving that item on a purchase order or shipment receipt, the markup percentage function will (i) flag the cost increase and (ii) recalculate the new price based on the new higher cost. Without a markup percentage entered, any cost increases will not be passed along to clients without manually increasing the price.

This system works particularly well within many of the server-based PiMSs and a few of the cloud-based software systems. Once a purchased order is received, any costs will be recalculated using the markup percentage. Take note that with most practice management software systems, prices will not go down if costs decrease. It will only suggest a price increase! If you are not sure about your software, I recommend finding out as a first step.

While performing inventory analysis and audits for clients, it's common for me to find products where costs have not been updated. As a result of not leveraging the "autocalculate price function," the products are priced lower than what the item costs.

7.4.3 Pricing Model: Total Cost Pricing Model (Including Your Indirect Costs)

The second method uses formulas that include a more holistic picture of your costs to price your inventory. This is much more precise and takes into account indirect costs and production to provide a more accurate picture. Using a formula also helps you be more strategic rather than applying a blanket markup percentage to all items. The downside of this method is that it requires each inventory item to be calculated by hand. In addition, once any prices increase, they must be manually recalculated and updated. As it stands now, there are no PiMSs that have an automatic way to accomplish this.

Let's revisit the southern resident orca pod: With Kelp's method for figuring out how much to eat by including variables like water temperature and activity level, more factors are accounted for and therefore it is the most precise method available. But, as he realized, it could take a long time to calculate the exact amount of salmon for each and every whale. In your practice, pricing using a formula is potentially the most precise method, but it might take up a lot of time and be unsustainable in the long run. If Kelp had been able to put a spreadsheet calculator in place (and had opposable thumbs and computer access), the process could have become more streamlined.

The specific formulas will be outlined later in this chapter, but typically, the formulas will be similar to the following two-step process.

Step 1: determine the total product cost.

$$Product\ Cost \times Indirect\ Costs = Total\ Product\ Cost$$

Step 2: calculate the price.

$$Total\ Product\ Cost \times Profit\ Margin \times DVM\ Production = Selling\ Price$$

7.4.4 Pricing Model: Margin Pricing

The third method is margin-based pricing, in which a specified dollar amount is added to the cost of the item to find the selling price. This method is particularly helpful for expensive injectables or other pharmaceuticals where the cost might be reasonable for smaller patients using the markup model but is uneconomical for larger patients.

Revisiting the orca pod from earlier, using Tahlequah's method for calculating how many prized squid to eat, some whales might eat too much or too little depending on their size. The larger whales might quickly become hungry again because they did not get enough to eat. In your practice, the margin method might have too little profit (especially for larger patients) for some items, especially when overhead costs, your team's time and expertise, and veterinarian production are considered.

Let's explore an example. Convenia® is an injectable and has a cost of $27.00 per ml. Your desired profit margin for this product is $35.

The formula for margin pricing is:

$$Price = product\ cost + margin$$

This means that for 1 ml of product, the price would be $62. The price for 3 ml of this product would be $116 (Table 7.6).

Using the margin model, your profit will always be the specified margin no matter what quantity of product you are dispensing or administering.

Let's examine an example of the markup pricing versus the margin pricing model. In this example, the markup percentage is 150%, the desired profit margin is $35.00, and the product cost is $19.00 per ml. Additionally, for the markup model, the injection fee is $20.00.

- **Example using product quantity of 0.6 ml** – Table 7.7 outlines a cost, price, and profit information comparison using the markup and margin model.
- **Example using product quantity of 3.2 ml** – Table 7.8 outlines a cost, price, and profit information comparison using the markup and margin model.

From the margin and markup examples, with a quantity of 0.6 ml, the final selling price is similar but the most significant difference is with larger quantities. With the markup model, the price to the client would be $172.00 for the injection versus $95.80 with the margin model. The profit, in dollars, is $111.20 with the markup model and only $35.00 with the margin model.

Table 7.6 An example of the cost versus selling price using the above example.

Quantity administered	Total product cost ($)	Practice profit ($)	Final selling price ($)
1 ml	27.00	35.00	62.00
2 ml	54.00	35.00	89.00
2.5 ml	67.50	35.00	102.50
3 ml	81.00	35.00	116.00

Table 7.7 A cost, price, and profit information comparison using the markup and margin models for a product quantity of 0.6 ml.

	Markup model ($)	Margin model ($)
Product cost	11.40	11.40
Cost + markup	28.50	—
Additional fees	20.00	35.00
Total price	48.50	46.40
Profit	37.10	35.00

Table 7.8 A cost, price, and profit information comparison using the markup and margin model for a product quantity of 3.2 ml.

	Markup model ($)	Margin model ($)
Product cost	60.80	60.80
Cost + markup	152.00	—
Additional fees	20.00	35.00
Total price	172.00	95.80
Profit	111.20	35.00

With the margin model, the injection is more cost-effective for the client, thus potentially reducing the barrier to care and increasing the chance of compliance. This might allow clients the opportunity to opt for more expensive injectables and the patient care team to feel more comfortable recommending an expensive injectable to a large dog. On the flip side, the profit margin is significantly less, so each injection will not be as profitable.

Bear in mind that the profit margin includes the team's time and expertise for calculating and administering the injection, the cost of drawing it up, including the syringe, needle, and any other costs associated with administration.

With the margin pricing model, there are two other factors to consider: The first is the indirect costs and overhead costs of your practice. Due to the structure of the margin model, any indirect costs will eat directly into the profit of the practice. Each practice has different indirect costs and overhead expenses, and it's key to keep these in mind to ensure that your profit margin is appropriate and genuinely profitable.

The second consideration is veterinarian production. With the margin model, a large percentage of the total price is actual product cost, so it's important that the production is based upon the profit margin only and not the entire client price. Production should not be based only on the total client price. I find that with expensive injectables, margin pricing is more common. With that, I've noticed during my work with practices that the production is being calculated based on the entire client's price. So, most practices are losing money each time an injection is administered to a large or extra-large dog.

To take into account the indirect costs or production for your practice, you can use the following formula. Keep in mind that indirect costs typically range between 25% and 40% for most practices (Heinke 2014). Adjust the percentage in this formula to reflect your practice's unique situation.

$$Price = total\ product\ cost + indirect\ cost\ \% + margin$$

$$where\ Total\ Product\ Cost = product\ cost \times quantity$$

$$Total\ Product\ Cost = \$19.00 \times 3.2\ ml$$

$$Total\ Product\ Cost = \$60.80$$

$$Price = total\ product\ cost + \left(total\ product\ cost \times indirect\ cost\ \%\right) + margin$$

$$Price = \$60.80 + \left(\$60.80 \times 25\ \%\right) + \$35.00$$

$$Price = \$60.80 + \$15.20 + \$35.00$$

$$Price = \$111.00$$

7.5 Pricing Formula Overview

Markup pricing formula – this formula is the easiest to implement and maintain with your PiMS. It's also the most commonly used method I've noticed for pricing in veterinary practices. Keep in mind that the cost multiplier is not the same as a percentage increase. For example, if you want to 3× the cost for an item, it will not be a 300% markup.

$$Selling\ Price = cost + \left(cost \times markup\ \%\right)$$

Standard pricing formula – this formula is the most precise and allows you to account for your desired profit margin, as well as any indirect costs and production paid. If this formula looks slightly terrifying, that's understandable! The first step is to find the total product cost by finding your indirect costs. Once that's done, you'll add on your desired profit and any veterinarian production.

Both the standard pricing model and overhead cost formula in this text are from *Practice Made Perfect* by Heinke (2014).

$$Product\ cost + \left[product\ cost\left(labor\ \% + facility\ \%\right)\right]$$
$$= total\ product\ cost + \left[total\ product\ cost\left(profit\ \% + DVM\ pay\right)\right] = Price$$

Step 1: find the total product cost.

$$Total \ Product \ Cost\left(TPC\right) = product \ cost + \left[product \ cost\left(labor \ \% + facility \ \%\right)\right]$$

$$TPC = product \ cost + \left(product \ cost \times labor \ cost \ \%\right) + \left(product \ cost \times labor \ cost \ \%\right)$$

Step 2: find the selling price.

$$Price = total \ product \ cost + \left[total \ product \ cost\left(profit \ \% + DVM \ pay\right)\right]$$

$$Price = total \ product \ cost + \left(total \ product \ cost \times profit \ \%\right) + \left(total \ product \ cost \times DVM \ pay\right)$$

Overhead cost formula – this formula is similar to the standard pricing formula and can be used if the exact labor and facility costs for a particular practice are unknown. This model uses the idea that, generally, overhead costs are approximately 40%. This formula is helpful when you want to be more precise with your inventory calculations and include indirect costs but are unsure what they actually are.

$$Product \ cost + \left(product \ cost \times 40\%\right) = total \ product \ cost +$$
$$\left[total \ product \ cost\left(profit \ \% + DVM \ pay\right)\right] = Price$$

Step 1: find the total product cost.

$$Total \ Product \ Cost\left(TPC\right) = product \ cost + \left(product \ cost \times 40\%\right)$$

Step two: find the selling price.

$$Price = total \ product \ cost + \left[total \ product \ cost\left(profit \ \% + DVM \ pay\right)\right]$$

$$Price = total \ product \ cost + \left(total \ product \ cost \times profit \ \%\right) + \left(total \ product \ cost \times DVM \ pay\right)$$

Margin pricing – this formula is helpful when pricing expensive items, especially expensive pharmaceuticals.

$$Price = total \ product \ cost + margin \ \left(\$\right)$$

If you want to use margin based pricing but also want to account for indirect costs or veterinarian production, the formula below can be helpful.

$$Price = total \ product \ cost + \left(total \ product \ cost \times indirect \ cost \ \%\right) + margin$$

7.5.1 Example Calculations

In this section, each formula will be demonstrated with the same two products to give an idea of how each pricing model functions. Product A will be a tablet and Product B will be a full bottle. Whenever I'm working with a formula, I always follow the same routine so that each calculation stays organized and I can keep track of my work. I start by writing out the formula in full. Then, I make a list of each variable that is required for that formula. Finally, I input the variables into the formula and perform the actual calculation.

Product "A" cost: $0.36 per tablet.

7.5.1.1 Markup Formula

$$Selling\ Price = \cos t + \left(\cos t \times markup\ \%\right)$$

Variables required.

Product cost = $0.36
Markup % = 250%

$$Price = \cos t + \left(\cos t \times markup\ \%\right)$$

$$Price = \$0.36 + \left(\$0.36 \times 250\%\right)$$

$$Price = \$0.36 + \$0.90$$

$$Price = \$1.26\ per\ tablet$$

Based upon a cost of $0.36 and a markup percentage of 250%, the price of the item is $1.26 per tablet. From here, a dispensing or prescription fee can be added as well.

7.5.1.2 Standard Pricing Formula

$$Product\ \cos t + \left[product\ \cos t \left(labor\ \% + facility\ \%\right)\right] = total\ product\ \cos t +$$
$$\left[total\ product\ \cos t \left(profit\ \% + DVM\ pay\right)\right] = Price$$

Variables required.

Product cost = $0.36
Labor costs (%) = 22%
Facility costs = 15%
Desired profit % = 75%
DVM production pay = 5%

With the standard pricing formula, it's often easiest to break it into two different sections. For the first step, you'll determine the total product cost and for the second step, you'll calculate the price.

Step 1: calculate the total product cost (TPC).

$$Total\ Product\ Cost\left(TPC\right) = product\ \cos t + \left[product\ \cos t \left(labor\ \% + facility\%\right)\right]$$

$$TPC = product\ \cos t + \left(product\ \cos t \times labor\ \cos t\ \%\right) + \left(product\ \cos t \times labor\ \cos t\ \%\right)$$

$$TPC = \$0.36 + \left(\$0.36\ \times\ 22\%\right) + \left(\$0.36\ \times\ 15\%\right)$$

$$TPC = \$0.36 + \$0.08 + \$0.05$$

$$TPC = \$0.49$$

Step 2: calculate the price of the product.

$$Price = total\ product\ cost + \left[total\ product\ cost\left(profit\ \% + DVM\ Pay\right)\right]$$

$$Price = total\ product\ cost + \left(total\ product\ cost \times profit\ \%\right) + \left(total\ product\ cost \times DVM\ Pay\right)$$

$$Price = \$0.49 + \left(\$0.49 \times 125\%\right) + \left(\$0.49 \times 5\%\right)$$

$$Price = \$0.49 + \$0.61 + \$0.02$$

$$Price = \$1.12\ per\ tablet$$

With the standard pricing formula, based on a cost of $0.36 and the variables listed above, the price of the item is $1.12. From here, a dispensing or prescription fee can be added as well. Note that with the standard pricing model, depending on your goals, the profit percentage can be adjusted up or down. With more competitively priced items, such as flea and tick or heartworm prevention, a lower profit percentage should be used in order to stay competitive with online pharmacies.

7.5.1.3 Overhead Cost Formula

$$Product\ cost + \left(product\ cost \times 40\%\right) = total\ product\ cost + \\ \left[total\ product\ cost\left(profit\ \% + DVM\ pay\right)\right] = Price$$

Variables required

Product cost = $0.36
Profit % = 125%
DVM production pay = 5%

As with the standard pricing formula, it's easiest to break this formula into two different parts. In the first step, you'll calculate the total product cost. In the second step, you'll calculate the price.

Step 1: calculate the total product cost.

$$Total\ Product\ Cost\ \left(TPC\right) = product\ cost + \left(product\ cost \times 40\%\right)$$

$$TPC = \$0.36 + \left(\$0.36 \times 40\%\right)$$

$$TPC = \$0.36 + \$0.14$$

$$TPC = \$0.50$$

Step 2: calculate the price.

$$Price = total\ product\ cost + \left[total\ product\ cost\left(profit\ \% + DVM\ pay\right)\right]$$

$$Price = total\ product\ cost + \left(total\ product\ cost \times profit\ \%\right) + \left(total\ product\ cost \times DVM\ pay\right)$$

$$Price = \$0.50 + \left(\$0.50 \times 125\%\right) + \left(\$0.50 \times 5\%\right)$$

$$Price = \$0.50 + \$0.63 + \$0.03$$

$$Price = \$1.16 \; per \; tablet$$

With the standard pricing formula, based upon a cost of $0.36 and the variables listed above, the price of the item is $1.16. From here, a dispensing or prescription fee can be added as well. Note, as with the standard pricing model, the profit percentage can be adjusted up or down depending on your goals. A lower profit percentage should be used with more competitively priced items, such as flea and tick or heartworm prevention.

7.5.1.4 Margin Pricing Formula

$$Price = product \; cost + margin \; (\$)$$

The margin pricing formula is slightly different from the other formulas because the margin encompasses these fees rather than calculating the price and then adding any prescription or dispensing fees. If you want to take into consideration any veterinarian production or other fees, you can adjust the formula accordingly.
Variables required.

Product cost = $0.36
Margin ($) = $30.00

This means that if one tablet or 100 tablets are dispensed, the $30 profit margin will be applied in addition to the product cost. For this example, let's use one tablet and 50 tablets to demonstrate how the margin formula works.

Example A: one tablet.

$$Price = \left(product \; cost \times quantity\right) + margin \; (\$)$$

$$Price = \left(\$0.36 \times 1\right) + \$30.00$$

$$Price = \$30.36$$

Example B: 50 tablets.

$$Price = \left(product \; cost \times quantity\right) + margin \; (\$)$$

$$Price = \left(\$0.36 \times 50\right) + \$30.00$$

$$Price = \$18.00 + \$30.00$$

$$Price = \$48.00$$

"Best Practice" Exercise
An action step for you: Experiment with an easy product in your inventory and try calculating the price of the product using the different pricing models. What did you notice? What model was the most helpful for that product? Was there anything unexpected that came up in this process?

7.6 Pricing Concept: Flat Fee or "Weight Bucket" Injections

There are some cases where it might be best to set prices as a flat fee for a certain weight class. Pricing a product like this can be helpful, especially when it comes to discussing pricing with clients or preparing estimates. This could look like this.

- Injection A : 0–25 lb $50.00
- Injection A : 26–50 lb $75.00
- Injection A : 51–100 lb $100.00

Generally, though, pricing all of your injections like that can be cumbersome to maintain, and cost increases may get missed and not passed along appropriately.

In most cases, I also do not recommend setting a flat fee for any prescription or injection unless you know for certain that the price will not fluctuate much or at all if the quantity changes. Although pricing an injection with a flat fee makes things very easy to discuss with your clients, it can be hard to monitor your profit margin. Let's explore an example together.

Let's say that Tank's Animal Hospital has an injection, carprofen, that costs $5.00 per ml and the price is currently set to $23.00 for an injection. Let us review what this could look like for three different patient sizes (Table 7.9).

After reviewing the sales information, Tank's Animal Hospital found that most patients receive between 3.0 and 3.5 ml, which translates to only $5.50 and $8.00 of profit per injection. A patient would only need 4.6 ml for the practice to lose money. Not only is the profit per injection less than ideal, but it's challenging day to day to know if a specific injection might be costing you money!

If you'd like to set up any injections as a flat fee, I invite you to run through a few different scenarios (like the example above) to see what your product cost and profit would be for various patient sizes. For any products you'd like to set up with weight classes, I also invite you to calculate the product cost and profit for the highest weight or largest quantity for that particular class.

7.7 Profit Goals

You might be thinking "That all sounds great, but what should my profit margin be for my inventory?" That is a great question but unfortunately, there is not a simple, one-size-fits-all answer. I highly recommend working with a veterinary-specific accountant to help determine what your overall profit margin and income-to-expense ratio should be for your inventory.

Table 7.9 An example of the total product cost, price, and profit for three different quantities of carprofen injectable.

	0.7 ml used ($)	1.9 ml used ($)	3.2 ml used ($)
Product cost	3.50	9.50	16.00
Price	23.00	23.00	23.00
Profit	19.50	13.50	7.00

7.8   Pricing with Your Practice Management System

Pricing strategies can be integrated with most PiMSs, although how this looks and functions depends on the software system and how it operates. As a baseline, your PiMS should have a place to enter the price to charge a client. Most software systems have a field in the individual item setup to enter a markup percentage. Once a purchase order or receipt is received, and the cost has increased since the last purchase, the price will be recalculated based on the markup percentage entered. It will typically prompt you if you approve the new price before making the change. Having this markup percentage entered is a helpful way to ensure prices are increased appropriately because it is an automated process and does not rely on you or a team member remembering to increase prices manually.

Pricing and receiving at a glance.

- In your software, there will likely be a function to enter or "receive" inventory into your PiMS. This tells your software the items you have purchased, the quantity, cost, and potentially more information like lot numbers and expiry dates.
- Entering in orders in your software will increase the quantity on hand for everything you have ordered and update cost, lot number, and expiry date information.
- If you have entered a markup percentage into the individual item, as your cost increases, your price will automatically be recalculated with the new highest cost and the markup percentages.
- Most PiMSs will allow you to confirm or reject the new pricing. Additionally, most PiMS will only increase the price and not decrease it if your costs go down.

Depending on which formula you use for calculating and setting your prices, the setup and maintenance in your software will be different. The markup model is the easiest to set up and support in the practice management software. The chosen markup percentage is typically entered into the inventory item setup screen and a dispensing/prescription fee is either entered or assigned to that particular item. Once this is completed, it's important that all orders are received into the system using a purchase order or receipt function so that if the cost increases, the price will be recalculated based on the entered markup percentage.

For both the standard pricing formula and the overhead model, the calculated price based on the formula should be entered into the inventory item screen and a dispensing/prescription fee should be either entered or assigned. The key with using the standard pricing formula or the overhead model is that as costs increase, you'll need to have a manual system in place that (i) recognizes that costs have gone up so that (ii) a team member can recalculate the price using the formula.

That's why I always recommend entering a "threshold" markup percentage that you never want to fall under whenever you are using a formula to calculate your prices. That way, if the manual price increase system gets missed or forgotten, the markup percentage entered will act as a safety backup measure. When receiving purchase orders or receipts, most software displays the cost you most recently purchased an item for, so it's easy to identify if the cost has risen.

When using the margin pricing model, the most effective way to set it up in your PiMS is to set your markup percentage as the indirect costs that are included in the formula (Figure 7.1). Then, set the prescription/dispensing fee as the desired profit margin. As an example, let's say that for a particular injectable medication, your practice wanted to calculate 20% of the cost as indirect/overhead costs and then wanted a $40.00 profit margin on top of the total cost of that

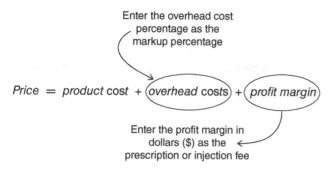

Enter the overhead cost
percentage as the
markup percentage

$$Price = product\ cost + (overhead\ costs) + (profit\ margin)$$

Enter the profit margin in
dollars ($) as the
prescription or injection fee

Figure 7.1 An example of how to set up margin pricing in the practice management system.
Nicole Clausen.

item. So 20% should be entered as the markup percentage and $40.00 should be entered as the injection fee.

Most software systems allow dispensing fees per item but in some cases, such as AVImark®, only one dispensing fee, injection fee, and handling fee can be set. In AVImark, if you are using the margin pricing formula for only a few items and are already using the other fees in different capacities, you can use the "special fees" table as a workaround. Adding an entry to the special fees table and assigning it to the item will allow for a fee to be added, similar to a prescription or injection fee. If your practice management software system allows for different fees to be set per item, you'll enter the profit margin in dollars as the fee.

Note: Software is always changing and by the time you are reading this book, maybe AVImark has wised up and allowed these changes. I can offer examples from what I know to be true right now, but if you are using AVImark in your practice, do not take what I say as gospel. Go and check! Maybe they have changed things.

7.9 Increasing Prices as Your Costs Increase

One of the key pieces of your pricing strategy is to create a method and system for increasing prices as your cost increases. Generally, procedure prices should be reviewed and increased annually or at regular intervals throughout the year (i.e., every quarter or every six months). On the other hand, inventory prices should increase whenever there is a cost increase. Note that if costs go down, your prices should not decrease. Your dispensing, prescription, handling, and controlled substance fees should be evaluated every six months to make sure they are still in line with your practice goals.

Some products (like flea and tick prevention, vaccines, diets, heartworm prevention, and manufacturer's branded or unique products) typically only increase in price once per year. The manufacturer will send out an announcement alerting practices to when the increase will happen and what the new prices will be. If you receive a new price list, these products' costs should be updated and their prices recalculated *before* the manufacturer increases go into effect.

Keep in mind that vaccine prices are a whole separate conversation (because they are considered a service or treatment), and do not follow these recommendations. Also, this information should be relayed to your team so they have any information about the new prices. If the client service team has any "cheatsheets" for flea and tick or heartworm prevention prices, these should be updated as well.

For other products, like generic pharmaceuticals, prices can fluctuate throughout the year depending on supply and demand, availability, and demand in human medicine, among other things. The most effective way to ensure costs get updated and prices are recalculated for these items is with your PiMS. It's best practice to use the purchase order or receipt to receive these items into your software system. During the receiving process, the markup percentage will recalculate the price depending on the increased cost. Or, if you are using a formula to calculate your prices and do not use a markup percentage, highlight on your invoice or packing slip the products that increase in price. Then, once that order is received into the software, the highlighted products can be recalculated and manually updated.

7.10 Putting It into Practice

Creating a pricing strategy or, at the very least, evaluating your prices is an important but often overwhelming task. If you have yet to establish a pricing strategy for your practice or if you are not sure where your pricing falls, there are several steps to start the process. Where to begin will all depend on your current system. If all costs have been updated and entered correctly through a purchase order or receiving process in the PiMS, the first step will not apply to your situation so start with step 2.

7.10.1 Step 1: Update your Inventory Costs

If you have not updated the cost of your inventory items in a while, this step will be especially important (and potentially time-consuming – plan accordingly). Ensure that each item lists the correct cost and the price that you are currently selling it for. There are several ways to do this. If you are short on time, you can go through each item in your normal weekly order and ensure it's updated when it's received. Through this process, eventually, all your products will be updated and accurate. If you have more time to spend on this process, go through each category alphabetically and enter either the last price you paid for the item or the current cost, whichever is most accurate.

The goal for this process is to have an inventory list in your PiMS that has a complete and accurate list of all products, prices, and costs of all items. **Take note: be sure that the cost matches the unit sold**. For example, if your PiMS is set up as per tablet for a particular item, ensure that the unit cost is per tablet. If a particular item is priced per bottle, ensure that the cost entered is per bottle.

7.10.2 Step 2: Survey Your Current Pricing

The next step is to evaluate your current pricing strategy. This involves several different aspects and will help to determine a clear picture of where you are with your pricing. The first part is to identify some important information. What are your current dispensing, prescription, injection, and other fees set at? Do they vary by category or is it the same across the board? When was the last time these were evaluated and/or increased? Write all your findings down and list out any current fees, the categories they apply to, and any other helpful information. Next, test several random products to ensure the fee is being applied properly.

After surveying the fees, the next step is to look at each individual item. Are there any markup percentages set in your software? Does the markup vary depending on the category or do they vary wildly depending on the item? How and when are prices increased as costs increase? It's helpful to run a "product setup" report in your software that lists all inventory items, the cost, price, and markup percentage entered for each product. This is just the information-gathering stage: We want to know how things are currently priced, how prices are increased, how new items are getting priced, and the different processes surrounding pricing in your practice.

7.10.3   Step 3: Calculate Your Current Markup Percentages

The next step, depending on your practice management software system, will be to calculate the current markup percentages for all items. For most software, the cost can be adjusted and the markup percentage will not recalculate the price automatically. It's highly recommended that you calculate your current markup percentage to ensure that you do not have any negative markups (items that cost more than what you are charging) or any exceptionally low markups. In my career as an inventory management consultant, it's incredibly common for me to find items that have a negative markup or items priced significantly lower than ideal while completing an inventory and pricing audit with a client.

7.10.3.1   Markup Percentage Calculation Formula

$$Markup\ Percentage = \frac{\left(Selling\ Price - Unit\ Cost\right)}{Unit\ Cost} \times 100$$

Variables required.

Selling price = $1.42 per tablet
Unit cost = $0.79 per tablet

$$Markup\ Percentage = \frac{\left(Selling\ Price - Unit\ Cost\right)}{Unit\ Cost} \times 100$$

$$Markup\ Percentage = \frac{\left(\$1.42 - \$0.79\right)}{\$0.79} \times 100$$

$$Markup\ Percentage = \frac{\$0.63}{\$0.79} \times 100$$

$$Markup\ Percentage = 0.797 \times 100$$

$$Markup\ Percentage = 79.7\%$$

"Best Practice" Tip
Calculate markup percentages in an Excel or similar program spreadsheet to save time.

Once you have calculated the markup for all your inventory items, review the markup for each item and ensure that it's at an appropriate level. If you are using a spreadsheet program, you can sort the table in ascending or descending order to view the lowest to highest markup or vice versa. First, identify any negative markups, which are immediate concerns because this means that the price is lower than the cost. Addressing these is a top priority because this essentially means we are paying a client to take that item. Next, ensure the remaining products have the appropriate markup. Keep in mind what your desired profit is and the hidden indirect costs for your practice.

7.10.4   Step 4: Decide on a Pricing Method

After calculating your current markup percentages to see where you stand, the next step is to decide on a pricing strategy based on the goals of your practice. Decide if you want to mark up products based on the markup model, margin model, standard pricing formula, or overhead cost model. There is not one best answer or fit here. The key is to determine what will work best for your goals and your profitability with your PiMS. Your pricing strategy could also include a mix of the different formulas.

What's your preferred method? When it comes to determining which pricing strategy to use, it's important to (i) protect the profitability of your practice, (ii) have a system in place for increasing prices as costs increase, and (iii) build trust with your clients for competitive, frequently priced items (Table 7.10).

7.10.5   Step 5: Implement Your Pricing Strategy

Once you have decided on a pricing strategy, the next step is to implement it into your practice. As with every task, I always ask the same questions.

Table 7.10   An example of a pricing strategy brainstorm. Document what fees you'd like to charge and how items will be priced.

Fees	Fee or strategy ($)
Prescription fee	15
Injection fee	25
Additional controlled substance fee	4
Prescription fee for bottles	5
Pricing	
Competitively shopped items	XX% above online pharmacies/retailers or minimum advertised price
Diets – *markup model*	45%
Select injections – *margin model*	Costs + $35 margin
Injections – *markup model*	200%
Pharmaceuticals – *markup model*	>$0.05 per unit – 500%
	$0.06–1.00 per unit – 200%
	<$1.01 per unit – 100%
Over-the-counter/retail items – *markup model*	100% or MSRP

- Who does it involve?
- What specific tasks need to be completed?
- What can be delegated?
- How can it be measured? How will the process be documented?
- What is the goal and deadline?

In this situation, who will ultimately be in charge of implementing this pricing strategy, and who will ensure that price increases happen as costs increase? What specific tasks need to be completed? What needs to be updated in your PiMS? Does a spreadsheet need to be created for the standard pricing formula? Answering the above questions can help implement this pricing strategy effectively into your practice.

8

Selling and Consuming Your Inventory Appropriately

8.1 Why Selling Your Inventory Appropriately and Accurately Matters

Selling, using, and dispensing your inventory accurately is a key piece of your inventory ecosystem. When inventory is not sold correctly for one reason or another, it tends to have a snowball effect. You might have missed charges, products that were not invoiced correctly, mishandled employee accounts, codes that were not set up correctly, and more headaches than you signed up for. As a result, you could experience a loss in revenue or have an inaccurate quantity on hand.

As an example, if an item is filled with the incorrect quantity, there is a loss of revenue and the on-hand quantity in the practice management system (PiMS) is now inaccurate. With an inaccurate on-hand quantity, the software will not flag reorder points correctly which could result in a stockout.

When items are not dispensed, used, or sold correctly, on-hand amounts will become inaccurate, negatively impacting our ability to use reorder points in our PiMS. It also leads to inaccurate reports, like sales and usage data (which, again, impacts our reorder point calculations) or the on-hand value report for tax purposes. We can even experience medication errors and mistakes! Ultimately, running out of items negatively affects our ability to fulfill our "why" and provide our patients with the best care possible.

The take-home? Dispensing, using, and selling our inventory accurately helps ensure our PiMS or other electronic reorder points are flagged when appropriate so we are not running out of things and can rely on reports and data from our PiMS when making data-informed decisions.

8.2 Impact of Missed Charges

Imagine that on every single paycheck, your employer missed paying you anywhere from two to five hours each week. Not realizing it, you have less money to pay your bills and expenses or to enjoy life with. Because you have less take-home pay to work with, you are not able to put enough away into your savings or retirement account, and it's harder to make ends meet. Not only that, but your income should be higher.

It's the same with missed charges in your practice. You should be generating more revenue but you are not. That means you have less money for raises, bonuses, and new team members. There's

Inventory Management for Veterinary Professionals, First Edition. Nicole I. Clausen.
© 2024 John Wiley & Sons, Inc. Published 2024 by John Wiley & Sons, Inc.
Companion website: www.wiley.com/go/clausen/inventory

Table 8.1 Effects on revenue if there were no missed charges for the year, if two boxes per week were missed, and if four boxes per week were missed.

	No missed charges	Two per week	Four per week
Boxes dispensed	894	894	894
Boxes missed	0	104	208
Total costs ($)	71,520	71,520	71,520
Total revenue ($)	107,280	94,800	82,320
Total revenue missed ($)	0	12,480	24,960

less money to pay bills and other expenses. Depending on the scale of missed billing or discounts, it can significantly negatively impact the practice's profitability.

Here are three ways missed billing can impact your practice.

- Missed charges reduce the amount of revenue generated, which leads to less money available for team wages or bonuses.
- Missed charges mean that inventory is not deducted properly, the on-hand quantity is inaccurate, and the reorder point likely will not flag at the accurate time, which can lead to a stockout.
- Missing laboratory tests could have a snowball effect of bloodwork getting missed on a patient and a serious client service "miss" when the patient needs to come back for another blood draw or the client does not get a call back about lab work results.

Let's explore an example of how missed charges might impact your inventory. Tank's Animal Hospital sells Simparica Trio™. After running some reports, they realized that they had sold 894 boxes last year. They purchase this product for $80 a box, have a markup of 50%, and a selling price of $120. Table 8.1 shows that forgetting to charge for four boxes per week means that Tank's Animal Hospital missed out on almost $25 000 in revenue. Imagine if this happened to 10 products. What about 20 products? What could your practice do with $25 000? $250 000?

"Best Practice" Questions to Consider
- Does your practice struggle with missed charges?
- Do your heartworm prevention, flea/tick prevention, vaccines, or other expensive items always seem to be off, and you cannot figure out where they're going or why?
- Have you ever audited your practice's medical records to see if you had missed billing? What did you find?

Throughout this chapter, we'll be reviewing some tools and techniques you can use to leverage your PiMS or other invoicing systems to sell your inventory accurately. We'll also review some of my favorite "checks and balances" to use to investigate missed billing.

8.3 Leveraging Your Practice Management System

If you are using a PiMS, you can set it up to help deduct the quantity on hand for a particular item once it has been sold. Leveraging your PiMS software can help automate this process and keep the on-hand amounts of inventory items more accurate. Why is this helpful? Keeping the quantity on hand accurate throughout the year can:

- help know what you have on hand so you can identify waste or theft more quickly
- accurately flag reorder levels or minimum product levels to help make ordering easier
- keep track of the value of inventory on hand (aka your carrying costs) to see if you are over-stocked or have an excessive amount of cash flow tied up in inventory
- allow for much easier and more efficient end-of-year inventory counts.

If you do not use a PiMS or your software does not have an inventory module, this may not apply to you. I invite you to continue reading just in case the information will apply to any of the technology or software that you use in your practice. Additionally, you can also read more in the Appendices section on "Frequently Asked Questions" to explore more about not having a PiMS.

An excellent starting point for leveraging your software system is to make sure each item is set up correctly. This will serve as the base for the rest of your billing, invoices and inventory tracking. Remember "The Princess and the Pea?" When the princess had a horrible night's sleep because there was a tiny pea under all those mattresses, it caused quite a disruption for her. It's very similar to our inventory! The tiniest little pea (like not having the unit of measure set up correctly) can wreak havoc on the on-hand quantity. Not having some of these little details added correctly can translate into major headaches and a lot of extra work in your PiMS.

Each software system functions a little differently with some nuances but generally, there are some key pieces of information to add.

- **Item name, description, and item code**.
- **Package quantity or buy/sell ratio**: this lets your software know the difference between how it's purchased and how it's sold. As an example, if you set up gabapentin with a package quantity of 500, then for each bottle that's received, the software knows you received 500 capsules.
- **Unit of measure**: this tells your software in what unit of measure you are selling the item (i.e., ml, tablet, bottle, etc.). I recommend entering this as the lowest unit that you sell it. As an example, if you sell heartworm prevention per dose (and not per box), I recommend setting up the item as per dose. If you set it up as per box, then each time a single dose is sold, then a quantity of 0.16 would need to be entered.
- **Markup percentage**: as mentioned in Chapter 7, setting a markup percentage can help increase your prices as costs go up.
- **Dispensing and other fees**: adding any dispensing or necessary fees will help charge clients appropriately.
- **Reorder points or min/max levels**: as mentioned in Chapter 3, adding reorder points into your software can help flag when an item needs to be ordered.

"Best Practice" Question to Consider.
- In addition to the pieces mentioned above, what other information should be added to each item for your specific software?

Once individual items are set up and have the correct unit of measure information, they can be used to create various "bundles." Creating and using groups, packages, and linked items can be an excellent way to help deduct inventory effectively while charging your clients appropriately. Depending on the PiMS, it can also help review and analyze your profit margins for a particular service.

I like to think of groups, packages, and linked items as three different "buckets" or categories for setting up items. Let's explore them together.

Groups: I consider "Groups" a collection of services or items you want to bundle together, but you want the client to see each item individually.

- Benefit: these can minimize mistakes (like a team member forgetting to charge for something).
- Examples.
  - Blood transfusion group.
  - Chemotherapy group (might include any specialty supplies, a chemotherapy administration charge, any monitoring, etc.).
  - Hospitalization group (might consist of IV fluid administration, IV pump fee, a hospitalization charge, IV catheter, etc.).
  - ACTH stim group.
- These are slightly smaller versions of template estimates. They can be used to make charging more efficient while ensuring everything is included. Groups might also help in cases where a procedure or service is not performed often.

Packages: I consider packages as a service with inventory items linked/associated in the backend. These are set as a "choose your own adventure" style so the team can select the quantity used. The item will be deducted from inventory but the client does not see this on their invoice. Note: A package does not necessarily need to have a price. As an example, in the case of "preanesthetic medication," the price might be included in anesthesia or as part of the surgical procedure.

- Benefit: these can help keep your inventory more accurate and provide a more complete medical record. They can also help keep an electronic controlled substance log to make reconciling paper logs easier.
- Examples.
  - Preanesthetic medication.
  - Euthanasia/end-of-life care.

Linked items: I consider linked items as an inventory item or service that has one item linked in the backend. Clients do not see this and your team does not either. A prespecified quantity is deducted from the linked inventory item whenever the inventory or service is charged for.

- Benefit: helps keep your inventory more accurate and tracks the quantity sold.
- An example would be a vaccine. The vaccine is linked so that every time it's added to an invoice, it's deducted from inventory automatically.

Setting up groups, packages, and linked items in your PiMS can make it easier and more streamlined to charge appropriately and keep track of what's on hand.

"Best Practice" Questions to Consider
- Does your PiMS have the capability to set up groups, packages, or linked inventory items? How does it function in your software?
- Are there any procedures or services where it would be helpful to create any of the different types of bundles above? Brainstorm a list of the top five you'd like to create.
- Check in with your team. Are there any procedures, treatments, or services where the charging is confusing? Do they have any ideas or suggestions on what could be improved?

8.4 Auditing Medical Records

When I was younger and trying to learn better financial management, I was working with a financial coach to help me with that process. At the end of each week, I sat down with a worksheet and listed every transaction I made, the amount I spent or made, and categorized each expense. I spread out the papers and my favorite calculator (I know...) on my desk, hot tea in hand, and I examined each and every transaction. Through that process, I found subscriptions that no longer served me, transactions that did not align with my values, and more. I also found quite a few surprises, like how much I spent on skincare or crystal and mineral specimens. Whoops!

Sitting down each week to do that process was much less about the actual categorization of each transaction and more about intentionally evaluating where and how I spent my money. Did all the transactions make sense? Where was my money going? Did anything need to be changed, canceled, or updated in some way?

Auditing medical records in your practice is a similar process and should be done for a number of reasons. In this chapter, you'll learn how to audit your medical records and ensure your inventory is sold accurately and clients are charged appropriately. When reviewing medical records, finding individual instances where a charge was missed can be helpful. Still, looking at the overall picture to see if any trends or patterns emerge is even more beneficial.

As an example, when I started auditing medical records in my practice, I was not only able to find services, inventory items, or laboratory tests that were missed, but I also noticed the following.

- The appropriate level of hospitalization was rarely correctly charged for. There were three different levels of hospitalization, and usually, only level one was charged for. Levels two and three were just as common, so it was a cause for concern that wasn't reflected.
- There was often confusion about how to charge a patient for fluids on their second (and following days) of fluids and monitoring.
- When a patient was hospitalized for multiple days, injectables and medications that were administered regularly.
- Extractions, extra anesthesia time, and other services related to dental cleanings were occasionally missed, especially during longer procedures.

As I noticed these trends and patterns, I clarified and redefined how various services and procedures were billed. Not only that but by doing so, I had the opportunity to retrain the team and empower them to capture charges more accurately.

As a result of auditing medical records, I created and documented various charging guidelines that the team could use. Over time, I saw if the guidelines were helpful (fewer missed charges) or if I needed to refine the guidelines further.

By quantifying and providing examples and situations for exactly when one service or another should be charged, you can help set your team up for success!

8.4.1 Putting It into Practice: Auditing Medical Records

There are a few different methodologies for auditing medical records. Let's put them into two different categories.

- Wellness and exam room appointments.
- Hospitalized and surgical patients.

Depending on the category, you'll handle auditing the records differently. Ideally, wellness and exam room appointments should be double-checked or quickly audited before the patient leaves.

"Best Practice" Example Workflow for Wellness and Exam Room Appointments Depending on your client and team workflows, this will likely look different, but it's helpful to have charges reviewed before the client leaves the building. As an example:

1) the veterinary technician for that appointment enters the charges
2) the veterinarian and veterinary assistant verify the charges
3) during checkout, the client service representative verifies the charges again.

It can be helpful to pull a random selection of wellness or exam room patients from each doctor and/or doctor and technician team to see if there are any patterns for what or when charges are getting missed. Over the years, I've spoken to practice owners or managers who have such a pervasive challenge with missed charges that they have one person dedicated to ensuring everything is invoiced correctly and appropriately. Having someone specifically in that role has had a significant impact and return on investment.

Keep in mind that I always approach auditing medical records from a place of curiosity or investigation to see what and where charging overall can be improved!

Hospitalized and surgical patients are a whole different can of worms! For these cases, it works well to pull two to three extensive cases for each veterinarian from the previous month. If you work in an emergency or large practice, adapt this to your own unique practice. For each case, print off or view the following.

- Invoice
- Subjective, Objective, Assessment, Plan (SOAP) medical record
- Treatment sheets
- Surgical or dental records

If you are a paperless or paper-lite practice, access any attachments or scanned documents that might provide a sense of what was administered, provided, or services performed for that patient. Then, compare all the records. Was everything that was administered charged for or removed out of inventory? Was the appropriate number of extractions or anesthesia time invoiced? Was the correct examination or hospitalization charge entered? Were there any services, procedures, or inventory items that were either not appropriately added to the invoice or inappropriately discounted?

As an example, if a Cerenia® injection was administered, was the proper amount charged? If the patient needed a syringe pump for metronidazole, was both the medication and the appropriate equipment billed for? If the patient received five extractions, were they all charged for? The gingival flap that was performed? What about all the suture materials and bone grafts that were used?

I'll piece together the different records to see if anything was missed. It can be such a helpful process to (i) see if you have any major revenue leaks with missed billing and (ii) see what patterns and areas of opportunity arise from that information.

"Best Practice" Questions to Consider
- Do you currently audit medical records in your practice?
- If so, is there anything you'd like to change or improve about this process? With how you are currently auditing, what does the process look like after you have audited the records?
- If you are not currently auditing records, would you like to start this process? Do you think it would be helpful for your practice? Who on your team would excel in this role?

8.5 Using Barcodes in Your Inventory

Using barcodes in your inventory is (sometimes) more helpful in thought than in execution. It sounds like using barcode scanners in your inventory would make everything so much easier and be a helpful concept. Sometimes, it is. . . and other times, you are limited by your software capabilities. Some PiMSs and software systems allow you to use barcodes throughout the inventory process, including receiving and dispensing. Others are much more limited in their scope, and barcodes only work when dispensing.

Other times, the limiting factor is because an item or product does not even have a barcode!

One area or category tends to work well with barcodes across most PiMSs: prescription and retail diets. Let's explore what this might look like.

First, barcodes work using (typically) some sort of universal product code (UPC) or barcode on a product and a scanner. The UPC or barcode number is entered into the PiMS and assigned to a specific item. Let's say that Tank's Animal Hospital has barcode scanners at every client service representative's computer workstation. When a client wants to purchase a bag of food, rather than typing in the food, the bag (or can) is scanned and the appropriate food automatically comes up.

Using a barcode scanner, especially with prescription or retail diets or the retail area in general, can be helpful in making sure the appropriate food is invoiced. It can also reduce the number of errors with the incorrect food or the incorrect product being accidentally charged for. This is especially true with diets because sometimes the bags only look slightly different and are easily confused.

One of the nice things about barcode scanning is that it is relatively easy to set up. The barcode or UPC needs to be entered into the specific item in your PiMS. That's how your software will know what barcode belongs to which product. Then, barcode scanners are fairly universal, like a keyboard, and are often "plug and play."

If you are interested in adding barcode scanners to your practice, check with your PiMS support team to see what's possible for your specific software. What are the limitations? What are the possibilities? Where should the unique UPC be entered into each item? What will the workflow look like for your practice? What about the workflow for the inventory manager versus the reception team, for example?

Next, check with your IT specialist(s) or team to see what barcode scanners work best for your unique technology setup and your current workstations. What equipment will need to be purchased? Is the investment worth the expense? Is there an inexpensive "starter" scanner that you can try out to test the process before rolling it out to the entire practice?

"Best Practice" Barcode Setup

Depending on your software capabilities, here are some starting points for using barcode scanners.

- Move inventory to and from different locations, like interdepartmental transfers or transferring from a main storage location to a mobile vehicle.
- Set up barcodes on a sheet (like produce barcodes at a grocery store) and your top groups or bundles for easy, on-the-go charging for common appointment types.
- Using barcode scanners for receiving or building a receipt in your software.
- Selling diets or other retail items accurately.

How might you use barcode scanners in your practice?

8.6 Inventory Dispensing Cabinets

An electronic dispensing cabinet is a sophisticated (and expensive) piece of technology used in veterinary practices (and other healthcare facilities) to manage and dispense medications and occasionally medical supplies efficiently. These cabinets serve as automated medication dispensing systems to streamline dispensing and improve patient safety.

Here are some common features.
- Dispensing cabinets electronically track inventory levels of medications and medical supplies in real time. The inventory team can easily monitor stock levels, expiry dates, and usage patterns.
- Access to the medications stored in the cabinet is restricted through various authentication methods such as biometric verification, PIN codes, or proximity cards. This feature is especially useful for controlled substances and high-value items.
- When a medication is added to the electronic medical record, the care team can access the electronic dispensing cabinet to grab the specific medication. The cabinet contains drawers or compartments where medications are stored, each equipped with sensors and locking mechanisms. Only the drawer for the medication or injection prescribed will open after authentication by a team member.
- Electronic dispensing cabinets maintain detailed transaction logs, providing a comprehensive trail of all medication dispensing activities. These records and analytics are helpful for controlled substance logging and regulatory compliance, as well as data and information on inventory performance.

Inventory dispensing cabinets can be another helpful tool in your inventory management toolbox. Dispensing cabinets typically integrate with your PiMS and can help reduce missed charges, dispensing errors, and disappearing inventory. But, as with most things, it's not a perfect solution and there are some downsides to consider.

8.6.1 Inventory Manager Spotlight

Meet Jennifer Yacovazzi, BS, MBA, CVIP, Director of Inventory and Communications! She has had the privilege of serving as the Inventory Manager at AAWC for the past 3.5 years and has thoroughly enjoyed the journey. She has always had a fondness for inventory management and finds fulfillment in ensuring her shelves are well stocked for patients.

Jennifer's practice uses Cubex® electronic dispensing cabinets. When I wrote to her about including her experience in this book, she was quick to respond.

"Utilizing Cubex has been instrumental in keeping our inventory organized and readily available. With a large pharmacy to manage, Cubex has become an invaluable tool for me to track our stock levels efficiently. I receive my purchase orders via email every Monday and Thursday morning, allowing me to stay proactive in identifying any items that may need replenishing.

I've recently refined our system further by adjusting our minimum and maximum stock levels based on Cubex's dispensing frequency insights. However, one area where I've encountered challenges is with reporting functionalities. Although Cubex offers some reporting capabilities, it falls short when it comes to analyzing specific metrics like the top 20% of dispensed items or monitoring medication dispensing frequency accurately.

Nevertheless, I prioritize maintaining the accuracy of our inventory by conducting monthly cycle counts and ensuring that Cubex remains up to date. With a large team relying on our inventory numbers, this practice helps us maintain precision in our stock management processes.

To fellow inventory managers, I offer this advice: be kind to yourself and acknowledge that mistakes are inevitable. What truly matters is how we respond and learn from those mistakes. I've learned to grant myself grace for being human and focus on implementing positive changes moving forward.

In conclusion, effective inventory management is a continuous journey of learning and adaptation. By leveraging tools like Cubex and embracing a mindset of growth and resilience, we can ensure the seamless operation of our inventory systems for the benefit of our patients and team."

8.6.2 Electronic Dispensing Cabinet Considerations

I've seen dispensing cabinets most successfully used with controlled substances and varying degrees of success with other inventory items. Often, I find that the big cabinets become merely really expensive storage closets.

The success of the dispensing cabinets often depends on how much training the company gives and who sets up and maintains the cabinets. Other times, it's just not a great fit for a particular practice. I've seen some inventory managers who were incredibly knowledgeable and capable when it came to their cabinets, and they worked like a dream. For some practices, though, it's not a helpful tool and the investment is not worth it.

There can be tech challenges and workflow slowdowns with dispensing cabinets. If teams are used to being able to grab whatever they need, especially in an emergency or urgent situation, there can be slowdowns when adding in a dispensing cabinet. Additionally, there can also be challenges with the fingerprint scanner, code input, or little bin access.

"Best Practice" Dispensing Cabinet Considerations
If you are considering adding a dispensing cabinet to your practice, here are some questions to consider.

- What items would you like to put in the cabinet? Controlled substances? Flea, tick, or heartworm prevention? What injectables, supplies, or pharmaceuticals would be worth adding to the cabinet?
- Who do you envision being the main "administrator" for the cabinets? Who would be in charge of maintenance, product selection, reconciling errors, and running reports?
- If you keep certain items in the cabinets, would you also try to maintain the quantity on hand in your PiMS or other inventory software? Or would you solely rely on the dispensing cabinet to monitor the amount on hand?
- If you do not plan on receiving items that "live" in the dispensing cabinets into your software, how will you increase your prices as your costs go up?
- What type of training and support is offered by the company you are interested in? What about initial onboarding training versus long-term support and maintenance?
- What will be your workflow if there is a tech issue during an emergency or urgent situation, especially regarding controlled substances?
- How will your current pharmacy and inventory management workflows change with dispensing cabinets? Who will be in charge of navigating these changes and updating any processes?
- How do you envision these cabinets working in your practice? What problems or challenges are you hoping that they'll solve?

Inventory dispensing cabinets can be a great addition to your inventory, but they might not work for everyone. As with most things with our inventory (and in life!), they aren't the magic solution we all hope is out there.

8.7 Using an Online Pharmacy

An online pharmacy is a convenient electronic platform where clients can purchase prescriptions and other over-the-counter or retail items. Think of them as an extension of your practice and a way for your clients to buy a wider selection of items than your practice carries. Depending on the online pharmacy company, there can be a link between what's purchased and the medical record for easy documentation.

Using an online pharmacy can be helpful for your practice, but that doesn't mean it's without a downside! An online pharmacy can be used to supplement your in-house pharmacy. Not only that, but it's a great way to meet our clients' needs for convenience, shopping outside business hours, and home delivery. Clients can purchase through an online pharmacy any special orders or items that do not make sense to carry in-house.

The downside, though? Your practice makes a significantly smaller profit margin. But that can often be outweighed because it means that less cash is tied up on the shelf with low-turning or high-risk products. However, it's important to weigh up the benefits of not needing to stock the product in-house versus the downside of smaller profit margins.

Here are some tips for promoting your online pharmacy.

- Create a QR code for your online pharmacy and add it to the client invoice template. Each time an invoice prints, there will be a QR code to take clients directly to the online pharmacy.
- Add the QR code and the link to your online pharmacy to stickers for pharmacy take-home bags for clients.
- Create laminated online pharmacy explainer sheets/detailers for exam rooms and the lobby area.
- Create a small handout with the QR code, the pharmacy link, and a discount code to hand out.
- Add your online pharmacy link to your website and the practice's email signature.
- When recommending a prescription or product, send it through the online pharmacy during the client's appointment.
- Create a price comparison chart for your practice versus other online pharmacies – do not forget to factor in any rebates or coupons your practice has for clients or to update these with price changes.
- Train your team on how to educate and discuss with clients the difference between authentic products and products where the origin is unknown (through other outside online pharmacies).

8.8 Tips for Keeping Your Practice Management System Accurate

Your PiMS or other inventory software can be a helpful tool in your inventory management toolbox, except if it's never accurate and is a little (or a lot) disorganized. Why does the PiMS get off track so easily? Sometimes, it's just the software. It wasn't designed for inventory management, so it's either cumbersome to keep track of or there is not the capability to do it efficiently.

It might also be because there is not a lot of training or support from your practice management software, so you or the inventory team aren't even sure how to use the functionality. It's not your fault, it's a common problem!! On the other hand, it can be challenging to keep the PiMS accurate. Veterinary medicine is a service-based business, so inventory is not only sold to clients but it's also used and consumed. That's a lot to track. Sometimes, having an accurate inventory in your software is out of your control. But other times (and hopefully, this is the case for you), it's something you can learn.

I like to think about your on-hand quantity with two levers: in versus out. I do not mean the "good data in, bad data out" sort of way. I mean that if the correct inventory is not being added IN correctly, then the on-hand quantity will always be inaccurate. On the other hand, if the correct inventory is not being taken OUT, then the on-hand quantity will still be inaccurate.

Before we dive in, what are some "symptoms" that tell you that your PiMS's inventory module needs some correcting?

- Inaccurate quantity on hand (this could be extreme, i.e., −9243 capsules).
- Reorder points are not flagging correctly or showing up on the "reorder report" at all.
- Your inventory carry or value of inventory on hand might appear to be extremely inaccurate. For example, you might see the value of inventory on hand in your software as −$298,015 or, on the flip side, $49,721,054.
- This could mean that your system thinks the cost of one pill is the cost of one bottle. For example, product A has a unit cost of $0.03 but in the software, the unit cost is $16.95 (and is only sold for $0.09 per unit).
- Your PiMS updates by the wrong quantity when receiving.

Sometimes, the extreme examples seem silly but I've seen PiMSs do some pretty wild things! So, how do these issues occur? There are a number of reasons but it's important to note that it's incredibly common so, if you resonate with some of the examples above, you certainly aren't alone. Here are some examples of why your inventory quantity on hand might be inaccurate.

- Incorrect set-up of the individual item.
- Items that were used during a procedure but not documented.
- Items that were broken and not taken out of inventory.
- Treatments (with linked inventory items) or inventory items not getting charged for or invoiced appropriately.
- Items that have been returned or wasted and not entered.
- Mishandled employee or rescue accounts.
- Anything that affects the IN or OUT of inventory.

Let's dive more into the "in versus out" of your inventory. Essentially, if the quantity on hand is OVER, it's not being taken OUT correctly or too much is being added IN. If the quantity on hand is UNDER, it's likely not being added IN correctly or too much is being taken OUT.

Let's first explore the IN. Thankfully, as the inventory manager, adding inventory into your software through the receiving process is something you have control over. Receiving your inventory correctly and accurately is the first step to keeping your software accurate. Otherwise, you are off before you have even gotten started!

Questions to consider.
- Who enters purchase orders? What does this process look like? How often is it completed?
- Do you use the purchase order/receipt function in your software, or is the on-hand quantity manually updated?
- Do you have a way of double-checking if anything was entered incorrectly?

With the OUT process, you have slightly less control as your team is more involved with inventory being taken out. The biggest reason that I've found is either inventory is not charged for appropriately (theft or missed billing) or services are performed that have linked inventory items that aren't charged for appropriately. For example, a team member once charged a quantity of 0.5 instead of 1 for an "IV catheter placement." So, only 0.5 of a t-port, catheter cap, and catheter were taken out of inventory. Needless to say, I was fairly confused when the system said there were 13.5 t-ports in stock!

The biggest question when it comes to the OUT is ensuring that inventory and invoicing, in general, are as accurate as possible. Earlier in this chapter, you learned that setting up groups, packages, and linked items to leverage your software makes this easier. What other systems or structures of support could you add to help your team capture charges more easily? How confident does your team feel about charging accurately? Are there any areas of growth opportunity that you see?

One aspect that you do have control over is setting up the individual item. As you learned in the last chapter, I typically recommend setting up the item in the lowest unit that you sell it. For example, if you sell cephalexin per capsule, set the item up with a unit of measure per capsule. If you sell an item per bottle or per tube, set the item up with a unit of measure per bottle or per tube.

Sometimes, this can get a little tricky with flea, tick, and heartworm prevention. Ideally, I recommend setting it up as "Heartworm prevention A (25–50 lb) per dose," and if a box of six is sold, a quantity of six is entered. It does not work well to set it up as a box: "Heartworm prevention A (25–50 lb) per box," and if a single dose is sold, a quantity of 0.16 is entered. It will be extremely difficult to keep your inventory accurate!

Now, you might be thinking "Nicole, what if people accidentally send home a box but only charge for one dose?" That is certainly a concern that I do not want to minimize! You'll have to weigh that concern for your unique practice against alternative ways to ensure accurate charging. Can you hang a reminder note at the receptionist's desk? In the multistep verifying process, does that likelihood go down? What about a sticky note on the stock items? But, if setting up "per dose" is a method that you want to move toward, setting up a prescription double-check system is a great idea not only for accurate charge capture but also to minimize any medication errors.

When starting a prescription double-check system, I like to remember the "five rights" of medication administration: the right patient, the right drug, the right time, the right dose, and the right route (Grissinger 2010).

Another example is with packets of probiotic powder. Let's say that in your software, it's sold as "per box." However, a veterinarian decides to send home a seven-day course instead of the full box of 30 packets. They would need to figure out the correct quantity (in this case, 0.2333333) to enter. So, at the end of the week, you discover that you have 4.76666666 boxes remaining. Setting up this item as "per packet" would help to keep your inventory more accurate and hopefully reduce any team frustration.

8.9 Putting It all Together

Throughout this chapter, we have discussed several strategies to limit and reduce missed billing and help empower your team to confidently charge more accurately.

- Set and establish clear charging guidelines.
  - Does everyone on your team understand how and when to charge for certain procedures? As an example, does everyone know when to charge a Level One hospitalization versus a Level Three (Table 8.2)?
- Set up groups, packages, and linked items.
  - After reviewing this chapter, what are some groups, packages, or linked items that you'd like to set up in your software?

Table 8.2 An example of hospitalization charging criteria.

Hospitalization level	Level one	Level two	Level three
When to charge	IV catheter *or* Less than five treatments while hospitalized	IV catheter and on fluids **or** Between 5 and 10 treatments while hospitalized	IV catheter and on fluids, urinary catheter, or blood transfusion *or* In an isolation ward or greater than 11 treatments while hospitalized

- Train your team to look for areas of improvement (potentially with the help of auditing medical records).
  - Playing "The Price Is Right: Inventory Edition" is a fun game to help your team understand how expensive inventory is and why it's important to invoice accurately.
- Implement charging "double-checks."
  - Is there a process in place to review the charges before the client is checked out? Does this process differ for hospitalized patients or patients with extensive surgeries/workups?
  - Could medication double-check systems to check the "five rights" help prevent medication errors or missed billing?
    - As an example, Dr Tank wants to implement prescription double-checks at Tank's Animal Hospital. Georgia, a registered veterinary technician (RVT), is getting ready to administer a patient an injection of carprofen. Before drawing up the medication, she enters the charge into the medical record. Then, she has a fellow RVT check the dose, the amount drawn up, and the medication. Before administration, she confirms with Dr Tank the route, the patient, and the timing of the injection.
    - Alternatively, for a prescription that's being sent home with a patient, Georgia counts out the prescription according to the label. Dr Tank verifies the medication, the dose, the quantity dispensed, and the patient. He confirms that it's correctly entered into the medical record and affirms the instructions. They both add their initials to the prescription label and the medical record, noting who it was filled and witnessed by.
- Barcode scanners.
  - Could the addition of barcode scanners help with inventory management in general or at least help sell your inventory accurately?
- Would electronic dispensing cabinets be beneficial for your practice?

9

Optimizing Your Inventory

9.1 What Does It Mean to Optimize Your Inventory?

What does it mean to optimize your inventory? I like to think of it as a big red sign that says, "Pause. Does this make sense?" When we are buzzing around in the day-to-day busyness of our practice, we often fly from task to task to task and lose track of the big picture. Optimizing your inventory is really about being intentional about what you carry and continuously improving your inventory and processes.

According to the Oxford Dictionary, the official definition of optimization is "to make the best or most effective use of (a situation, opportunity, or resource)." What does that mean for you and your inventory? Essentially:

- you do not just want to spend less, you want to make the most of your spending
- you do not want to stock every item possible; you want to intentionally stock what's best for your patients
- you do not want to order based on shaking a bottle to see when it's low; you want to use demand forecasting to make the best use of your inventory investment.

Throughout this chapter, you'll learn structures and strategies that can help you be more thoughtful and intentional with your inventory so that you can see the day-to-day tasks and the bigger picture simultaneously.

9.2 Evaluating Your Products and Items

Routinely evaluating the products and items that you stock in your practice is so important in the quest for optimizing your inventory. Stale inventory items or items that are "sleeping" on the shelf can keep costs high (you are paying for the item but not selling it) and tie up cash on the shelf. In the day-to-day busyness of your practice, it can be easy to add a product here or there. Maybe members of your team came home from a fun conference where there were a lot of great promotions, new featured products, and "conference specials."

Or a veterinarian joins your practice and requests a number of products that you do not normally keep on the shelf. Or maybe evaluating your current formulary is not high on the priority list because there are new products being released and your team is significantly short-handed. There

Inventory Management for Veterinary Professionals, First Edition. Nicole I. Clausen.
© 2024 John Wiley & Sons, Inc. Published 2024 by John Wiley & Sons, Inc.
Companion website: www.wiley.com/go/clausen/inventory

are many reasons why evaluating your products may not happen for a while, but it's a step you cannot skip when you are optimizing your practice.

Intentionally evaluating your products ensures that the products you carry are the best fit for your specific practice. I highly recommend setting up a system or process so evaluation happens on a regular basis using one of the methods outlined in this chapter.

To start, what products should you evaluate? I would suggest starting with a category that has a lot of similar products. For example, you might start with your flea and tick category, which has a plethora of options and brands. Or you might choose a category that has not been reviewed lately. Alternatively, you might choose a category where the products are all expensive (like supplements or prescription diets).

To start evaluating your products, try the following questions.

- On what date was this product last sold?
- What is your average monthly sales for this product?
- What is the average inventory turnover for this product? What is the average number of days on the shelf?
- Where does the product fall on the profit margin versus sales quadrant spectrum (see below)?
- Is this item an A, B, or C product (for more information, see section 9.4 later in this chapter)?
- Is there a significant difference between your monthly usage and the package quantity?

    For example, your practice might only sell four doses of product A per month, but you need to purchase a carton of 60.

These questions can generally be answered using data from your practice management system (PiMS). Even if you are not currently using your PiMS for inventory, most practices will still have reliable sales data because of how clients are invoiced for their appointments. To find the information for the questions above, use a sales report from your PiMS to determine when the product was last sold and the average monthly sales for the product.

If you are not using a practice management software, look at the software or method you are using to invoice your clients. Is there a way to review the date of an item was last sold? Are there other analytics and reporting tools that you could use to answer the above questions? Alternatively, you could use your purchasing platform to see when an item was last purchased and how much is typically purchased at a time.

9.2.1 Profit Margin Versus Sales/Use Quadrant

Another helpful tool is to view these items using a profit margin versus sales/use quadrant. When viewing these products through the lens of this quadrant, it can be helpful to see where they fall. Does the item in question have both a low margin and a low sales volume? Or does it have a high margin and an average sales volume?

Helpful Definitions
- **Profit margin**: the amount of money a practice (and a business in general) makes after subtracting all its costs and expenses from the revenue it generates.
- **Low-margin product**: when a practice only keeps a small portion of the revenue for a particular product as profit after covering the costs.
- **High-margin product**: when a practice keeps a larger portion of the revenue for a particular product as profit after covering the costs.

For example, items that are considered low margin and low use should likely be questioned. You might ask yourself: Is this item critical for patient care? Could it be moved to an online pharmacy? What is our "why" for carrying this product?

Table 9.1 The profit margin versus sales/use quadrant.

High sales/low margin "Watch"	High sales/high margin "Winner"
Low sales/low margin "Questionable"	Low sales/high margin "On guard"

For items with high margins but low use (except for necessary emergency medications), you might have a healthy profit margin but if they aren't selling frequently, money is tied up on the shelf. Think of these as "on-guard" items that you should regularly evaluate and be vigilant about, especially if they are high-cost items. If any of these items are high cost, they are likely responsible for keeping your cost of goods elevated.

Alternatively, items that are low margin but high use are considered "watch" products. These might include highly competitively shopped products or items with manufacturer's suggested retail prices (MSRPs). How you decide to stock these products will likely depend on your unique practice and goals.

Lastly, items that are high use and high margin are "winner" products. Unless there are safety or efficacy reasons, these products are likely to be high-performing products in your inventory (Table 9.1).

The profit margin versus sales/use quadrant can be a helpful "lens" and quick assessment to see how effective a product is in your inventory. The downside of using a quadrant like this is that it's subjective. One practice's "low sales" might look different from another so it's helpful to keep your unique practice in mind as you are going through this process. If having a subjective tool is not helpful, I recommend calculating the average number of days on the shelf before an item sold, categorizing it using an ABC analysis (see below), or using the sticker dot challenge (this concept is introduced in Chapter 10).

9.2.2 A, B, or C Classification Using an ABC Analysis

Categorizing items in your pharmacy as A, B, or C products is similar to the profit margin versus sales/use quadrant but isless subjective. With an ABC analysis (see section 9.4 for instructions), items are designated a category (A, B, or C) using Pareto's Principle, also called the 80:20 rule, which states that "80% of the outcomes are controlled or decided by 20% of the activities." In this case, 20% of your products generate 80% of your sales. These are called "A" products and are similar to the high-margin/high-sales "winner" products mentioned above.

These "A" items are the most important to your practice. They are items that you never want to run out of! Note, because this is based on revenue generated or quantity sold data, it does not account for items that are critical to your patients for medical reasons (like euthanasia solution).

At the opposite end of the spectrum are your "C" products. These are the bottom 50% of your products that generate only 5% of your revenue. Your "C" items are a great place to start evaluating products, especially if they must be purchased in bulk.

Comparable to the "watch" and "on-guard" items above, your "B" class items are the middle 30% of your products that only generate 15% of your revenue.

As an example, let's say that a certain supplement needs to be purchased in a six-pack. After putting together an ABC analysis, you realize that this product is a "C" item. To top it all off, you review the sales history and find that only one bag is sold every three months. This means that purchasing one six-pack of this supplement will theoretically be over a year's supply!

9.2.3 The MERIT Model

The next lens that's helpful for evaluating your products is the MERIT model. This consists of five factors to consider for each product (markup, exclusivity, risk, immediacy, and turnover). It can be used for assessing a single product or for comparing multiple similar products (Figure 9.1).

9.2.3.1 Markup

High-markup (or high-margin) products that serve your client's needs are better to stock and resell than products with low markup potential. Low-markup products are not worth keeping on your shelf. Note that more expensive products of equal markup and demand are more profitable. For example, let's say that you have two products on the shelf that are fairly similar. Product A has a markup potential of 50% and product B has a markup potential of 175%, so product B is a preferable product to stock in house.

- Note: Examining both the markup percentage and the dollar value is beneficial. For example, a product that costs $100.00 might have a markup percentage of 50%, which equates to $50.00 each time it's sold! That is very different from a $5.00 product that has a 200% markup (which equates to $10.00).

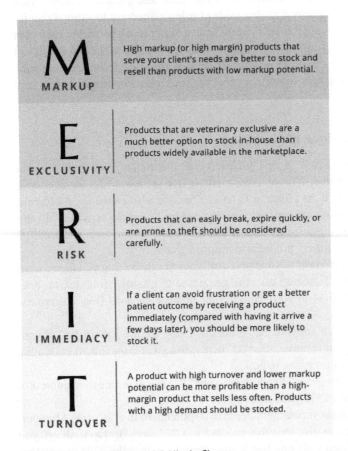

Figure 9.1 The MERIT model. Nicole Clausen.

9.2.3.2 Exclusivity

Products that are veterinary exclusive are a much better option to stock in house than products widely available in the marketplace. If a product line is veterinary exclusive and not sold by online pharmacies, you can often charge more. Offering these products provides a unique value to your clients, which encourages them to purchase from you. A great example of this is supplements; some supplements are sold exclusively through a veterinarian and cannot be purchased through an online pharmacy. Another great example is injectable medications versus topical or oral products. Topical and oral products are typically available through online pharmacies while injectables are not, which makes injectables the clear preference to stock in house.

9.2.3.3 Risk

Products that can easily break, expire quickly, or are prone to theft should be considered carefully. When products purchased by the practice cannot be sold due to these factors, there is a smaller overall profit margin, which makes it a less viable product to carry, even if the markup percentage is high. An excellent example of examining the risk of a product is tramadol. Many practices are questioning whether to stock tramadol in house or exclusively script to a human pharmacy due to the risk of keeping it in stock, regulatory requirements, and often high labor costs due to prescription monitoring programs. It's important to be conservative with high-risk products, whether the risk is from theft or diversion, a short shelf life, or a medication/product that is easily contaminated or preservative free.

Helpful Definitions

- **Prescription monitoring program**: a system that helps track the prescriptions people and animals receive for certain medications. It's a database that healthcare and veterinary professionals and authorities submit to and use to monitor the prescribing and dispensing of controlled substances.

9.2.3.4 Immediacy

When evaluating your products, it's key to stock medications where speed matters. If a client can avoid frustration or the care team can get a better patient outcome by receiving a product immediately (compared with having it arrive a few days later), you should probably stock it. This includes treatment for acute conditions and conditions where treatment plan adherence is key. An excellent example of this is prescription diets. A growing trend in veterinary practices is only stocking diets in house for acute conditions (like gastrointestinal, urinary, and kidney diets) while utilizing direct-to-home shipping options for nonacute diets.

9.2.3.5 Turnover

A product with high turnover and lower markup potential can be more profitable than a high-margin product that sells less often. Products with a high demand should be stocked. For example, gabapentin, trazodone, and enalipril are relatively inexpensive items so they do not have a huge profit margin per unit. But, because they often have a very high turnover and sell often, they are profitable.

Fun fact: For 95% of the inventory analysis and audits that I run for clients, gabapentin and trazodone are within the top five, or even the top three, products sold (by quantity).

"Best Practice" MERIT Model Questions

- What is the markup (both the percentage and in dollars) for this item?
- Is there an item on the shelf that's similar and has a better markup potential (for example, brand name Baytril® tabs versus generic enrofloxacin tablets)?

- Is this product only available from veterinarians or can it also be purchased through online pharmacies?
- Does this product expire shortly after opening?
- How long is the shelf-life for this product?
- If it expires, is there any return policy or credit available from the vendor?
- Is this item prone to breakage (glass bottle, heavy, etc.)?
- Is this product high- isk and prone to theft or diversion?
- Can a patient get a better outcome by starting this product immediately?
- Will the patient be negatively affected if they have to wait for this product to be delivered?
- What is the turnover like for this product? Is there a similar product that has a better turnover?

The MERIT model is a great evaluation framework and can help to intentionally consider whether a particular item best fits your practice and patients.

9.2.4 Product Evaluation Example – Putting It all Together

Let's take the three different methods for evaluating your products (ABC ranking, MERIT model, and profit versus sales/use quadrant) and explore an example together. In the initial evaluation, we'll use the ABC ranking and the profit versus sales/use quadrant, and investigate the sales information. Then we'll use that information to consider the MERIT model.

Tank's Animal Hospital realized that it had been quite a while since they reviewed what was on the shelf and their formulary. So Georgia decided to create a list of products they'd like to evaluate. The first product is a joint supplement that used to be popular but its sales have declined in the last year.

Initial evaluation.
- Date last sold: June 27th.
- Average monthly sales: one bag (it sold an average of four bags per month two years ago).
- Average number of days on the shelf: 35.
- Where does the product fall on the profit margin versus sales/use quadrant? Low sales and high margin.
- ABC classification: C product.
- Is there a significant difference between your monthly usage and the package quantity? No, it can be purchased by the bag.

The MERIT model.
- Markup potential: the markup potential for this item is on the lower side. The average markup is 75%, which equals $30.
- Exclusivity: this product is not veterinary exclusive and can be purchased over the counter and at online pharmacies.
- Risk: there is no risk in stocking this product; it always has good dating and no theft concerns.
- Immediacy: the patient will not get a better outcome whether they start this product today or in four days.
- Turnover: compared to other joint supplements, this product has a relatively low turnover rate.

Ultimate decision: due to the declining sales for this product, the relatively average markup potential, and the fact that we stock other more effective and efficacious joint supplements, this product will be discontinued and moved to the online pharmacy.

Using the different "lenses" for assessing your inventory can help you intentionally evaluate which products should be stocked, which ones should be moved to an online pharmacy or special order item, and which should be eliminated altogether.

"Best Practice" Questions to Consider

- When was the last time you evaluated the products in your inventory?
- Going forward, how often would you like to evaluate your inventory ideally? What will this process look like? Who will be in charge and who will participate?
- As you read through this section, what products came to mind that you'd like to evaluate first?

9.3   Adding New Products

Personally, one of my favorite things to purchase is skincare products. I love a great moisturizer that is full of natural ingredients and great benefits, especially if the packaging is beautiful. I have little to no willpower with the product trifecta: beautiful branding and packaging, clean ingredients, and excellent benefits!

I have to be careful, though, because I can easily get carried away. I get excited about a new product, forget I have almost a full tub of moisturizer sitting on my bathroom counter, and bring the new one home in a trendy compostable tote. It has happened so many times that my sister has come to expect a skincare overstock gift at least once a year. (You're welcome, Heather.)

We have to watch out for the same habits with our inventory! After all your hard work evaluating the products that you currently stock, you need to have guidelines and processes in place for how you'll choose to add new products. Otherwise, you might get carried away until you suddenly realize that you now carry nine different types of ear cleaners on the shelf. The guidelines for adding new products are very similar to the questions you considered when evaluating your current products earlier in this chapter.

I highly recommend setting up an approval process for when team members request new products. An approval process with a written request form can circumvent pressure coming from team members to purchase specific products, allowing the management team or veterinarians to be intentional about what they buy and function less reactively throughout the process.

"Best Practice" Questions for Adding New Products

- Why is this product being requested? Is it for a specific patient or is this a new formulary addition?
- Is this product replacing another similar product that's currently on backorder or has been discontinued?
- Does this product have benefits that other products currently stocked do not offer?
- Does this product have a better or a greater range of benefits than a product that is currently stocked?
- How many team members are comfortable with the product and willing to use, sell, and recommend it?
- How does it stack up against the MERIT model? What is the markup potential? Is it veterinary exclusive? Does the product have any risks or theft concerns? Does stocking this product affect patient outcomes? What is the anticipated turnover or sales volume?
- What will the storage and security requirements look like for this product? Does it take up a lot of space? Is it a controlled substance? Does it require refrigeration or a specific temperature?
- Are there any other concerns or considerations with this product?

Once you have decided to carry a product, there are some other considerations and product guidelines to help set the product up for success.

- Set up the product in your PiMS or invoicing software, priced, and ready to be sold before it ever arrives. Ideally, all the required setup, marketing, and planning are complete before it arrives, so once it does, it just needs to be received and stocked.
- Prior to the product arriving in the practice, fully train the team on how to use it, dosing information, contraindications, how to charge and invoice, and what to expect. Give the opportunity for the team to ask questions and provide feedback. A "lunch and learn" or product demo is a great place to start!
- Set up an alert or communication to let your team know as soon as it's in stock and ready to be used or sold.
- If the new product is replacing a previous product, order it around the previous product's reorder point to ensure you do not have too much of the old product sitting on the shelf, expired, and collecting dust. If the product is being ordered due to a backorder, safety, or efficacy concern, it can be ordered at any time.

One of the main goals when adding new products is to avoid "product creep" and be intentional about what is carried in your practice. You want to limit the negative financial impact on your practice that comes from carrying six types of flea/tick prevention, nine kinds of joint supplements, and an overwhelming number of options on the shelves.

9.4 Cycle Counting Your Inventory

Cycle counting is such a helpful task in your inventory toolbox. You might be thinking, "Nicole, the very last thing I want to do is count a bazillion pills." I know it's not the most fun part of inventory management but it's incredibly beneficial. The good news is that there are ways to make it easier, and it often gets easier the more often you do it.

Perhaps the tiniest mention of counting draws up images of long hours in dimming light counting pills, needles, and gauze pads until your brain is fried. If you already feel the panic or your eyes are glazing over, you are not alone. You've already done a lot of work in your practice to make sure that you do not get trapped in the back, individually ticking through everything until the process hypnotizes you.

So what actually is "cycle counting"? Cycle counting is the opposite of the long, drawn-out process we tend to think of. With cycle counting, you count small amounts of inventory throughout the year on a rotational basis. For example, you might count a few products every day, a handful every week, or a section every month. It can be set up to be both sustainable and helpful!

There are numerous benefits to cycle counting. First, it's a really easy and efficient way to identify inventory that has gone missing. This is also called **shrinkage**: Any difference between what is on the shelf versus what your PiMS says is there. The difference can be due to something as small as a receiving error or as frightening as theft or diversion. Unless it's a software or setup error, that shrinkage is a potential loss of revenue. Cycle counting is helpful because if you are counting an item once a month versus once a year, you can identify and investigate any discrepancies sooner.

Helpful Definitions
- **Shrinkage**: when items or products go missing or are lost without an easy explanation, causing a decrease in inventory. This can be due to theft, errors, damage, evaporation, missed charges, or other reasons.

- **Diversion**: when someone with authorized access to the pharmacy or other inventory storage areas takes or steals the item for unauthorized purposes.
- **Cycle counting**: counting small amounts of inventory frequently rather than all at once.

For example, let's say that you count cephalexin 500 mg once a month, and between February and March you are short 15 tablets. On the flip side, let's say that you only count Product A once a year and you are short 832 tablets. It will be much easier to identify what happened to the 15 cephalexin tablets in the last month versus the 832 Product A tablets in the last year. Not only that but because you are counting once a month, you will be able to notice any patterns of ever-increasing discrepancies and differences.

In an example of theft, someone might steal 50 capsules of Apoquel® to see if anyone notices that they had gone missing. If you used cycle counting, you would recognize that difference quickly. If you only count once a year, the thief may have continued stealing in larger quantities, encouraged because no one realized it was missing.

There are three main ways to create a cycle count schedule: ABC analysis, by item category, or by inventory zone. Above all else, the method you choose needs to be sustainable for your practice. Cycle counts are most beneficial when the schedule is maintained to count on a semiregular basis.

This is also your permission slip to start small if needed. You can always start with a particularly important category (like flea/tick/heartworm prevention) and expand as you have time and capacity.

9.4.1 ABC Analysis for Cycle Counting

One of my favorite ways of creating a cycle count schedule is based on an ABC analysis. This way is more labor intensive to set up but can provide you with a lot of great insights into your inventory.

Earlier, you learned that the Pareto Principle (80:20) states that, generally, the top 20% of your inventory makes up for 80% of your inventory dispensed. This means that 20% of your inventory is critical to your practice and should be counted more frequently than other items in your inventory. The time and effort devoted to counting gauze squares are not as impactful as counting controlled substances or expensive injectables. Examples of the Pareto Principle in action include the following

- 80% of your revenue comes from 20% of your services.
- 80% of your client visits comes from the top 20% of your clients.
- 80% of your inventory sales comes from the top 20% of your products.
- 80% of your revenue comes from the top 20% of your clients.

Now we are getting to the meat and potatoes, my friend! The best way to classify your inventory into the different A, B, and C categories is by utilizing your PiMS or your purchase history. If your software system does not do this for you, you can calculate them from your PiMS's usage or quantity sold reports. Some software systems have a report that calculates this information for you, although it's less common than doing it yourself.

The first step in this process is to determine what report you need to access from your software. The information that you'll need includes:

- each inventory item listed that generated a sale
- the quantity used or sold in a particular time period.

Note: It's helpful if you are able to select a time period for this report (a 12-month period will give you a nice average usage for all products).

Once you have found the report that you'll need, the next step is to export or "print" this file to Excel. For some software systems, you will export it to Excel by selecting "Excel" as your printer. Once it's in an Excel or spreadsheet format, you will likely have to do some formatting cleanup first. Remove anything that is not inventory related, like treatment or service codes. Delete any columns that are unnecessary. The only information that you need is the inventory name or description and the quantity used or sold. It's sometimes helpful to have the item ID or code, but it's not a necessity. Your Excel or spreadsheet file should look similar to Table 9.2.

The next step in this process is to create a filter to sort the data. You'll want to attach the filter to the column labels so you can easily sort by quantity. Once you have applied the filter, the next step is to sort your spreadsheet. Sort the quantity used or sold column from most sold to least sold. Tip: Make sure that the filter is applied to the whole table so as your quantity column gets sorted, the item name stays with the corresponding quantity. Now that the table is sorted, you'll be able to see what items you sell the most. Sometimes, it's surprising to see how much of a particular item you sell throughout the year!

Your Excel or spreadsheet file should now look similar to Table 9.3, with your most sold/purchased products at the top of the list.

Now that you have exported the report into Excel or another spreadsheet program, removed any rows or columns that aren't necessary, and sorted the table by quantity from most dispensed to least dispensed, the next step is to assign an A, B, or C classification to each item. As you recall, the ABC classifications are as follows.

- "A" products are the top 20% of your products that make up 80% of your usage and unit sales.
- "B" products are the middle 30% of your products that make up 15% of your usage and unit sales.
- "C" products are the bottom 50% of products that make up only 5% of your usage and unit sales.

Table 9.2 An example sales history report exported to Excel or another spreadsheet program.

Product name	Quantity sold	Classification
Product A	3,570.0	
Product B	136.8	
Product C	9,832.0	
Product D	8.0	
Product E	239.0	
Product F	721.0	

Table 9.3 An example of a sales history report exported to Excel after sorting by quantity sold.

Product name	Quantity sold	Classification
Product C	9,832.0	
Product A	3,570.0	
Product F	721.0	
Product B	136.8	
Product E	239.0	
Product D	8.0	

With this information, use the total number of items to determine how many products are 20%, 30%, and 50% of the total. Once you have determined these numbers, you can classify the top 20% of your products as "A" items, the middle 30% of your products as "B" items, and the bottom 50% of your products as "C" items. I find it best to add a column to the spreadsheet table and add in the A, B, or C classification.

Your Excel or spreadsheet file should now look similar to Table 9.4, with your most sold/purchased products at the top of the list and your A, B, and C products identified.

Once your products are classified into A, B, and C (nice work!), you can now create a cycle counting schedule based on each category. A good rule of thumb is to count Class A items once per month. You can break this down even further into four equal sections and divide it into Week 1, Week 2, Week 3, and Week 4. The top 25% of the products should be counted in week 1 of the month, the second 25% counted during week 2, and so on. If you'd prefer, you can break it down even further into days of the week. For example, count products 12–15 on Tuesday (Table 9.5).

Class B items can be counted once per quarter by breaking the category out into three equal sections and assigning a time period to be counted. Class C items should be counted every six months. **Controlled substances are an exception and should be counted at the very least once per week.** Some practices will need to count every shift, some every day, and some might be able to count once weekly. How often you count controlled substances will depend on your practice, your records' accuracy, and the volume of controlled substances used.

Table 9.4 An example of a sales history report exported to Excel after sorting by quantity sold, with the ABC classification added to each item.

Product name	Quantity sold	Classification
Product C	9,832.0	A
Product A	3,570.0	B
Product F	721.0	B
Product B	136.8	C
Product E	239.0	C
Product D	8.0	C

Table 9.5 How you might spend your time differently with an "A" product versus a "C" product.

"A" product	"C" product
More time and effort managing	Less time and effort managing
Pricing strategy evaluated more often	Pricing strategy evaluated less often
Counted more frequently	Infrequently counted
Reorder points are recalculated more frequently	Reorder points adjusted infrequently
Watch for demand changes or shifts in seasonal demands	Demand rarely changes or shifts
Overstock is locked up	Overstock is in central storage

Creating a cycle count schedule by classifying your inventory items based on the relative impact and importance they have on your practice is an excellent way to make sure your time is spent as wisely as possible. With that being said, the ABC method has downsides. Because there is no rhyme or reason to what products are in the "A" category (besides how often they sell), they will likely be all over your practice and stored in different locations. If you have a large practice, you might find that you are spending too much time going to different locations to count.

The other downside to this method is that because it works off quantity sold, your vaccines, expensive injectables, and flea/tick/heartworm prevention might be "B" products, even though they are very expensive and valuable. If you are advanced in Excel or another spreadsheet program, you can create a weighted column to sort by quantity sold and sales volume, and dollars. You can also just decide to classify all vaccines, flea/tick/heartworm, and expensive injectables as "A" products.

"Best Practice" ABC Analysis Calculation Review

1) Export the sales report or purchase history information into Excel.
2) Remove unnecessary rows or columns.
3) Sort the table by quantity from most dispensed to least dispensed.
4) Assign A, B, or C classification to each item (remember the Pareto Principle!).
   - Consider the expensive and valuable items that will not classify appropriately based on sales data and manually assign.
5) Create a cycle count schedule following these general principles.
   - Count controlled substances weekly at minimum.
   - Count Class A products once per month.
   - Count Class B products once per quarter.
   - Count Class C products every six months.

9.4.2 Inventory Manager Spotlight

Meet Bree Henry, CVIP, an exceptional and wonderful inventory manager!

"Cycle counting, though it may appear tedious, forms the cornerstone of my inventory management system. The accuracy of these counts holds significant importance as discrepancies can have a cascading impact on various aspects of inventory management. We conduct bi-annual, quarterly, monthly, every other week, and weekly counts to maintain precision.

On Mondays, I initiate the week using Inventory Ally, an inventory management software that analyzes purchase history from Vetcove and product usage from our PiMS. This generates a list of items for counting. By uploading purchase history to Inventory Ally, printing the counting checklist, and physically counting by purchase unit (e.g., bottles on the shelf rather than exact tablets), the process becomes quick and efficient while ensuring a comprehensive inventory check throughout the hospital. After inputting the count into Inventory Ally, it facilitates order generation.

Later in the week, typically on Thursdays, I perform a more detailed count based on quarterly ABC analysis. This involves counting vaccines, preventatives, and a quarter of "A" items per unit of measure (e.g., tablet, capsule, dose). The comparison of this count to the quantity on hand in our PiMS is crucial for maintaining system accuracy. It directly influences reorder points, highlights potential issues like team confusion or organizational needs, and addresses concerns such as theft.

Ensuring the total quantity of inventory on hand is as accurate as possible serves as the foundation for my entire inventory management system, influencing reporting, reorder points, purchasing strategies, and team communication. This meticulous approach is aimed at fostering efficiency and reliability in the management of our inventory."

9.4.3 Cycle Counting Based on Item Category

Another method for creating a cycle count schedule is establishing a rotation through different categories of items. This method is helpful because high-value items are still prioritized, but it does not require as much effort to set up as with an ABC analysis. With this method, some categories should be counted monthly: Vaccines and biologicals, diets, heartworm and flea and tick prevention, and any other category that is valuable or has a consistently high turnover in your practice.

Start by assigning important categories to weeks during the month. So, for example, a small-animal general practice will:

- during week one, count diets
- during week two, count vaccines, biological products, and expensive injectables
- during week three, count heartworm and flea and tick prevention.

During week four, rotate through the remaining categories in your inventory. Separating them into several categories is beneficial depending on how many tabs, pills, and liquids are carried in your practice. An example of the remaining categories might be:

- ophthalmics
- otics
- over-the-counter (OTC) and retail items
- injectables 1
- injectables 2
- tabs and pills 1
- tabs and pills 2
- liquids
- dental supplies
- surgical supplies
- lab supplies and pharmacy supplies
- hospital supplies.

Helpful Definitions
- **Biological products**: medications or products made from living organisms or their parts. This umbrella term can include vaccines, blood products, gene therapies, or other medications derived from cells or tissues.

You can (and should!) adjust these categories depending on what makes sense for your practice.

9.4.4 Inventory Manager Spotlight

Introducing Shelly Chadwick, CVT, VDT, CVIP, inventory manager rockstar! Shelly was also crowned the veterinary Inventory Manager of the Year in 2023.

When I asked her what she was most proud of in her inventory; it was her cycle counts! "I was very proud of getting my inventory to a completely "live" count [year-round]. Gone were the days of quarterly counts and adjustments that nobody wanted to do! I ran an "ABC" report for two six-month spans, one for spring and one for fall. I created count sheets from these reports showing each item's location and how exactly to count them (by the tablet, bottle, box, etc.).

New sheets were hung in the hospital tech station every Monday. Each tech had to count three to four items a week (one a day!). Not only did this negate having to do quarterly counts, but it also made my counts more accurate by making the process only take a few minutes a day. I would 100%

recommend that this be one of the first things you do with your inventory system. From this, you can adjust your reorder points, track lead times, and hopefully cut back on times you "run out" of medication or supplies."

She added, "My biggest piece of advice would be to not try to 'fix' everything all at once. Keep a big-picture idea of where you would like to see your inventory, but do not set unrealistic time-frames/goals. Set small goals and celebrate yourself for even the smallest accomplishment! Remember, without you, there would be no supplies or medication to help your patients!"

9.4.5 Cycle Counting Based on Item Location or Inventory Zone

The third method for creating a cycle count schedule involves crafting a counting schedule based on where an item lives in the practice. For example, you could count everything in the refrigerator during the first month, everything in the pharmacy during the second month, and so forth. This method is helpful because there is a low barrier to getting started. It is also easy to delegate by assigning team members to specific zones they always count. The downside of this method is that it does not prioritize high-value or high-turnover items as well as the first two methods.

There are other methods for creating a cycle count schedule but remember, you are searching for the most sustainable method for you and your practice. A method that I've noticed is doing a full practice-wide inventory count once a quarter. I do not recommend this method. In my opinion, I think high-value and high-use items should be counted more frequently. Also, white goods and hospital supplies (think tongue depressors and cotton swabs) do not necessarily need to be counted quarterly. My preference is to prioritize your important items and spend more time and effort focusing on those particular products.

"Best Practice" Cycle Counting Questions
- What method of cycle counting would work best for your practice?
- Have you ever cycle counted before? What lessons did you learn or what would you like to improve upon from that experience?
- Will your counts be delegated to another team member? Will they also make any adjustments necessary in the software? What will that workflow look like?
- Do you anticipate any roadblocks or challenges when cycle counting?
- What are some "safety nets" you could build in so that if you are on vacation or short-staffed and have less time, your cycle counts continue?

The three guiding rules for cycle counting are:
1) follow a routine schedule
2) count the product
3) update the product amount in your PiMS.

9.5 Creating a Routine with Your Cycle Counts

Once you have determined which method you'd like to use and calculated your cycle count schedule, the next step is to implement it into your practice and start making it a part of your routine. As I mentioned before, I recommend counting your "A" products or those very important to your practice once per month. To make it even easier, I like to break those products into weekly sections. The top 25% of the products should be counted in week 1 of the month, the second 25% counted during week 2, and so on. You can even break it down further so that you are only counting two or three products per day. The key with cycle counting is to create a schedule and system that becomes routine and is a manageable task. One of the key benefits of cycle counting is to catch theft, errors, or missed charges swiftly, and to make end-of-year counts less daunting.

After your routine is set, it's time to count the product. Remember to keep your units consistent. For example, if you sell Proin® by the bottle and it is entered as "per bottle" in your PiMS, you should only count by the bottle. If you sell a medication by the tablet and it's entered into your software as per tablet, you should count the number of tablets on hand. This might be second nature to you but if you are delegating your counts to another member, they must understand the nuances or remember to check the PiMS for how something is accounted for.

After a product is counted, update the actual on-hand amount in your PiMS. Depending on your software's terminology, this can be completed using an adjustment or variance.

Critical note: Before updating the on-hand amount in your software, check to see if any medications are waiting to be picked up but not paid for. These items will not be included in your physical on-hand amount, but your software system may still be counting these in your on-hand amount. For example, AVImark® will take them out of inventory and list them as an "Allocated Quantity," but once the client checks out, the quantity will be deducted from the on-hand amount. Before embarking on this adventure, reach out to your software support team to see how your on-hand quantity will be affected by prescriptions that have been filled but not checked out yet.

For example, you counted 60 tablets of enrofloxacin but there were 21 tablets, unpaid, waiting to be picked up by a client. Your PiMS might display an on-hand quantity of 81. In this instance, do not make an adjustment because as soon as the client checks out, the PiMS on-hand quantity will drop to 60 and match the physical on-hand quantity.

9.6 Monitoring and Interpreting Discrepancies

One of the important benefits of cycle counting is to catch and evaluate any discrepancies in your on-hand counts. A discrepancy is when there is a difference between what is on the shelf and what your PiMS says you have. This difference is also called inventory shrinkage.

Reasons outside your software that can cause discrepancies include:

- receiving errors
- theft and diversion
- employee accounts not handled properly
- missed charges or not charging appropriately
- evaporation
- expiry
- broken or damaged items.

As an example, let's say that on November 1st, you counted gabapentin 100 mg and had 310 capsules on the shelf, but your PiMS said you had 340 capsules. That means there was a difference of 30 capsules. That difference might represent a missed opportunity for revenue (theft or missed charges) or a protocol/training issue (receiving error or PiMS error). The next month, on December 1st, you again counted gabapentin 100 mg and had 131 capsules on the shelf, but your PiMS said you had 580 on hand. That's now a significant difference of 449! Both of these situations should warrant an immediate investigation to find out why this discrepancy exists.

Trying to find where your inventory went missing can certainly be frustrating and feel a bit like trying to find a needle in a hay stack. It's helpful to have a system in place and a documented process for investigating and monitoring variances or discrepancies when you are performing cycle counts. If you note a discrepancy, immediately perform a recount. If you still have a mismatch, involve a management team member and investigate further why that inventory went missing, and where it is if it's not on the shelf. There are three things that you can immediately start with.

- Pull an inventory variance or adjustment record since the last count. Identify if any other adjustments were made, the amount, reason, and who performed the adjustment.
- Next, match your PiMS purchase order receipts with any invoices to see if it was received correctly.
- Pull a "who-got" report and reconcile it with dispensing records (this might be any surgical or medical records, treatment sheets, or Subjective, Objective, Assessment, and Plan [SOAP] medical records) to see if any charges were missed.

Starting with these three tasks is a great way to help you find the reason behind the missing inventory. If these turn up short, you can dig deeper by pulling more reports in your software, talking with team members, or using other investigation methods you have in your toolbox. There may come a time when, no matter how hard you try, you cannot find the source of the missing inventory. Mistakes can and do happen; we are only human after all. But if a particular item continues to go "missing" or you notice trends or patterns, it's probably time to add safety measures such as the following.

- Implementing new protocols.
  - Hospitalized patient charging guidelines.
  - "Canned" or template estimates for surgeries or treatments not routinely performed.
  - Patient charge approvals by another team member or a member of the management team prior to the client checking out.
- Adding additional security measures (security cameras, lock and key, etc.).
- Double-checking systems for prescriptions. These double-check systems could be for either dispensing or selling inventory items or for receiving and the management of your pharmacy. Examples include:
  - regularly review purchase orders and invoices or statement reconciliation
  - two team members to sign off on all orders received
  - all prescriptions must be double-checked and/or witnessed.
- Creating an approval process and standard operation procedure for discounts and returns.
- Ensuring that every item always leaves the practice with a label. Especially if you are using a PiMS for billing, a label cannot be printed without it being added to the medical record and/or invoice.

Depending on your practice management or inventory software, you can monitor these variances within your software, but you might need or want to use a spreadsheet to keep track of them manually. The minimum amount of information you should track is:

- the inventory item
- the date the count was performed
- the quantity on the shelf
- the quantity on hand in your PiMS
- any reason for the adjustment.

Although not essential, it is helpful to track the value of the adjustment (i.e., an adjustment of 31 capsules of gabapentin cost the practice $1.34 but had a client price of $32.78).

"Best Practice" Quick tips for Cycle Counting in Your Inventory

- Try to make a habit of counting just a few items every day or weekly.
- Delegate if you need to! Even though items need to be counted, it does not necessarily mean that you need to be the one to count.
- As soon as you count the item, make the on-hand adjustment before the item is sold again.
- Make sure that all invoices, packing slips, or purchase orders for items that have already been stocked in the practice are entered before making any adjustments.
- If you notice a large, odd, or problematic number of units missing, investigate it immediately!
- Tip: Keep track of any adjustments made. This is especially true for large or expensive products.
- Do not forget to check and account for any medications that are waiting to be picked up by clients but have not been checked out yet.

9.7 End-of-year Counts

I vividly remember the first time I did an end-of-year count. Dogs were barking, the whir of the dental machine was loud in the background, and the team was buzzing in and around the treatment area, seeing patients. Over the dogs whining as they woke up from anesthesia, music playing in the background, and the occasional waft of anal glands, it was a challenge to focus!

Prior to this, inventory had never been counted in years. I was still fairly new to inventory management and had no idea what an adventure I was in for! I counted everything by myself, and the practice opted not to close for the counts, so I counted during business hours while appointments were being seen. So, every time a member of the care team needed something, they would come in and interrupt me, and I'd have to start counts over again. Or someone else would ask me for a favor, not realizing how busy I was. I also had to navigate medications being sold while I was trying to count.

Then, while I was counting, I discovered a lot of products or items that had never been added into the systems, codes that had never been inactivated or cleaned up, and there were unit of measure issues galore.

I spent so much time getting AVImark cleaned up, adding new codes, inactivating old ones, fixing unit of measure and description issues, and adjusting the quantity on hand. I felt like I was in a race against time, trying to get it all situated before the end of the year. I had not anticipated how much time was necessary for "cleanup" and it took much longer than I thought it would!

I learned a lot from that first inventory count! The second year, it was much easier. The practice had grown and added new team members and another doctor, so this time, it was decided that we would close for half a day and all team members would help count (yay!). Prior to the count, I prepped the count sheets and cleaned up items in the software system. I assigned different categories to specific team members and walked them through the process.

At the very beginning, I also started counting but I quickly realized that everyone had a lot of questions about where items lived, how they should be counted, how to recount any big off-counts, and more. Anything they could ask about, they did. I ended up delegating my counts to someone else and spent my time answering questions and entering the counts as soon as they were finished with a count sheet. The process was smoother and faster than the first year. We were finished in an afternoon (plus an evening for me) rather than the weeks it took me by myself in the first year.

The following year, I took it one step further and started cycle counting. Through that process, I was able to keep counts accurate throughout the year. Each year, I was able to experiment and learn what worked best for that particular practice and fine-tune it even further for the next year.

So, why spend all this time and effort counting at the end of the year? Why does it even matter? If you are a practice in the United States, it's a very different reason from our cycle counts. With cycle counts, we want to quickly identify theft, missed charges, or otherwise missing inventory. Our end-of-year counts are mostly for tax purposes. This will vary depending on the business structure of your unique practice, but many need to give their accountant the value of inventory on hand at the end of the year for tax preparation and calculations.

9.7.1 An Example End-of-year Count Protocol

If you use a PiMS or other inventory software, it will likely have a report that lists each item in your inventory, the current quantity on hand, the unit cost, and the total cost for each item. It will often total the value up by category and provide a grand total at the very end of the report. If your software does not have such a report or if you do not use a software, you can do this with Excel or another spreadsheet program. You'll need:

- the item name
- the total quantity on hand
- the unit cost
- the total cost on hand for that item.

Exactly what needs to be counted tends to vary by accountant. Before the end of the year, I recommend checking with your accountant or practice owner to find out exactly what needs to be counted and how equipment, especially smaller pieces of equipment, will be handled. Some equipment will technically be considered an asset and handled differently from inventory, so it's important to understand what should or should not be included in your specific calculations.

Similarly to cycle counting, it is helpful and important prior to counting to make sure that all invoices, packing slips, or purchase orders have been received into the system, if the inventory has been already stocked in the practice. It's also important to check for any outstanding client invoices and see if any medication is waiting to be picked up.

Once your inventory has been counted, the next step is to make the appropriate adjustments in your PiMS to reflect what's currently on hand. If you are using a spreadsheet, you'll want to update the item cost and current quantity to calculate the totals for each item and then the grand total.

Here's an end-of-year count checklist to give you some ideas and inspiration.

Prep work.
- Set the date and time for your inventory counts.
- Let your team members know about the schedule and counting plan..
- Make sure all the necessary equipment is in order (counting apps, scale, barcode scanners, pill counters, etc.).
- Train any new team members on the inventory counting process.

End-of-year counts.
- Organize the space: Clean and organize any storage areas. Tip: Make sure everything is properly labeled and arranged for easy counting.
- Receive any outstanding purchase orders, receipts, invoices, etc. into your PiMS.
- Assign specific sections or categories to different team members.
- Double-check any off-counts or large discrepancies.
- Set aside items that are expired or damaged. Make note of any overstock. Later, determine whether to write off, discount, or dispose of these items.

- Reconcile discrepancies between physical counts and what's in the software. Analyze reasons why (errors, theft, missed billing, etc.) and take action, if necessary.
- Generate the end-of-year report and set aside an extra copy for safe keeping.
- Summarize your findings, discrepancies, and action steps for improvement.
- Evaluate how this year's count went and note areas you'd like to change or improve upon for next year.

After you have completed your counts, do not forget to celebrate yourself and your team! This can be a big process!

9.8 Prioritizing Your Inventory and Using an ABC Analysis

In this chapter, we have discussed how to put together an ABC analysis to categorize your products into A, B, and C categories. We also discussed different ways in which you can use this information to help evaluate your products and create a cycle count schedule. But there are other ways an ABC analysis can be helpful as well! It really is the Swiss Army knife in your inventory toolbox.

Once you have classified your products into A, B, or C categories, you can use that information to help prioritize your time, energy, and efforts. Your "A" items (which might be vaccines, cephalexin, gabapentin, or heartworm prevention) will be used more frequently and be more valuable to your practice than your "C" items. As a reminder:

- "A" products are the top 20% of your products that make up 80% of your usage and unit sales
- "B" products are the middle 30% of your products that make up 15% of your usage and unit sales
- "C" products are the bottom 50% of products that make up only 5% of your usage and unit sales.

Prioritizing your items can help you focus more on the products that are your "movers and shakers" and spend less time on the items that aren't. For example, the time and effort you spend managing vaccines should be greater than the energy spent managing tongue depressors, silver nitrate sticks, or cotton swabs.

Prioritizing and optimizing your inventory can help you focus your time on what matters most. It's a great way to pause and reflect "Does this make sense for our practice right now (and not necessarily in the past)?" When we are buzzing around day to day in our practice, going from task to task to task, sometimes the bigger picture can be lost. Optimizing your inventory is really about being intentional about what you carry and continuously improving and refining what's working well.

10

Why the Wheels Come off the Bus and How to Fix It

In the previous chapters in this book, you learned about the flow and cycle of inventory in your practice. You learned about demand forecasting and how to plan your purchases. You learned about efficient ordering, receiving, pricing, and many other systems and structures you can set up in your practice. In these next chapters, you'll focus on how you can start implementing this knowledge and systems into your inventory. This chapter teaches you how to get your inventory back on track.

10.1 What is an "Out-of-control" Inventory?

Things snowball when your inventory tactics aren't efficient and effective, and there's no control or management of inventory. It may begin as feeling unsure of what to order, but it quickly affects areas of the practice outside inventory. Maybe items start to run out, so products or supplies aren't available for patient care (which can snowball into a service miss for clients, causing mistrust in how the practice operates).

Maybe the inventory purchaser panics about running out and orders way too much (which affects the practice's financial performance). Too much cash is tied up in inventory, leaving little room for raises or hiring new team members. Cash flow becomes tight and affects how the practice functions.

Having the "wheels come off the bus" in inventory can negatively affect the practice in almost every way. But the exciting part is that once we know better, we can do better. You can learn to manage inventory effectively and make your role more enjoyable, but you also become the hero of your practice! You can shrink your giant runaway inventory snowball and see your hard work pay off.

10.1.1 Signs that Your Inventory is Functioning at a Less than Ideal Level

When your inventory is out of control, it can be summarized in one word: Chaos. What does chaos look like?

- Items constantly running out of stock.
- People asking where things are hundreds of times a day.
- Receiving texts about inventory on your days off.

Inventory Management for Veterinary Professionals, First Edition. Nicole I. Clausen.
© 2024 John Wiley & Sons, Inc. Published 2024 by John Wiley & Sons, Inc.
Companion website: www.wiley.com/go/clausen/inventory

- Free-for-all pharmacy shelves.
- No protocols for storing supplies or pharmaceuticals
- Cringing about running inventory reports in PiMs.
- Confusion about what's actually in stock.
- Overwhelm (anxiety, nervousness, guilt, fatigue, and flailing).
- The feeling of failing at your job.

When your inventory is set up properly, it is like a well-oiled machine; you feel confident, empowered, and comfortable in your skillset and systems. This chapter is a great place to start getting your inventory set up. I'm cheering you on every step of the way!

10.2   Is "Fixing" Your Inventory Worth It?

Perhaps you are thinking "Should I really fix my inventory? Is it even worth it to put in all that effort? What if I put in all this effort and nothing gets better? What if it gets even worse?"

Those thoughts and fears are a normal part of the evaluation process. Throughout this process, thinking about your "why" and checking in with what you are hoping to achieve and your overall goals can be helpful.

If you are not really sure what's possible, here are some aspects I focus on improving as I work with my clients to better their inventory:

- **Increase your skills and competence as an inventory manager**: when inventory is not set up, it can feel like you are trying to pull a giant boulder up a raging river in the middle of a snowstorm – unsettling and extremely challenging. You might question yourself and your role on the team or struggle with feelings of unworthiness and doubt. Your team might seem constantly frustrated with you, and you feel like you cannot do anything right. I've personally been there and know many other inventory managers who have been in the same situation. Helping you feel more confident in your inventory is the most important aspect for me as an educator and a consultant. So, we focus on the specific skillsets, protocols, and practices that help you own your role and responsibilities in a way that feels like "I've got this!"
- **Reduce the cost of goods sold (COGS) and inventory costs**: high inventory costs and COGS can jeopardize the practice's financial health and negatively impact profitability. Lowering your inventory costs opens up possibilities for growth and investment in your practice: Bonuses or raises, new equipment, and a secondary location. The opportunities are endless.
- **Decrease time spent managing inventory**: when systems and processes aren't set up in your inventory, managing them takes longer than necessary. The goal is a streamlined inventory system that frees up time and allows you to attend to other aspects of your practice, like your patients. If your role is solely focused on inventory, fixing your inventory can help make the day-to-day tasks easier. It frees up your time to focus on big-picture projects, like optimizing inventory, continuous improvement, and moving toward operational excellence.
- **Improve the financial performance of your practice**: streamlining your inventory can have other positive financial benefits. By decreasing the amount of inventory you carry, which reduces the value of your inventory on hand, you free up and improve cash flow. A lot of stale inventory on the shelf means money tied up in inventory. Imagine stacks of hundred-dollar bills frozen inside cubes of ice. Improving your inventory turns and reducing how much you carry on the shelf greatly impacts your bottom line.

Helpful Definitions
- **Cash flow**: the money that moves in and out of a business. Money flows in from income and payments collected from clients. It flows out for expenses like facility costs, payroll and labor costs, inventory costs, and other expenses. When there is more money coming in than going out of a practice, that creates a positive cash flow.
- **Inventory turns**: how many times a practice sells and purchases inventory in a given time period. High inventory turns are generally better because it's a sign that a practice is efficiently selling or using its products and not letting them sit on the shelves for too long.

Do you remember your "why" from the beginning of the book? Has it shifted? Knowing and remembering your why is like looking up to see light at the end of the tunnel. It will help you keep going when you have hit a rough (or frustrating!) patch.

10.3 Fixing Your Inventory

I think that managing inventory sometimes feels like trying to put an octopus back in a box. As soon as you figure out one thing, a bazillion backorders appear. As you sort those, you discover the reorder points are a huge mess or you are running out of something (again!). It seems like no matter how hard you try, you'll never fold all those suctioning, windy legs into the box.

If managing inventory has always felt like trying to put an octopus back in a box, it might be hard to imagine that it could feel differently. How do you get from "I do not even want to go in to work today because I'm terrified about what we are going to be out of" to "I feel confident in my skills and abilities as an inventory manager"?

First, focus on one octopus leg – it's easier than wrangling all eight legs simultaneously. If your inventory has been out of sorts for years (or decades), sorting everything out will not happen overnight. It will take time, research, trial and error, and maybe even tears, but it will be worth it. Streamlining and setting up your inventory helps your patients, team, and sanity today while leaving a lasting legacy in your practice for years to come.

So, how do we set up your inventory and "put the octopus in the box"? Let's dive in together.

10.3.1 Step 1: Evaluate

First and foremost, you must understand where your current inventory is and how it's functioning.

- What *is* working?
- What needs to be improved or adjusted?
- How do you feel about your skills and abilities with inventory?

Surveying the current systems and processes, your skillsets, the team's capacity, and your bandwidth for change will provide direction and insight into where you should start first and the desired end result.

10.3.2 Step 2: Audit

Auditing your inventory has two parts. Part one focuses on the bird's eye view of your inventory, while the second part focuses on what systems are and how they function. The process of tackling and setting up your inventory is very much like gardening.

Imagine you purchase a new house and there is a very overgrown garden with a lot of potential. You look at the weathered garden beds full of weeds, some flowering plants, and overgrown vines – the whole space smells faintly of lavender and you can see the dried purple buds scattered throughout the tangle. At first glance, it's overwhelming to look at. Where do you start? There is so much overgrowth that it's hard to imagine it ever functioning as a garden.

You take a deep, grounding breath and survey the situation. It's hard to see exactly what is what, but beneath old ivy are sunflower stakes, runaway blackberry bushes, and countless grasses and weeds that hide a stone garden path. There are bird feeders swaying empty in a light breeze and deteriorated bags of seed leaning up against the wall. The hose needs a new sprayer, and the cherry tree is so wide and wild that little sunlight breaks through the branches to reach the vegetable boxes. Once you have *audited* the overgrown garden, you can break it into more manageable, bite-sized pieces and tasks.

The first step is to get the pruners and cut away what's dead, dying, or invasive. You have a plan, there is hope, and it feels better already.

When we are just starting to fix our inventory, it can feel like a giant, overgrown garden. Auditing our inventory allows us to survey the current situation and uncover what's most important to start tackling first. When surveying your inventory, I recommend setting some uninterrupted time aside so you can focus and really think about where you currently are and where you want to be.

"Best Practice" Auditing Questions
As you are auditing the big-picture view of your inventory, here are some questions to help jump-start the process.

- What part of your inventory works best?
- What part needs the most work? Or what aspect seems the most stressful?
- How do you feel about your skills and abilities?
- How often do you run out of things? Why does that tend to happen?
- How often do nonemergency meds expire?
- What would it look like if you could wave a magic wand with your inventory?

Once you've reviewed some of your inventory's bigger themes and structures, it's time to zoom in and look at specific systems. Are there any processes or systems you have learned in this book that you want to set up right away? Is there a particular aspect that you want to address first? Ask yourself these questions.

- Do you have well-designed and organized inventory location "zones," and are all or most items clearly labeled?
- Do you use reorder points and reorder levels to know when something is low?
- Do you know what you have on the shelf? Do you have accurate(ish) counts of all your items and their locations, and do you know if any are soon to expire?
- Do you have an ordering routine and schedule that works with your other roles?
- Do you have documented policies and procedures for all phases of inventory management?
- Do you use intentional and consistent descriptions of your items? Does your team regularly charge correctly or is there confusion often?
- Do you have processes for receiving your inventory (especially controlled substances and temperature-controlled items)?
- Are units of measures defined in your PiMS (for example: per ml, per capsule, per weight class, per bottle, etc.)?
- Do you have a system for increasing your prices as costs go up?

This is a great time to meet with your team, practice owner, and management team to get their feedback on what to tackle and what could be improved from their perspective. It helps you understand their desires and helps them know what you'll be trying to accomplish and achieve through the inventory setup process.

When meeting with your team, you could ask the following questions.

- Ask about their preferences and any specific supply, product, or equipment questions. For example: Do you like this brand of IV catheters? What about the syringes and needles we purchase?
- What's frustrating for you when it comes to inventory?
- Do you have any ideas or suggestions on how we could improve our inventory?
- If one thing about our inventory could be improved, what would it be?

After answering some of these questions and surveying your inventory, what jumps out at you? What are the areas that need immediate attention? For example, if you find that you are always running out of items, you are placing orders every single day, or products are expiring left and right, that would signal to me that your reorder point and demand forecasting processes should move to the top of the list. If your team constantly cannot find what they need and it feels like inventory is all over the place, organization and adding in physical reorder points (like reorder tags or reorder bins) might be a great place to start.

"Best Practice" Example Priority List
- Evaluate our pricing – "What are our dispensing fees and current markup percentages? What is the process for increasing prices as costs go up? When was the last time our pricing structure was evaluated?"
- Calculate reorder points and set up reorder flags for our top items.
- Reorganize the central and treatment room storage areas.
- Organize the refrigerator and freezer, paying special attention to vaccines and in-house lab testing supplies.

Now that you have a more solid understanding of where you want to go and a path forward, set time aside to devote to reestablishing your inventory. If, after auditing your inventory, you still feel overwhelmed and are unsure where to start, below are some activities and action steps you can take to start building momentum.

10.3.3 Step 3: Identify Slow-moving Items

Before you start adding in reorder points or creating solid pricing structures, it's beneficial to identify your slow-moving items (you know, those dusty ones at the back of the shelf). One of my favorite activities for this is called the circle dot challenge or color dot quest. I'm not sure who originally came up with this, but a fellow inventory manager told me about it when I just started. I've been using and recommending it ever since! This activity is a great way to visualize how quickly (or slowly) items come in and leave your practice.

In this activity, you place colored sticker dots on everything in your inventory. You can do it for a few specific categories, but I recommend you do your *entire* inventory. Sometimes, the daily tasks of inventory management keep you from seeing the big picture. You might think you know how quickly products are used but in my experience with clients, it's hard to have an accurate picture when your focus is split. However, if you want to first "trial" this activity, I recommend starting with your prescription and retail diet category.

Table 10.1   An example worksheet you can use to note which products still have colored dot stickers.

Day 15	Day 30	Day 60	Day 90
Product A	Product A	Product B	Product B
Product B	Product B	Product C	
Product C	Product C		

What you'll need:
- colored circle stickers (one color is all that's needed)
- a piece of paper or spreadsheet for taking notes.

To complete the color dot quest:
1) add a color dot sticker to every item in your inventory on day one. This should include every bottle, every tray of vaccines, and every bag of dog food. Make a note of the date as "day one" or your starting date
2) after day one, do not add any more stickers
3) after 15 days, make a note of all the products that still have a colored dot sticker. If your goal is to stock a 30-day supply at a time, it's likely that most of your products will still have colored dots. You can skip this step and check after 30 days instead
4) then, note all the remaining products after 30, 60, and 90 days (Table 10.1).

Ideally, there should not be any sticker dots left, depending on your turnover goal, after 60 or 90 days. If any products still remain, it tells you that the item has not sold in over 90 days. There are practices that have done the challenge and called me a year later to say that some products *still* have stickers!

This activity is one of my favorites because it easily gives you so much information (no calculations necessary!) about what products are selling and which aren't. After you have identified your "slow movers," you can use this data to decide if you (i) need to update your order point or the bottle size that's purchased, (ii) discontinue selling the item and move it to an online pharmacy, or (iii) discuss the results with your team.

"Best Practice" Questions to Consider
- Would the circle dot challenge be helpful for you?
- Are there specific categories you'd especially like to check for slow-moving items, or would you prefer to start with your entire inventory?
- Brainstorm some ideas for when you'd like to complete this activity, who you'd like to have involved, and what the process will look like.

10.3.4   Step 4: Unearth Inventory Discrepancies

Using inventory counts and discrepancies can be a great diagnostic tool for your inventory. Looking at the difference between what you have on the shelf and what the on-hand quantity is in your PiMS can give you a lot of insight. For example, if you have 124 capsules of doxycycline 100 mg but your software says that you have −9,482 units on the shelf, you know there is some work to do. Alternatively, if you are looking at Douxo® Calm shampoo and have three bottles on the shelf but your software says that you have four, there is different work to do. Knowing what inventory you have on the shelf is important because you cannot manage what you do not know is there.

Without monitoring on-hand amounts, it's nearly impossible to detect if products walk out the door, charges are missed, or inventory is mishandled.

"Best Practice" Unveiling Inventory Discrepancies

To start unveiling inventory discrepancies, take a small cross-section of your inventory items.
1) Pick a handful of items from various categories.
2) Count how many units are on the shelf and compare that to what your software expects you to have.
3) Ask:
   - Are there significant differences? Small differences? Or is it basically the same?
   - Are the levels of discrepancies similar for each product or category, or are there big inconsistencies between the categories?

Let's explore an example together. The team at Tank's Animal Hospital is going through the process of fixing their inventory, and they want to understand how "off" their software system is and dive into analyzing the discrepancies. Heather, one of the inventory managers, and Dr Tank work together to make a list of five different products, and Heather counts what's on the shelf. Here are the results.

Item	Category	What's on the shelf	What's in the software	Difference
Product A	Otic solutions	3	−17	20
Product B	Supplements	8	−92	100
Product C	Vaccines	37	389	352
Product D	Antibiotics	749	−9,842	10,591
Product E	Heartworm prevention	57	−256	313

Based on the results from the investigation, Dr Tank and Heather realize that some categories and some products have significantly greater differences than others. Knowing that information, Heather can dive into investigating the categories with more extreme differences first.

Once the "problem" items or categories are identified, explore further.

- Are there receiving problems? Do receiving protocols and systems need to be established or is retraining necessary?
- Are charges getting missed? Can we audit medical records to verify?
- Has it been an extremely long time since items were last counted, and a "reset" needs to happen?
- What other reasons can you think of to explain the discrepancies you found?

Once you start pulling back the layers, you can identify what needs your attention and what you should tackle first.

10.4   A Surefire Way to Keep Your Important Items in Stock

When you are short-handed or your inventory is "in transition" and you are working on setting up your systems, it can feel chaotic and ungrounded. Some items have reorder points on them but some do not, so you cannot rely on those quite yet. You're short-staffed and split between your roles as a client service representative (CSR) and veterinary assistant, and you are just trying to place an order quickly in between appointments. No matter what is keeping you from feeling competent or confident in your role, it's important to have a system for keeping your most important items in stock.

Rather than trying to keep your most important items at the top of your mind all the time, create a secret weapon in the inventory toolbox: A VIP (Very Important Products) checklist! A VIP checklist is a list of all your most important items (Tip: include the reorder levels for easy reference). Having a list of your most critical and popular items builds in a double-check when placing an order. You can quickly review the products on this list to make sure enough is in stock.

A VIP checklist can also be leveraged as a tool to delegate responsibility in your inventory. If you have limited time while "holding down" the front desk or trying to submit payroll, another team member can review the products on the VIP checklist and mark any key items that are running low. The list can also be used for critical emergency meds in your portable emergency kit or "crash cart."

Common important or top-selling items to use as inspiration for your VIP checklist include the following.

- Vaccines
- Controlled substances
- Paper towels or toilet paper
- Carprofen
- Apoquel®
- Rx labels or dram vials
- Cytopoint™
- Euthanasia solution
- Dexmedetomidine
- In-house laboratory testing supplies (clips, rotors, reagent kit, etc.)
- Antisedan®
- Premedication and/or induction agents
- Cephalexin
- Cerenia® injection
- Heartworm prevention

I know it can feel like *all* of your inventory is critical to patient care, but making a list of the most valuable, most important items gives you a quick reference cheat sheet, just in case. It's extremely valuable, and many of my clients have one separate from their PiMS as an emergency backup measure.

Turn building this list into a fun group activity to get your team members' insight and help them feel involved. This discussion can take place with all your practice members at once, or you can speak with different departments or sections of the care team individually. To help facilitate participation, partner different groups together to brainstorm what their list would be. Then, bring everyone back together and write all the options on a large whiteboard. Once each group gives their suggestions, everyone can work together to determine what are the VIPs for your practice.

"Best Practice" Steps for Creating a Group Activity and Getting the Team Involved

1) Gather all team members who will be involved in this activity.
2) Start the meeting off by providing background. Then, connect with their "why" and explain why it impacts the practice and patient care. Explain the activity.

3) Break everyone into groups of four or six, depending on the size of the team. If you have a practice with lots of team members, you could meet with each department separately or use larger group sizes for this activity.
4) Set a timer for 10 minutes and have each team brainstorm all the critical products for your practice.
5) At the end of the 10 minutes, have a spokesperson from each team give their VIP list.
6) Write each group's list on a whiteboard (or something similar).
7) Then, work together to narrow down the list and conclude what should be included in your practice's VIP list. Try to aim for 15–30 products.

Whether you create a VIP checklist yourself or involve your team, the end result is a quick reference list to make sure your most important items are in stock and do not get forgotten (no matter what happens during the day).

10.5   Why the Wheels Come off the Bus

The wheels on your "inventory bus" can come off for a number of reasons. When your inventory starts to feel out of control, it can seem chaotic, not only for you but the rest of your team as well. The good news is that it is possible for you to set up your inventory and take control back. You can feel empowered and confident in your skills. Your inventory can move from putting an octopus back in a box to a flourishing garden. The first step is to audit your inventory and understand where you are at. Then, you can start fixing your inventory and set up systems and processes that make managing inventory so much easier.

The core challenge of managing inventory is that there is not much education on exactly *how* to manage inventory in a veterinary practice. It's not taught in veterinary school and is rarely covered during veterinary technician training. Even many practice manager programs do not effectively teach inventory management! Many current inventory managers were inadequately trained by the person before them.

So, we have this situation where there is not much training or education available on how to set up effective inventory systems, compounded by the fact that there aren't a lot of intuitive, easy-to-use tools to make it easy. Then, we add gasoline to the fire by often not having enough time or person power in the practice to manage inventory. As inventory managers, we often wear many hats and there's a strong desire to help our practice – which sometimes comes at the expense of our own well-being and mental health.

If that sounds familiar, it's not a personal or practice-level failing that your inventory got a little sideways. The fact that you are reading this book right now speaks to the exact opposite of that. If your inventory feels way too overwhelming and you are embarrassed about how out of control it feels, you are in very good company here.

Wherever you are in your inventory journey, I invite you to think about how you can celebrate yourself along the way. It can be a long road getting your inventory in order and your systems set up, plus you are simultaneously ordering, receiving, and managing at the same time. It can be hard for our teams to understand how much time, effort, and brain power goes into it all.

Here are some ideas and inspiration for celebrating yourself along the way and reminding yourself how far you have come.

- Take before-and-after pictures of spaces that you organize so you can remember how things looked before you started.

- Keep a favorite treat (like peppermint tea or apples and peanut butter) in the breakroom and enjoy it after you have finalized an order.
- Take a quick walk outside and get some sun on your face after deep cleaning or organizing a space.
- Keep a file (either physically or digitally) and save all the thank you notes and kind words that you get to remember how awesome you are.
- Join a community of inventory managers, like the Veterinary Inventory Strategy Network or the Veterinary Inventory Management Group on Facebook, to be connected with other folks who see you and genuinely care about you.
- Keep some words of affirmation on a sticky note on your computer monitor or on your phone's lock screen as a reminder to yourself.
- If you have an office or other dedicated space (if you are able to), make it comforting, cozy, or another favorite vibe/atm.

"Best Practice" Personal Care Questions
- How can you celebrate your small wins?
- What about your big wins and checking off big projects or milestones?
- How else can you support yourself (or ask for support!) through this process?

As you continue, you may find that one common theme is frustration from your team. Their main focus is patient care, so while you are working on overhauling your inventory, your focus is not patient care. It might appear to them like you are just sitting around doing computer work. Meanwhile, you aren't just playing solitaire – you are fixing every single item in your software, pouring your brain into setting up codes, making adjustments, and fine-tuning your inventory. But your team likely does not realize how much work this process involves (Figure 10.1).

Not only that but, as you are working through your pricing or reorder points, prices will likely change; you might be stocking less of a particular item or have discontinued some items

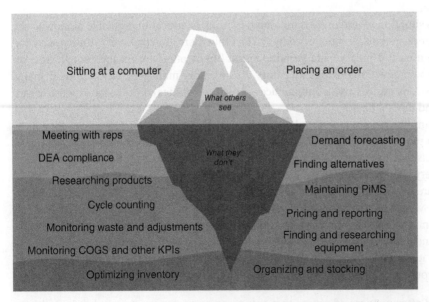

Figure 10.1 What your team can see versus what they do not always see as you manage inventory. *Source:* Iceberg graphic by Valerie Bodnar. Reproduced under license from Creative Market.

completely. This process will involve many changes, including changes your team can and cannot see. Setting expectations and involving your team in what's happening is helpful. I know it can feel discouraging and disheartening to put in all this work for your practice and feel like you are getting nothing but disrespect or contempt in return. The inventory managers who work through this phase well focus on communicating clearly and respecting themselves and their boundaries throughout the process.

The practice owner or manager can explain the changes to the team and empower the inventory manager to start this process. An inventory manager can work with their management team to discuss goals, vision, and projects they are working on so management can also communicate any necessary information to the team.

Just because you are not directly involved with patient care does not mean you are any less valuable or important in your practice. You can gently remind people of this: "Thank you for valuing my work with patient care, but right now, I need to focus on making sure that the patient care team has everything that we need and that the profitability of the business stays healthy. I know that may feel like you are carrying more work for the time being, but trust that this is an important process for the entire business." Focusing on inventory, operations, or systems really enables patient care and allows it to thrive. I invite you to keep one of my favorite affirmations in mind:

There is space for me to grow.
I am not confined to my current situation or inventory systems;
there is a season for everything, and no season is permanent.
I can let go, and I can embrace change with an open heart.

11

You're Brand New... Now What? How to Set Up Your Inventory

If you are a brand new inventory manager, welcome to the world of inventory! If you are just starting, the section below outlines some important considerations for you. If you are a veterinarian who recently purchased a practice or is starting up a de novo practice, there are sections later in this chapter to help you get started.

Helpful Definition
- **De novo practice**: a brand new practice that is starting from scratch. Instead of buying an existing practice, a veterinarian builds or establishes it independently.

11.1 You're a Brand New Inventory Manager ... Now What?

First off, congratulations!! Welcome to the world of inventory! You are in good company. If you have read the earlier chapters of this book, you may be feeling overwhelmed and wondering how you'll do it all. Do not worry, that is completely normal! Managing inventory involves many moving parts, and nobody wants to let their team down. Take a deep breath. Remember that this is why you are reading this book – to gain the tools you need to do the job well.

People enter inventory management from a lot of different places. I moved from a receptionist/care team helper to also wearing the "inventory manager hat" for my practice. Others are hired as inventory managers already possessing the skillset (through on-the-job training). Some come fresh-faced straight from school. Others are given the task of inventory management after the previous person left the practice. Whether you are shifting into a position of inventory management in your current practice or a brand new hire as an inexperienced or experienced inventory manager, this section is helpful to start on the right foot.

If you are new to inventory versus new to the practice or new to both at once, your first steps will look different but have the same goal: To assess your inventory and understand the nuances of your unique practice. This focus will help you in managing inventory today and down the road. Here are some areas to evaluate and (hopefully) ask the person training you about.

11.1.1 What are the Current Inventory Policies?

How does your practice currently manage inventory? Find out from whoever is training you what the current processes are and how they work. What information is critical or important for you to know? Ask your team members how inventory seems to be working. Is there anything they have a hard time finding? Do products run out often? Is there anything frustrating for them?

Inventory Management for Veterinary Professionals, First Edition. Nicole I. Clausen.
© 2024 John Wiley & Sons, Inc. Published 2024 by John Wiley & Sons, Inc.
Companion website: www.wiley.com/go/clausen/inventory

As a brand new inventory manager, my training was extremely limited, and I was never told that I needed to order rabies tags toward the end of every year. In my first year as inventory manager, I did not even think to buy rabies tags for the new year. After a very dear fellow receptionist asked about them, I realized much too late that I needed to order them. They did not arrive until two weeks into the New Year, creating quite a backlog of new tags to be issued. Ask as many questions as you can to help understand what your role is and what your responsibilities are. Doing so will help you in the long run.

11.1.2 What are the Current Inventory Zones?

Where are items currently stored in the practice? Where are the pharmacy, the backup, or the secondary pharmacy storage areas? Where are hospital supplies and white goods currently stored? Learn as much as you can about where everything is stored, and make a list so you have a reference handy in the future.

11.1.3 What are Your Top 20 Products?

Talk with your veterinarians, practice owner, management team, and the rest of the care team, and find out what they consider to be the top products in the practice. This will help you to know what products to focus on and ensure you do not run out. If your practice utilizes a practice management system or another software system, you can often run a report to see the top products. You can also use your vendor reps and ask them for a report of your practice's top purchased items. Afterward, I invite you to create a list of your top products for easy reference (think VIP [Very Important Product] checklist!).

11.1.4 Who are Your Vendors?

Next, find out what vendors your practice uses and who the preferred manufacturers or distributors are. If your practice orders specialty supplies or medications, find out what those items are and where they are purchased. Are there any other special orders that you should be aware of? It's helpful to find out if you are part of any buying groups or group purchasing organizations that give you extra savings or preferred pricing. Knowing your vendors and any unique purchasing incentives guides you on where to order from.

11.1.5 What are the Shipping Times and Other Important Shipping Information?

After discovering your vendors, it's important to understand shipping speeds. Are there vendors that are faster than others? Do you have order minimums or shipping charges you should know about? How do they handle items that must be kept cold, and how reliable are their delivery dates? Knowing the shipping speeds and if there are any order minimums can help you navigate purchasing and plan for ordering.

Once you have surveyed your new role and learned as much as you can about how inventory works currently in your practice, it's time to master the art of inventory ordering. How does your practice know when something is running low? What's in place now to help plan for what needs to be purchased? Are there reorder points already in place that you can use or will you need to rely on other methods? If your practice does not currently use reorder points or has no minimum thresholds for items, you must understand what "low" means for each item.

Depending on the level of training you received, knowing what is "low" will probably be a little difficult in the beginning, and you may have to lean on your team. This will be especially true if you are brand new to the practice. If you have worked at the practice for a while, even if it was in a different position, you might already have a sense of what "low" means for each item. Additionally, as you order and discover what's low, you can view sale reports in your practice to see how much has sold recently to help guide the replenishment of that product.

If your practice does not have a system for calculating reorder points, start there. Calculating those order levels and setting up "flags" to know when something is low changes the game! It makes ordering much easier, and you'll feel more confident you are ordering the right products each week. You'll know what's running low and have a reference point for how much to order. To learn more about calculating and setting up reorder points, review Chapter 3.

While becoming familiar with your practice and inventory management, you should walk around with this book under your arm to refer back to the chapters that will help. You'll look nerdy (in the best way), and inventory managers are a nerdy bunch. Embrace it!

Managing inventory can be challenging (especially when there aren't many systems set up), but it can also be fun and rewarding. Knowing that you enable patient care and are the inventory rockstar that helps set your team up for success is a great feeling. There will always be challenging or difficult days, especially when a rogue backorder pops up on a very important item. Still, the more competence you have in inventory management, the easier it is to handle these situations skillfully and gracefully. And I also want you to know that you are not alone if you are struggling and feeling discouraged.

I've certainly experienced my fair share of negative time periods, and many other inventory managers (friends, colleagues, and clients) have too. Your fellow inventory managers are rooting for you even during the hard days or the frustrating times. My hope is that you remember how valuable and important your role is (you care for the health of the entire ecosystem of your practice) and that there are lots of resources and tactics throughout this book to make managing inventory easier for you.

Whether you are starting a new practice, you are a brand new practice owner, or you have been newly appointed to the role of inventory manager, you can do it! At first glance, it might seem daunting and overwhelming, but setting up systems and structures in your practice to guide and support inventory management will be a game changer for you (and your team, patients, and your practice)!

11.2 Author's Note

Starting any new adventure is a wonderful mix of excitement, nervousness, and everything in between. I remember when I first started Veterinary Care Logistics, I thought I was going to be a "traditional consulting firm." And then life happened, COVID hit, and I leaned more into what brought me joy. Looking back at my five-year plan, it makes me giggle. When I started my business, I could never have imagined having five online courses, including an inventory manager certification program, hosting a podcast, being a co-founder of an inventory software, and working with most of my clients remotely.

I'm so glad things did not turn out the way I expected.

Part of the adventure is facing the unknown, embracing uncertainty, and trusting yourself. I think the same can be said for your inventory when starting a new practice. Much of this book has focused on improving your current inventory. But how do you do that when you are a brand new practice with no history? Later in this chapter, I'll share some strategies that can help if you are a practice owner who is purchasing an existing practice.

11.3   You're a Veterinarian Starting a Brand New Practice ... Now What?

When you are just getting started and opening a new practice, your path forward will vary slightly depending on whether you have an established clientele in the area or if you are starting fresh in a new territory. If you have clients that will follow you in the area or if you are more certain about the anticipated patient load or type of cases you'll see, you might have a sense of how much inventory you'll use during the "start-up" phase. You might have more questions if you are new to the area or do not know what you'll need.

First off, congratulations on starting a new practice or being part of a practice that is just starting out! There are probably quite a few questions swirling around in your brain about inventory and "how do I know what to order? How do I make this all work?" I am glad that you are here so we can walk through this process together.

"Best Practice" Getting Started Brainstorm
At the very beginning of this process, I invite you to consider a few questions before diving in.

- How do you feel about your performance and skills related to your inventory? Have you managed inventory before or seen it done well at another practice?
- What manufacturers or vendors are you certain that you want to work with? Do you know what brand of vaccines, heartworm prevention, flea/tick prevention, diets, in-house laboratory tests, or other brands you'd like to carry?
- Are you new to the area or do you have an established clientele? Do you have any thoughts on what the demand or patient load will be when you open?
- How quickly do you anticipate growing and adding new veterinarians?
- As you think about your practice, what are your mission and vision? What clients and patients do you want to serve? What are your values? In what ways will this affect your inventory?
    - For example, if you are a large animal rural practice, you'll need to stock much differently than a metro mobile practice. If you are a boutique specialty center with a very specific patient population, you'll also have very different inventory needs.
- Do you have a main distributor in mind that you'd like to work with? Or are you flexible and still need to find a "best fit" distributor?
    - Remember, a distributor (like MWI Animal Health) is like an online grocery store. They will carry most things you need to purchase and will have all your favorite products and brands that you can buy from; this saves you having to buy from each vendor individually.
- How familiar are you with the Drug Enforcement Administration (or similar organization if you are outside the United States) regulations for controlled substances? Do you feel confident about the requirements as the DEA registrant? For more information on controlled substance regulations, see Chapter 12.
- What practice management system are you planning to use?
- What have you discussed with the software team about the inventory module? Will you receive any training? Will there be any assistance adding or transferring inventory into the software?

Answering these questions gives you a solid foundation and understanding of where you are currently while showing you the gaps in your knowledge for where you want to go.

11.4   Getting Your Inventory Started Overview

One of the first things you'll (likely) need to do is open accounts with the vendors and manufacturers you'd like to use. Before you officially open an account, check with them on the timing of their "new practice program."

Many distributors and vendors have what's called a "new practice program." Depending on the company, they offer different promotions and special financing options for new practices. Some of these programs have timeline restrictions on what's considered a "new practice," so it's important to check with the vendors on time-frame restrictions before opening the account.

These programs typically offer significant discounts and promotions: "buy one, get one free" and "delayed billing." Your first instinct might be to buy "a lot" because it's cheap now and you'll use it eventually, right? I advise my clients to err on the conservative side and the anticipated demand or patient load. Suppose you have a very loyal client base already. In that case, you'll probably purchase very differently from someone starting a practice in a brand new area without an established client base.

I have talked with many veterinarians who have purchased too much through new practice programs and later regretted it! (Remember: overordering and underordering can be equally detrimental to the health of a practice.)

That said, the field representative for your chosen distributor can be a great resource. They often have lists of "new clinic recommendations" that outline everything from antibiotics to hospital supplies, which can be a helpful reference to ensure you do not forget something important to patient care! It's not beneficial if you have everything to place an IV catheter . . . besides the actual catheter or catheter cap! Distributors often have equipment teams to help ensure you purchase the equipment with the necessary and correct specifications.

"Best Practice" Tip

I find it helpful to create a list or spreadsheet of all the items, products, and supplies that you want to order. Then, set aside your list for a while and come back to it with fresh eyes. Is there anything that you are missing? Do you have any team members or colleagues you can check with to get their opinion? Depending on how your brain works, it might be helpful to start this list well in advance of the open date so that you have plenty of time to refine, add, and change things as you go.

11.4.1   Building a New Facility

If you are building a new facility, it's important to make sure that your architect, building designer, or whoever is on your team is leaving enough intentional room for the pharmacy and storage areas. I often encounter practices that did not build nearly enough storage and now, half of the treatment kennels are just used as inventory storage! It's also helpful to consider your long-term growth and vision. Do you anticipate just being a one-veterinarian practice or do you want to hire additional veterinarians in the future? There are plenty of veterinary-specific builders that can help make sure you are starting out on the right foot.

Whether you are building a new facility or renovating an existing building, creating inventory "zones" and deciding where products will be stored is helpful to make sure you have allocated enough space for inventory. Where will your pharmacy be located? What about secondary back-stock storage? Will that need a lock and key or some other restricted access? Review Chapter 6 for security, protection, and organization tips. Will you have a dedicated central storage or will the inventory organization run throughout the practice? Start planning your inventory zones so that when your first order arrives, you already know where items will be stored.

11.4.2 After Your First Opening Order

Once you have opened up accounts with all your vendors and decided on your first opening order, the next step is to decide what you'll do with all of your inventory!

"Best Practice" Considerations

- Who on your team will be in charge of ordering, receiving, organizing, or other individual phases of inventory management? Will it be you or will specific tasks be delegated to other team members?
- According to your estimated open date, when will the order need to be placed?
- How will the newly purchased opening order be recorded? Will it be entered into the practice management system or another inventory software?

Before placing your opening order, prepare an action plan for "what's next." A lot of inventory will arrive at your practice, often just before the open date, so it's important to have a game plan for navigating the arrival. If all the inventory will be received into the practice management system, set up the inventory and procedure/treatment codes before the order arrives.

Tip: If you have not used the software before or if there is no one on the team who is very familiar with the program, work with the software support team to understand exactly how to set up each code and then document the process. You'll likely need to add a lot of new codes, so it's important to remember the correct setup.

Often, I am called in when practice management systems go "sideways" because the codes were not set up correctly. Once you are in practice and working day to day, it is difficult to go back and fix (or reset) any setup errors. Setting yourself up for success means correctly setting up the codes before the doors open. You might need to decide how you'll want to charge for some things (which can always change as you go), but as long as the setup process is understood, you can update or change it later.

When you are thinking about your codes and how to set them up, I recommend creating a "new item guide" outlining the step-by-step process: What information needs to be added, linked, and entered for different codes. For example, you might have a treatment code with a flat weight range (ProHeart® 26–50 lb), but you want the inventory linked on the backend to record how many milliliters were used. How will that be set up in your system? What if you wanted one treatment code (like Premedication Administration, which is included in surgical procedures) to have a price of $0.00, but you want all the injection possibilities linked on the backend so your team can select what meds were used and the amount administered? How would you set this up?

Tip: Review Chapter 8 for tips on selling your inventory accurately and setting up your practice management system for success.

Now that your inventory and treatment codes are set up, linked together, and situated appropriately, the next step is to create a system of documenting all your received inventory. These documents can live in your practice management system, another software, a spreadsheet, or another manual process. Your practice, your choice. Just make sure it works!

As mentioned in an earlier chapter, when using a practice management system, it's helpful to receive invoices and packing slips to update the quantity on hand, increase prices as costs go up, track inventory counts, and leverage reorder levels and quantities. Whether you use software, other technology, or a manual process (Figure 11.1), have a log or list of all the inventory in your practice, how much you purchased it for, the quantities, the selling price of the item, and other pertinent information (like expiry date).

Expect a flurry of activity when the opening order arrives! Boxes to unpack, items to verify and put away, invoices and packing slips to check off and receive, and plenty more.

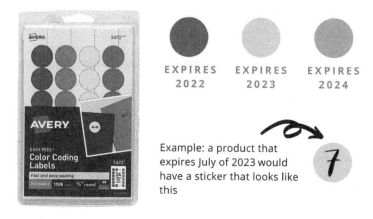

Figure 11.1 An example of a manual method for tracking expiry dates. Nicole Clausen.

Before your first order arrives, set time aside to brainstorm or outline several policies. You may have an idea prior to opening what policies you'd like to establish, but you can always fine-tune, improve upon, or change them as you go!

- What type of expiry date tracking system will you use? Can you use your software, or will you need to track expiry dates manually?
  - A note on expiry dates in your software: Some practice management systems do not manage expiry dates or lot numbers well. Some will assume which container you are dispensing from (and it's never accurate). Others only have the capacity to manage one at a time. Before deciding on a method, look into how your specific software handles this.
  - Expiry dates can be tracked manually using a color dot sticker, a spreadsheet, your practice management system or other inventory software, or a combination of the different methods. Ideally, you'll want to know if a product will expire in the next three months so you can plan how to handle it. Additionally, I recommend evaluating if a product has expired to see if it should still be stocked.
- How will items be shelved? Will you use the FIFO (first in, first out) rule on the shelf? Or will containers be stored according to their expiry dates?
- Decide on a good system and create a policy for discrepancies, wasted, or expired inventory.
- What will your emergency drug or crash cart situation look like? Ensure you have a properly stocked emergency kit that includes all emergency drugs, supplies, dosage charts, and other beneficial information or tools.
- Be sure to start your safety data sheet binder (or digital version, if approved by your state/area) and add all medications, cleaners, and any other required items to this binder for staff to know where to find the hazard and safety precautions of these items.

Once your practice opens and you start seeing patients, you'll likely have a good sense of growth and caseload. You will likely not be able to set reorder points right away. Typically, I like to start calculating reorder points around the three-month mark (this could be sooner or later, depending on your situation). Until then, a helpful way to order is to replenish and purchase how much you have sold. For example, if you notice that doxycycline is running low, you can review a sales report from your software to see how much you have sold in the last two weeks or 30 days. Based on that, you'll have an idea of how much to order. If you are growing at a very fast pace for very high-use or important items (like vaccines, for instance), you might consider adjusting that number to reflect the anticipated growth.

I wish I could say it will be perfect every time! But when opening a new practice, there are often unexpected changes or situations that you'll need to adapt to, and that's especially true for inventory. There might be times when you run out or forget to order something, but sometimes that is growing pains. If that happens, remember to be a detective rather than a perfectionist. How could you handle it differently next time to prevent that situation from happening again? What systems (like reorder tags or an order checklist) could you put in place?

Taking time before your practice opens (and continuing the process when you open) to establish systems, structures, and policies in your inventory can set you up for years to come!

11.5 Example: Setting Up Your Inventory Action Plan

This checklist contains various examples of action steps and systems you can use to set up your inventory. The section headers correspond to different chapters in the book, so if you'd like more information and guidance, please refer to that specific chapter to learn more.

11.5.1 Chapter 3: Forecasting and Purchase Planning

- Review how to set up reorder points in your practice management system.
  - You'll need more sales data information/history before calculating and setting up reorder points for your practice. But knowing how to accomplish this once you have enough history is helpful.
  - Tip: I recommend setting up reorder points around the three-month mark after opening. You know your practice, so adjust this timeline if needed!
- Create a list of product categories and determine what types of reorder points you'd like to use (for example, reorder tags for hospital supplies and electronic reorder points in your software system for things that are sold) (Figure 11.2).
- Identify any seasonal products and make a note to calculate seasonal reorder points when applicable.

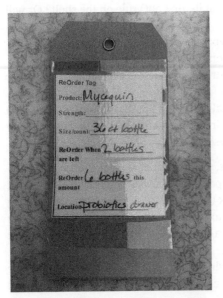

Figure 11.2 An example of reorder tags that Chrissy Mohr, inventory manager and Certified Veterinary Inventory Professional, has created for her practice. *Source:* Courtesy of Chrissy Mohr.

11.5.2 Chapter 4: Efficient Ordering and Replenishment

- Outline an ideal ordering cadence and schedule. When will you place orders? What vendors will you use (i.e., prescription diets, regular orders, specialty products, etc.)?
- Learn what report to run for products flagged low when it's time to order.
- Learn how to create a purchase order in your practice management system.
- Once an order has been placed, create a purchase order in your software so that receiving is easier and you can tell if something arrived incorrectly.
- Learn how to add and create new products in your inventory.

11.5.3 Chapters 5 and 6: Receiving and Organizing Your Inventory

- Learn how to receive purchase orders in your software. Note: I recommend receiving purchase orders within 24 hours of shipment delivery and updating the costs each time you order.
- Ensure that each item has a designated primary "home" and a defined backup or secondary location. Each location should be labeled with any helpful information, as well as the backstock location (Figures 11.3 and 11.4).

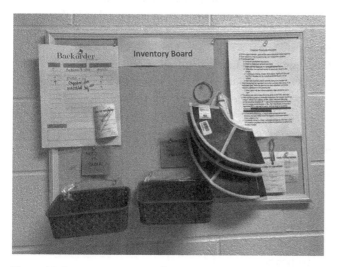

Figure 11.3 An example of an "inventory board" created by Lisa Sideropolis, Clinic Manager and RVT at Rescue Village. The board has a list of backordered products, an inventory receiving checklist, reorder tag bins, and more. *Source:* Courtesy of Lisa Sideropolis.

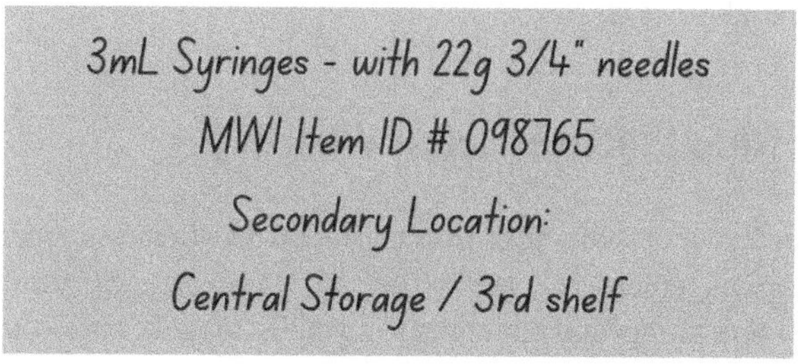

3mL Syringes - with 22g 3/4" needles
MWI Item ID # 098765
Secondary Location:
Central Storage / 3rd shelf

Figure 11.4 An example of a shelf label that includes the item name, code for ordering, and the item's secondary location. Nicole Clausen.

Table 11.1 An example outline of a practice's desired markup percentages by category. For your practice, create a document that lists your specific categories and the corresponding desired markup.

Category	Markup
Over the counter	100%
Diets	45% or manufacturer's suggested retail price (MSRP)
Injectables (can also have a sliding scale)	125–300%
Pharmaceuticals	Sliding scale (e.g., <$0.05 per unit –400%. Everything in between – 250% >$1.00 per unit – 125%)
Competitively shopped items	50–100%
Retail items	100%

11.5.4 Chapter 7: Strategic Inventory Pricing

- Document your current pricing strategy. Ensure that each item in your inventory has a markup percentage, dispensing/injection or special fees, and any other important pricing-related information.

11.5.4.1 Example Markup Percentages by Category

- Learn how to set up pricing exceptions and how to increase prices as costs go up. (This is typically done with a markup percentage when receiving items on a purchase order.) If you are manually pricing your items using a formula, outline a process and standard operating procedure so they are always calculated and increased appropriately (Table 11.1).

11.5.5 Chapter 8: Appropriate Inventory Sales and Consumption

- Link any relevant inventory items to procedure codes.
- Learn how to set up different bundles and packages so that inventory items can be linked to bundles to pull out of inventory appropriately.
- Test any complex codes, bundles, or packages before trying to add them to open invoices.

11.5.6 Chapter 9: Optimizing Your Inventory

- Brainstorm a cycle count schedule. Tip: Remember to start small if needed. The benefits of cycle counting are really seen when it's done consistently.
- Set up an expired product tracking system. Most practice management systems do not do this well, so it's often better to do this as a manual process.

11.6 You Just Purchased an Existing Practice ... Now What?

Suppose you are a veterinarian or practice owner who just purchased an existing practice. Congratulations! Operationally, inventory management is a key aspect of running a successful practice so, if you just purchased a practice, there are several elements to consider to make sure you are off and running smoothly.

The first step is to evaluate the current situation.

"Best Practice" Current Inventory Audit

Before making any changes or alterations, it's important to understand the current situation fully. The following questions will help kick off your audit.

- What is the state of the pharmacy? Are there any expired medications? Anything that you'd eventually like to discontinue? Do you see any medication "gaps" or products that you'd prefer to carry?
  - Create a list of all expired medications (if applicable) and talk to your distributor rep to see if there is anything that can be done.
  - Create a list of all the products that you'd like to discontinue. Depending on whether there are safety or efficacy issues, you might want to discontinue sooner rather than later. If there are no concerns with the product and depending on the team, a phased approach to changes might be helpful.
  - Create a list of products or supplies that you'd like to add to the formulary. Review Chapter 9 and the section on adding new products for tips.
- What is the state of the storage areas? Are they disorganized? Could the organization and storage be improved? Assess the layout and current inventory zones to see if anything should be shifted or improved.
- Assess the current inventory team. Who is currently in charge of inventory? Have them walk you through the process. How are they feeling about their skills and abilities in relation to inventory management? Are there any areas of opportunity for training or process improvement? Do they need more dedicated time to manage inventory?
- After working in the practice, how does inventory control feel? Does it feel chaotic? Are items constantly running out? Or does it run fairly smoothly?
- Next, assess any inventory metrics, key performance indicators, and financial performance of the practice. What is the cost of goods sold as a percentage of revenue? What about the value of inventory on hand? How does the inventory turnover stack up?
- Make a list of any processes or current policies you'd like to investigate and learn more about. What other aspects of the practice or inventory would be helpful to review?

The insights you gain from assessing and auditing the practices's inventory will help to map out areas of opportunity and improvement. Once you have outlined those areas, what feels most critical? If you are constantly running out and it's affecting patient care, start there. If items are disorganized and it's hard to find what you need, start there. I invite you to resist the urge to fix it all tomorrow (or even today!). If there have been long-term inventory challenges, getting them sorted out will take time and patience. (See Chapter 10 for more help with this.)

Plus, you'll likely have other areas of the practice that you'll need to focus on (including your patients). It's okay if it's not going to be fixed right away but with time and effort, your inventory will get there. I cannot overstate that a well-trained inventory manager is worth their weight in gold. If the person who is currently managing inventory does not feel like a "best fit" or there is a skill/values misalignment, who else might be a great candidate to take over inventory? Or what training could you provide the current inventory manager? (You can hire a consultant like me!)

Having a skilled, well-trained inventory manager, or at the very least someone who is eager to learn and grow into the role, will be an incredible asset for you. Delegate where you can and focus on your strengths and what brings you joy!

12

An Introduction to Controlled Substances

12.1 Author's Note

This chapter covers inventory management for controlled substances as well as a few Drug Enforcement Administration (DEA) regulations (one of the most important aspects of inventory management – and potentially the most confusing). One of the challenging things about controlled substance information is there is both a ton of (sometimes wrong) information out there and simultaneously none at all. I do not want to get it wrong for you. I'm not a DEA agent but I've learned from them, scoured the Federal Code of Regulations, and have lived experience as an inventory manager. This chapter feels much more vulnerable to write because I know how much is at stake when the DEA's regulations aren't properly followed.

This chapter is quite a bit more dense than others; many rules and regulations are included here. So grab a snack or a fizzy drink, and take your time reading through this.

In this chapter, you'll find specific inventory systems to have in place for your controlled substances. There are some important systems, tasks, and processes to be mindful of, and key federal-level regulations that you need to be aware of. With that being said, there are many state-specific regulations as well. I highly recommend utilizing your state Veterinary Board and Pharmacy Board to see if your state has particular regulations or rules that also need to be followed. Also, DEA regulations can and do change, so be sure to review the most current and up-to-date information! There are often controlled substance regulation webinars and online classes; this type of format will provide the most current and up-to-date information. You can usually find webinars through state veterinary associations, veterinary conferences, and other educators and consultants.

Ultimately, it's the responsibility of the DEA registrant to be fully aware of and adhere to all the necessary regulations. If your state regulations differ from federal regulations, you must follow whichever is more stringent.

This chapter is written from the perspective of controlled substance regulations in the United States. If you are outside the United States, your country will likely have different laws and regulations. So it's important to research your country's specific regulations and laws regarding controlled substances.

Inventory Management for Veterinary Professionals, First Edition. Nicole I. Clausen.
© 2024 John Wiley & Sons, Inc. Published 2024 by John Wiley & Sons, Inc.
Companion website: www.wiley.com/go/clausen/inventory

12.2 What is a Controlled Substance?

Under the Controlled Substance Act in the United States, "certain drugs, substances, and certain chemicals that are used to make drugs" (www.dea.gov/drug-information/drug-scheduling) are regulated and split into five different categories: Class I through Class V. These categories, or classifications, depend on the particular acceptable medical use for the drug in humans and animals as well as the potential for abuse in humans (Table 12.1).

Many controlled substances are necessary in veterinary medicine, often serving as the backbone of anesthetic and other pain management protocols. Unfortunately, many of these medications and substances are highly addictive and prone to theft. As a result, the Controlled Substance Act, part of Title 21 of the United States Code, outlines a list of controlled substances, regulations, and rules to prevent misuse, theft, and diversion and ensure proper handling.

Table 12.1 List of common veterinary controlled substance classes and examples. Class I substances are not included in this list because there are no current veterinary applications for these substances as of December 2023. Class or Schedule 1 (I) drugs, substances, or chemicals are defined in the Controlled Substance Act as drugs with no currently accepted medical use and a high potential for abuse, with potentially severe psychological or physical dependence.

Drug schedule	Definition	Examples
Class II	Substance has a high potential for abuse, with use potentially leading to severe psychological or physical dependence, but has currently accepted medical use, with severe restrictions	Codeine Demerol® Duragesic® Duramorph™ Fentanyl (injectable and patch) Hydrocodone Hydromorphone Morphine Oxycodone Oxymorphone Tussionex®
Class III	Substance has potential for abuse less than schedule I and II drugs and has accepted medical uses	Buprenorphine Ketamine Simbadol® Tilzolan®
Class IV	Substance has a low potential for abuse relative to drugs in schedule III and has accepted medical uses	Alfaxan® Alprazolam Butorphanol Diazepam Lorazepam Midazolam Phenobarbital Tramadol
Class V	Substances with lower potential for abuse than schedule 4 (IV) and consist of preparations containing limited quantities of certain narcotics. Schedule 5 (V) drugs are generally used for antidiarrheal, antitussive, and analgesic purposes	Lomotil®

Figure 12.1 Hydrocodone has a CII printed on the label, indicating that it's a Class II controlled substance. Nicole Clausen.

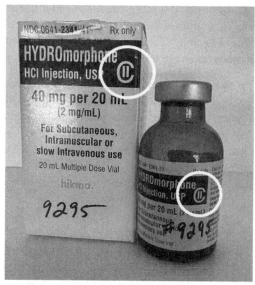

All controlled substances are categorized into different classes (or schedules; these terms are often used interchangeably) based on their risk: Class I (most risk) through Class V (least risk). The DEA places substances "in their respective schedules based on whether they have a currently accepted medical use in treatment in the United States, their relative abuse potential, and likelihood of causing dependence when abused" (www.dea.gov/drug-information/drug-scheduling).

The different classes of drugs will have different record-keeping requirements. The manufacturers are required to notate a large "C" with the corresponding Roman numeral to be printed on the packaging and the bottle itself to signal the class (Figure 12.1).

Substances can change classes, so it's important to monitor controlled substance regulations often. Additionally, some states have categorized substances into different classes than Federal regulations dictate. As an example, in Michigan, gabapentin is considered a Class V controlled substance (www.michigan.gov/opioids/nel/panel-news/news/gabapentin-scheduled-as-controlled-substance-to-help-with-states-opioid-epidemic). Gabapentin is not currently controlled federally under the Controlled Substances Act (DEA 2023a) but more and more states are considering it controlled. At the time of writing in 2023, gabapentin is considered controlled in the following states: Alabama, Kentucky, Michigan, North Dakota, Tennessee, Virginia, and West Virginia. Furthermore, many more states require gabapentin prescriptions to be processed through Prescription Monitoring Programs (PMP) (Sharkey 2023).

Controlled substances need to be handled differently from our regular inventory, so it's important to understand the regulations but also exactly what drugs are considered controlled.

12.3 Controlled Substances and the Cycle of Inventory in Your Practice

Think of your controlled substance log as a diary or journal. It should tell the whole story and journey of every milliliter and every tablet of controlled substance that came into your practice and how it left. How was it ordered? Who ordered it? Who was it ordered from? When did it arrive? When was the bottle opened? How and when did it "leave"? Was it waste, was it dispensed, was it administered? If it was given to the patient, tell that story. Who was it given to? What is the patient and client information? Who administered it? If the DEA were ever to come to your practice, they should be able to determine through your controlled substance logs and your records the exact journey for any of the drugs in your practice.

Proper record keeping serves as the foundation of DEA compliance!
Throughout this chapter, you'll explore the cycle and flow of inventory and how that specifically applies to controlled substances. The Code of Federal Regulations, 21 CFR 1301.71(a), states that "All registrants, including practitioners, shall provide effective controls and procedures to guard against theft and diversion of controlled substances" (www.ecfr.gov/current/title-21/chapter-II/part-1301/subject-group-ECFRa7ff8142033a7a2/section-1301.71). So it's important to not only follow the rules and regulations but also have proper procedures and systems in place to guard against any diversion or theft!

12.4 Forecast and Purchase Planning

Before ordering, you must first know when controlled substances are running low. This can look similar to how you calculate and use reorder points for the rest of your inventory, depending on what kind of drugs you stock in your practice. For example, Class III–V controlled substances can be purchased normally through your distributor's website and do not have any additional delays or processes.

On the other hand, Class II controlled substances must be purchased with a DEA Form 222 or the electronic equivalent. The DEA Form 222 can be requested by the registrant. This form must be completed and mailed to the distributor or vendor you are purchasing from. After the vendor receives the 222 Form, and as long as there are no issues with it, they'll ship out the order. As a result, Class II drugs can take longer to arrive than your other inventory. In this case, I recommend having a higher reorder point to account for the extra days. For more information on reorder points and safety stock, see Chapter 3.

Controlled substances are often related to anesthetic or pain management protocols as something a practice should never run out of, so I err slightly on the conservative side and do not run so "lean" for controlled substances in general. Additionally, I keep extra euthanasia solution in case a bottle breaks or gets contaminated for some reason. One of my biggest fears is running out of euthanasia solution.

12.4.1 DEA Form 222 and Class II Controlled Substance Ordering

A few important things to note about DEA Form 222.

- Once the DEA registrant (or the Power of Attorney) has completed the DEA Form 222, a copy must be made, and the original mailed to the vendor (www.ecfr.gov/current/title-21/chapter-II/part-1305#1305.13). You must keep a copy of the Form 222 for at least two years.
  - Note: You can only keep the copy; the original *must* be mailed in!
- When the order arrives, you must add on your (the purchaser's) copy "the actual number of commercial or bulk containers received and the date received" (www.ecfr.gov/current/title-21/chapter-II/part-1305#1305.13).
- You'll also need to keep in your records any fully executed/completed DEA Form 222s, as well as any copies of any unaccepted or defective forms with the statement attached (www.ecfr.gov/current/title-21/chapter-II/part-1305#1305.17).

- These records must be kept separately from all other records and on file for at least two years. Check with your state to see if state-specific guidelines are longer.
- If the DEA Form 222 has not been filled out correctly, is incomplete, is not legible, or shows any alterations, cross-outs, erasures, or changes to the form (www.ecfr.gov/current/title-21/chapter-II/part-1305#1305.15), it will be sent back, and your order will not be fulfilled. So it's important to fill out the form correctly!
- DEA Form 222 can be submitted electronically with the Controlled Substance Ordering System (CSOS) program. It saves a lot of time because there is no waiting for the physical copy to be sent through the mail, but the registrant must enroll and complete the registration process before any submissions are filed.

When I was just starting out, I wrote the date wrong on the DEA 222 Form, crossed it out, and put the correct date. I did not realize that was not acceptable. So the distributor sent the form back and did not fill the order. Thankfully, I had set my order points to where we did not run out of Class II drugs (which was one of the main drugs used for anesthetics), but it came close!

Depending on what controlled substances your practice stocks, consider changing your reorder points for Class II drugs to allow for the extra time related to mailing in the DEA Form 222 (and potential form rejection delays). Class III–V drugs do not require any special forms to purchase, so no extra time is needed in the reorder point calculations.

To know when your controlled substances are running low, you could use an electronic reorder flag by entering the reorder points into your practice management system or other inventory software. Some practices use automated dispensing cabinets (more information in Chapter 8), so reorder levels could be added if applicable. Because your controlled substances are all contained in one location (potentially in multiple safes), reorder tags or a reorder checklist work.

12.5 Ordering and Replenishment

Once you have identified that controlled substances are running low, the next step is to order them. In section 12.4, we reviewed how you'll order controlled drugs depending on the class they belong to. Class II drugs are handled a bit differently than Class III–V as they need to be ordered using a DEA Form 222.

Only team members who are authorized by the practice to order controlled substances should do so. Additionally, it's important for the DEA registrant to review what and how much is being ordered compared to what is being administered or sold by the practice. For example, if a practice only sells 10 ml of ketamine a month but they are consistently ordering 50 ml per month, that's a red flag. The DEA registrant should have a process in place to regularly review this information to ensure there is not a significant mismatch between what is being ordered and what is being sold. With that, the registrant can be on the lookout for any substance purchases that aren't normally stocked in the practice.

12.5.1 Drugs Lost in Transit

If any ordered drugs are lost in transit or if all or part of the shipment does not arrive, the supplier is responsible for reporting the in-transit loss to the DEA (www.ecfr.gov/current/title-21/chapter-II/part-1301/subject-group-ECFRa7ff8142033a7a2/section-1301.74). The purchaser and DEA registrant are responsible for notifying the loss of any controlled substances after signing for or taking custody of the shipment through a DEA Form 106 (www.ecfr.gov/current/title-21/chapter-II/part-1301/subject-group-ECFRa7ff8142033a7a2/section-1301.76).

As an additional layer of security, the person who orders should not be the same person who receives the controlled substances. Ordering and receiving controlled substances (and inventory, in general) should be completed by two or three different people. Having specific roles and responsibilities for these team members and checks and balances is critical.

"Best Practice" Questions to Consider

- Does every team member, from the CSR to the practice owner or DEA registrant, know and understand their responsibilities when it comes to controlled substances?
  - For example, do all CSRs know and understand that you cannot "take back" controlled substances from clients after they have left the building (unless you are a facility approved to do that) (DEA 2023b)?
- If a controlled substance procedure does not happen, or if there is a "miss," how will you know?
- What small checkpoints can be instituted so that if a process or standard operating procedure (SOP) is not working or being followed, it's immediately caught?
- Do you currently have controlled substance SOPs in place? If so, how often are they reviewed and updated to reflect any changes?

12.6 Receive and Organize

When controlled substances arrive in the practice, there are quite a few record-keeping requirements. As a reminder, only team members who are authorized by the practice to handle controlled substances should be part of the receiving process. Ideally, it should also be someone different from the person who ordered the controlled substances.

As soon as the controlled substances are delivered, they should be assigned a bottle number and logged in to an unopened container log. This is very important and beneficial because the bottle number allows you to track the "progress" or specific journey of the bottle in your practice. As an example: If you are a busy practice and you order 20 bottles of midazolam but do not immediately number the bottles or log them into an unopened container log, and one goes missing, how long would it take for you to realize that one has disappeared? How would you begin to investigate what happened?

Once Class III–V drugs are unpacked, the date must be recorded on the invoice or packing slip (www.ecfr.gov/current/title-21/chapter-II/part-1304/subject-group-ECFRed220d26113f6a5/section-1304.21#p-1304.21(d)). When Class II drugs are unpacked, the DEA Form 222 must be filled out with the quantities received (the number of bottles or containers) and the date. Personally, I prefer to add more information than that. I check off each item on the packing slips and invoices, notating that it was received, the date received, the initials of the person who unpacked the box, and a witness. That way, if there is ever a question about whether an item was received or who handled the shipment, the information is there to draw from.

The Federal Code of Regulations states that "The record must also contain the name of each controlled substance, the finished form, the number of dosage units of (the) finished form in each commercial container, and the number of commercial containers received" (www.ecfr.gov/current/title-21/chapter-II/part-1304/subject-group-ECFRed220d26113f6a5/section-1304.22#p-1304.22(a)(2)(iv)). Typically, all of this information is already contained on the packing slip, but it's your responsibility to verify that it is.

Once the controlled substances have been unpacked, the quantities verified, the packing slips or invoices notated, the bottle numbers assigned, and the bottles/containers added to the unopened container log, they can be restocked. Ideally, this whole process should be completed with one person restocking and another witnessing the entire process.

Make a copy of each invoice and packing slip and put the original in a binder or similar file that is readily retrievable if the DEA ever comes on site. **Class II original invoices and packing slips should be filed separately from Class III–V, and all records must be kept on file for at least two years unless your state requirements are longer**.

I'm often asked if electronic copies are okay. The simple answer is "yes" but I personally do not want to print off two years' worth of invoices and packing slips while a DEA agent is waiting. I'd rather be able to hand them a binder quickly and know everything is there and ready. How often does your printer sense urgency and decide to break?

The copy of the invoices and packing slips are what is used for receiving and book keeping.

12.6.1 Storage Requirements

The Code of Federal Regulations does not provide many details regarding the storage requirements for controlled substances. According to 21 CFR 1301.75(b), "Controlled substances listed in Schedules II, III, IV, and V shall be stored in a securely locked, substantially constructed cabinet" (www.ecfr.gov/current/title-21/chapter-II/part-1301#1301.75). You may have additional security requirements if your practice works with extra-large animals or wildlife (like elephants, moose, or other similar-sized creatures). According to the CFR, "thiafentanil, carfentanil, etorphine hydrochloride and diprenorphine shall be stored in a safe or steel cabinet equivalent to a U.S. Government Class V security container" (www.ecfr.gov/current/title-21/chapter-II/part-1301#1301.75).

Also, you might note that it does not mention anything about a double lock. A double-locked cabinet is not required (Teitelman n.d.) but is often recommended. A substantially constructed cabinet is, of course, subjective. But I tell my clients to think about it like this: If someone broke into your practice in the middle of the night, how likely is it that they could break into your cabinet with a hammer or walk away with it completely?

Depending on your practice, having a smaller safe for "working stock" works well, where each authorized user has their own safe combination. This smaller safe only has opened bottles plus one extra bottle of euthanasia solution. This only works if the protocols around security are followed (the safe door is not left open and the master keys aren't easily accessible).

All other unopened containers can be stored in a limited-access backstock safe. The backstock safe, which may only be accessed by the DEA registrant and a few authorized users, could be a repurposed gun safe. Distributors who offer equipment often have several appropriate safe options for sale as well.

Multiple DEA agents have recommended having a separate log book for each safe. I have not been able to find that specified in the regulations, but it's good practice because it makes the record keeping between safes more efficient.

Let's explore an example of managing the movement of inventory between log books. Tank's Animal Hospital has a large backstock safe as well as a smaller "working stock" safe. The backstock has an "unopened container log" because no drugs are dispensed out of this safe. The smaller working stock safe has a combination of log booklets, including an unopened container log and a dispensing log. Dr Tank needs to move an unopened container from the backstock safe to the working stock safe. He logs the unopened container OUT of the "unopened container log" and IN to the corresponding drugs' log book at the working stock safe as an unopened container. Once the container is ready to be opened, it will be logged out of the unopened container section and into the dispensing/open container section.

A reminder: Your log books should be a record or diary of the entire journey of a controlled substance from the second it arrives to the second it "leaves" (was either administered, dispensed, wasted, etc.).

12.7 Strategic Pricing

There aren't any specific regulations related to how you price your controlled substances in any of the federal or state regulations, but I recommend adding an additional controlled substance fee on top of your normal dispensing or injection fee. More on pricing in Chapter 7.

If your practice management system does not have the capability to add that fee, you can set up a "tier two" injection or dispensing fee that is higher than a "tier one" (which would be regularly priced items). This additional fee helps to offset the labor costs related to staying in compliance and for any state PMPs, as well as the cost of log books, automated dispensing tools, and software systems related to controlled substance regulations.

Helpful Definition
- **Prescription monitoring program (PMP)**: a system that helps track the prescriptions people and animals receive for certain medications. It's a database that healthcare and veterinary professionals and authorities submit to and use to monitor the prescribing and dispensing of controlled substances.

12.8 Appropriate Inventory Sales and Consumption

This is the phase of the cycle or flow of inventory in your practice where your controlled substances are administered, sold to patients, or (hopefully not) wasted. One of the key requirements for your controlled drugs is that the records are current, complete, and accurate. I think the requirement that *current* records must be maintained is really important here. As an example, let's say a ton of controlled substance pre-meds are pulled up before surgery, but they do not get logged until the afternoon. The log book would not be current (or accurate) and would not be considered to be in compliance. So, the logging and record keeping must be current, accurate, and complete!

One thing that the regulations do not specify is the design or layout of the logbook. There is a frequently parroted long-standing myth that log books must be in a bound format. Regulations do not specify the look or layout of the logbook (Seibert n.d.). However, regulations do outline what information is required in the log book.

According to the CFR, records must be maintained that include (www.ecfr.gov/current/title-21/part-1304/section-1304.22#p-1304.22(c)):

- the name of the controlled substance
- the quantity dispensed
- the name and address of the person to whom it was dispensed. Note: Some DEA agents have explained to me that the address and phone number can be maintained in the medical record, and only the client name, patient name, and client ID must be included in the log book
- the date dispensed
- the written or typewritten name or initials of the individual who dispensed the controlled substance on behalf of the practitioner
- the finished form (for example, a 20 mg tablet or a 10 mg/ml liquid) and the total number of units in a container (for example, a 500-tablet bottle).

Additionally:

- log books must be kept for a minimum of two years (some states require them to be kept for longer)
- they must be "readily retrievable"
- records for Class II and Class III–V should be kept separate from each other.

There is not necessarily a "best" log book. The best log book system is whichever one helps your team be the most accurate and have complete and current records!

"Best Practice" Tip

Do not forget to regularly review controlled substance requirements to see if anything has changed or if additional requirements are necessary to comply with Federal or state regulations!

12.8.1 Controlled Substance Refill Requirements

There are specific controlled substance refill requirements for all Class II and Class III–V drugs. However, they are always changing as states add different or more restrictive requirements with PMPs. I highly recommend researching your specific state and jurisdiction to determine the current requirements and schedule time yearly to update your practice to current standards.

12.8.2 Controlled Substance Disposal

There may come a time when you have controlled substances that have expired or been damaged, or you simply want to dispose of them. Although not required (DEA 2023b), you can send them to a reverse distributor for destruction (www.ecfr.gov/current/title-21/chapter-II/part-1317#1317.05). Reverse distributors are companies that handle the return and destruction of controlled substances and help manage their proper and lawful disposal.

Helpful Definition

- **Reverse distributor**: a company that helps handle the return and disposal of unused or expired controlled substances and processes them according to regulations and laws.

If you'd rather not use a reverse distributor, you must first contact the DEA, the Special Agent in Charge of the Administration, for approval and permission. If you decide to go that route, requesting a letter from the DEA that demonstrates proof and authorization for the destruction is important.

If you decide to use a reverse distributor, you will transfer the unwanted controlled substances to them. It's important to document in your records exactly which substances are being destroyed, the size, strength, quantity, and other pertinent information. The reverse distributor is responsible for completing the DEA Form 41 (www.deadiversion.usdoj.gov/21cfr_reports/surrend/41_form.pdf).

If you decide to get approval from the DEA Special Agent in Charge for alternative methods of destruction, the registrant is responsible for filling out the DEA Form 41 (www.ecfr.gov/current/title-21/chapter-II/part-1304/subject-group-ECFRed220d26113f6a5/section-1304.21). This form does not need to be submitted to the DEA, but it must be kept on file for at least two years at the registered location and be readily retrievable in case of inspection.

Note: It's important to remember that "as a DEA registrant, you are not eligible to dispose of controlled substances from your office stock using drop boxes designated for disposal of controlled substances by the general public, or during prescription drug take-back events" (DEA 2023b).

12.9 Biennial Inventory Requirements

A common misconception in vet med is that controlled substance requirements are only related to logging your drugs. In actuality, there are other record-keeping regulations and responsibilities, such as performing an initial physical inventory count of all the controlled substances that are in a DEA registrant's possession on the date that the registrant first starts dispensing controlled substances.

You are also responsible for doing biennial inventory counts (www.ecfr.gov/current/title-21/chapter-II/part-1304#1304.11). This is a complete physical inventory of all your controlled substances on hand and must be completed at least every two years. Your biennial count should be kept at the registered location and "readily retrievable" in case of inspection.

Helpful Definition
- **Registered location**: the business address provided during DEA registration. This location is where required records and controlled substances are kept (DEA 2023b, p. 13).

Remember, your records for Class II must be kept separate from your records for Class III–V substances.

You might be thinking, "Nicole, we already count way more often than that." That may be true, but a biennial count is different. The initial and biennial inventory counts require more information. In the initial and each following biennial count, you must include the following.

- The date of the inventory.
- Whether the inventory was taken at the opening or close of business.
- Whether it's an initial or biennial inventory count.
- The name of each controlled substance inventoried.
- The finished form of each of the substances (e.g., 10 mg tablet).
- The number of dosage units or volumes of each finished form in each commercial container (e.g., 100-tablet bottle or 3 ml vial).
- The number of commercial containers of each finished form (e.g., four 100-tablet bottles).
- A count of the substance (www.ecfr.gov/current/title-21/chapter-II/part-1304#1304.11; https://uscode.house.gov/view.xhtml?req=(title:21%20section:827%20edition:prelim)%20OR%20(granuleid:USC-prelim-title21-section827)&f=treesort&edition=prelim&num=0&jumpTo=true).

According to the *DEA Practitioner's Manual*, "Although it is not required by law, DEA recommends that registrants keep an inventory record that includes the name, address, and DEA registration number of the registrant, and the signature of the person or persons responsible for taking the inventory" (DEA 2023b, p. 38).

If you perform end-of-year counts for your entire inventory each year, performing a biennial count at the end of each year can be a good way to ensure you stay compliant. Your biennial inventory count can be completed more frequently than every two years, but not less than.

12.10 Auditing and Reconciling Your Controlled Substance Logs

While the DEA only requires that the controlled substance inventory count be conducted every two years, it is very important to count and reconcile log books more frequently than that! Your drug logs must be accurate and up to date at all times to stay in compliance so you'll likely need to audit your drug logs often. Some practices reconcile their log books after every shift, some at the end of every day, and others once a week.

You may encounter a situation where your log books and what you have on hand do not match. If that happens, immediately find where the difference is and correct it. It is important to have a standard method of determining how and where you are off.

The first step in this process is to ensure that every drug gets logged, every time, without exception. It is vital for everyone on the team to understand how important compliance is, what their particular role in compliance is, and what the potential negative effects are.

So, how do you resolve an "off" count? This is exactly why having a physical log in addition to your practice management software (or another method for medical records) is helpful. If you are off in your log books, reports from your practice management system or software serve as a great double-check.

The first step is to compare your practice management system item sales report or controlled substance reports to the controlled substance log and match up any missing entries.

The second step is to ensure all math is executed correctly. Make sure that all additions and subtractions are correct and that all drugs/strengths are recorded in the appropriate columns.

If necessary, the third step is to reconcile any surgical or euthanasia logs (depending on the substance). Then, search for any refills that were declined or potentially mishandled.

If a significant shortage cannot be explained or you suspect there is an off-count due to theft, the DEA requires registrants to notify their local DEA field office in writing of any significant loss due to theft or otherwise within one business day. In addition, the registrant should submit a DEA Form 106, "Theft or Loss of Controlled Substances."

Additionally, in addition reconciliation, it can be helpful to audit your controlled drug logs periodically to make sure that the amount purchased minus any quantities dispensed or reports of lost/stolen controlled substances is equal to the current quantity on hand.

For example, let's say that Dr Tank, the DEA registrant of Tank's Animal Hospital, wants to audit their controlled drug logs. First, he gathers the appropriate drug log and looks back to when he last audited the logs to find the "beginning balance." Then, he calculates the total number of units purchased and the total number of units dispensed, stolen, or lost. He adds the beginning balance and the purchases together and then subtracts the number removed from inventory (by dispensation, administration, theft, or loss). That number should equal the amount currently on hand.

The purpose of auditing and reconciling your drug logs is to ensure you are in compliance but, most importantly, that there is no theft, misuse, or diversion happening.

12.10.1 Theft or Significant Loss of Controlled Substances

As stated above, in the case of suspected theft or any significant loss of controlled substances, the DEA registrant must notify their local DEA Diversion Field Office within one business day (www.ecfr.gov/current/title-21/chapter-II/part-1301/subject-group-ECFRa7ff8142033a7a2/section-1301.76). Additionally, they must fill out a DEA Form 106 ("Report of Theft or Loss of Controlled Substances"), which is used to note the drugs and quantities involved as well as any circumstances regarding the theft or loss.

The DEA has provided some guidance and clarity around the DEA Form 106 and stated, "DEA has become aware of instances in which registrants have used a DEA Form 106 to document or explain minor inventory discrepancies, thereby 'balancing the books.' DEA wishes to stress that the DEA Form 106 should be used only to document thefts or significant losses of controlled substances. Minor inventory discrepancies, not attributable to theft, should not be reported to (the) DEA or recorded on a DEA Form 106. Rather, registrants should make appropriate notations of minor inventory discrepancies in their records, indicating the amount of variance between the physical count and the amount accounted for through records. Such discrepancies need not be reported to (the) DEA if they are not significant or actual losses. If a registrant is unsure of the significance of a loss after considering the factors described below, the registrant should file the report. Any continuing pattern of loss of seemingly insignificant quantities should always be considered significant" (www.federalregister.gov/documents/2003/07/08/03-17127/reports-by-registrants-of-theft-or-significant-loss-of-controlled-substances#p-16).

To help determine if a loss is significant, the DEA recommends reviewing the following factors.

- How much of the controlled substances was actually lost, taking into account the type of business.
- Which specific controlled substances were lost.
- Whether the loss can be linked to certain individuals having access to the substances, or if it's related to specific activities involving the substances.
- If there's a pattern of losses over time, how random they seem, and what actions have been taken to address the losses.
- If the specific controlled substances are likely to be diverted for unauthorized use.
- Consider local trends and other signs that could indicate the potential for diversion of the missing controlled substance.

This is a brief overview of the requirements for reporting any theft or loss of controlled substances. I highly recommend continuing your research and learning about the regulations to make sure you are up to date with all the most current requirements.

12.10.2   Employee Reporting of Theft, Abuse, or Diversion

According to the DEA, all employees are required to report any signs of theft, abuse, or diversion by other employees to their employer (www.ecfr.gov/current/title-21/chapter-II/part-1301/subject-group-ECFRbf5f8d39b8823bb/section-1301.91). It also states that the employer must take all reasonable steps to keep the information confidential as well as the identity of the person reporting the information. The DEA also states that any failure to report information on potential drug diversion will be considered when determining the employee's status or eligibility to continue working at the practice.

12.11   Other DEA Regulations

There are more regulations related to DEA registration, employee screening, and other topics that are outside the scope of this book. There are many fantastic resources, including books, live webinars, and self-paced courses, out there to learn more about controlled substance regulations. DEA regulations might seem overwhelming and scary, but many DEA agents say that as long as you are trying your best and doing everything in your power to be compliant, they are willing to work with you.

Finally, keep in mind that the *DEA registrant* is ultimately responsible for maintaining compliance! They should be aware of and follow *all* controlled substance regulations.

12.12   What Next Steps Should You Take?

After reviewing the various requirements for DEA compliance and identifying where your practice may have gaps, the next step is to create and outline all your SOPs, processes, and policies regarding controlled substances. At a minimum, this should include the various DEA regulations and what your practice does to be compliant with those. However, this document should also include any practice-specific policies for prevention against theft and diversion.

Ultimately, every team member in the practice should know and understand what their responsibilities are in their specific roles as related to controlled substance regulations. Not only that but there should be processes for checks and balances. If a particular regulation is not met, how will your practice know? How can any potential "misses" in compliance be brought to light right now? Think through how this might look for your unique practice.

Once your SOPs for DEA compliance have been documented and put into place, it's important to update them regularly. Review yours on a routine basis with a critical lens and evaluate the following.

- Where might there be gaps in regulation compliance?
- Where are there definitely gaps in regulation compliance?
- Have there been any updates to any state or Federal regulations that I need to respond to or react to?
- Looking at the cycle or flow of controlled substances in our practice, is there any potential for diversion? Do we have any gaps in our policies?
  - For example, how could I improve the security of controlled substances? Could I improve or add visibility by installing cameras, instituting witnesses, and double-checking when drawing up, administering, or counting controlled substance prescriptions? Can I add or leverage any technology to help reduce the risk of theft and diversion?

Controlled substance regulations outline rules and guidelines to ensure the proper handling, prescribing, dispensing, and record keeping of substances with the potential for theft, abuse, and misuse. DEA registrants must both understand and adhere to these regulations. Key aspects include maintaining accurate records, securing storage and handling of controlled substances, preventing unauthorized access, reporting thefts or losses promptly, and complying with prescription requirements.

The regulations also emphasize the need for registrants to stay vigilant, adopting measures to prevent diversion and misuse of controlled substances. Compliance with these regulations is crucial to prevent the unauthorized use of controlled substances and maintain the safety of our teams, patients, and communities.

12.12.1 Additional Resources

- *The Complete Veterinary Practice Controlling Controlled Drug Manual* by Philip J. Seibert, Jr., CVT of SafetyVet (www.safetyvet.com/pubs/manuals.html).
  - Phil is also an incredible resource for OSHA and other hospital safety concerns.
- *AAHA Guide to Safeguarding Controlled Substances* by Jack Teitelman and Kelley Detweiler.
- Controlled Substance Management in Veterinary Medicine, course by Lauren Forsythe, PharmD, DICVP, FSVHP (www.vetmedteam.com/class.aspx?ci=947)

12.13 Author's Note

You made it! Nice work reading through this chapter. I know there was a lot of material and information included here. I personally have never had the DEA audit or visit a practice I was working at. However, quite a few students, clients, and community members have undergone DEA audits.

In my experience, if you are doing the best you can to follow regulations and want to work with the DEA to resolve any issues, they'll work with you. With that being said, there are significant fines or other consequences for not following the regulations.

At the end of the day, it's our responsibility and duty as DEA registrants or professionals who handle controlled substances to be good stewards, for our patients, our teams, and ultimately, our communities.

13

Maintaining Your Inventory

13.1 Author's Note

When I was an inventory manager, toward the end of getting everything "fixed" and situated how I wanted it to be, it felt like I spent significantly less time each week, leading me to question if I was doing it wrong. By then, I had set up reorder points in AVImark®, cleaned up the inventory list, linked my treatment and inventory codes properly, and reorganized the pharmacy and storage areas until they were right. Everything was priced appropriately and I had workflows that made ordering and receiving a breeze. It felt so strange.

Throughout that period, I had invested much time and effort (and a few tears and a gray hair or two) into my inventory. Because the systems and workflows I had set up were working well, I could quickly place and receive my orders weekly. It was a strange sensation. I couldn't help but think "What am I missing? This feels too easy and good to be true. What am I doing wrong?" It dawned on me that this is what I had been working so hard for. I was experiencing the fruits of my labor. I had made it! I could finally transition from "fixing and adjusting" to maintenance mode.

13.2 How to Maintain your Inventory

How do you maintain all your hard work once you have spent all that time fixing and setting up your inventory? It will depend heavily on the systems and workflows you set up for your inventory. For example, suppose you mainly rely on your practice management system for reorder points. In that case, maintenance will look different from if you mostly utilize checklists that you delegate to different team members.

When it comes to reorder points, I recommend recalculating order points and order quantities for your high and medium turn (or your "A" and "B") items every six months. Recalculating every 12 months is sufficient for your low or "C" class items. Alternatively, reevaluate reorder levels three months after a veterinarian leaves or joins the practice. This gives enough time to capture any changes in demand and adjust your order points accordingly. Another consideration is whether your practice is in a period of significant growth. If your practice grows and your demand constantly increases, you'll likely want to reevaluate your order points more frequently.

Think back to the cycle or flow of inventory through your practice. What systems did you set up for each section? How will these be maintained? Does the process need to be documented? How will the steps and requirements be captured?

Inventory Management for Veterinary Professionals, First Edition. Nicole I. Clausen.
© 2024 John Wiley & Sons, Inc. Published 2024 by John Wiley & Sons, Inc.
Companion website: www.wiley.com/go/clausen/inventory

Let's explore an example together. Tank's Animal Hospital is almost done getting its inventory fixed and all the little moving pieces are practically settled. Georgia, the lead inventory director, wants to set up a maintenance plan for their inventory going forward. First, she outlines the projects she tackled and the systems and workflows she added to their inventory. Then, she outlines what needs to be done regularly to support and maintain those workflows. She outlines a snapshot of several aspects.

- **Reorder points** – recalculated for high/medium-turn items every six and 12 months for low-turn items. Additionally, order points will be recalculated three months after a veterinarian leaves or joins the practice.
  - A "reorder tag/shelf label tracker" spreadsheet will be updated as needed to track what products have reorder tags or shelf labels and what the corresponding reorder points are.
- **Formulary** – any new items that are requested will go through an approval process first before being added to the formula. At the end of every quarter, an inventory team member will review the inventory list to check for any redundant or slow-moving items that need to be discontinued.
  - A colored dot challenge will be performed every 12 months to visualize and monitor the turnover of the entire inventory.
- **Pricing** – inventory items will be priced using a markup percentage (for now), and the prices of items will immediately be increased as the cost goes up. This will happen by receiving purchase orders in the practice management system, and the software will recalculate the new price. Any items priced manually will be added to a spreadsheet tracker with the pricing method so these items can be monitored and prices can be increased as needed. Additionally, the various dispensing fees will be evaluated every six months.
- **Expiry dates** – at the end of each month, an inventory team member will check to see if any products are set to expire within the next three months. They will create a list of these items to discuss with Dr Tank to see if they should be reordered, discontinued, or moved to an online pharmacy.
- **Organization** – each "inventory zone" in Tank's Animal Hospital is organized according to the 5S Process (see Chapter 6 for more information). Each week, the team member in charge of each zone will compare how the zone should be organized to how it actually is. They'll also be responsible for tidying up the zone and resetting the space as necessary.

Once Georgia and Dr Tank outline the workflows that need to be maintained and the required tasks, Georgia adds all the tasks to a task management system or her calendar. Hence, she always has reminders for exactly what she needs to focus on. These "maintenance tasks," in addition to the regular tasks for inventory management, can help keep the inventory running smoothly through the practice ecosystem.

Another excellent method for maintaining your inventory is to document your various processes, systems, and policies into standard operating procedures (SOPs).

13.3 Creating Standard Operating Procedures

Our SOPs are frameworks for performing a specific task or aspect in our inventory or practice (as opposed to outdated, useless documents that don't reflect how things are actually done). They are mini guides that set the standard for accurately accomplishing different tasks. So, if you win the lottery, or you're short-handed and need to delegate tasks, someone could pick up a SOP and get it done without missing a beat (and not undo all your hard work and efforts).

You can get lost in the hundreds of different formats for SOPs and the many ways to make them work for your practice, but don't overcomplicate the process. At the end of the day, SOPs outline how to do a particular task or policies that team members should be aware of.

"Best Practice" List of Helpful SOPs

- **Reorder point SOP**: this outlines the different policies related to reorder points (for example, what method of calculation is used, what type of reorder flags are used, how often they are calculated, etc.) and the step-by-step instructions for calculating.
- **Hospital organization SOP**: outlines exactly what inventory zones are in the practice, how often they should be organized, and who is responsible for what. It can include pictures of exactly how each zone should be organized or a "plan-o-gram" that outlines where certain categories of items should be stored in each "zone."
- **New inventory item SOP**: outlines the entire process from when a team member wants to request something until it's on the shelf and ready to be sold. It can include the policies around filling out a request form, what tasks need to happen before the product arrives, step-by-step instructions for setting up an item in the practice management system, and any other helpful information.

At their worst, SOPs are documents that are written and forgotten about – wasted effort. At their best, SOPs are accessible, and the team in your practice has the habit of reaching for them when completing a task. It may take some time for them to be utilized appropriately, but they save so much time and make delegation a breeze. It's worth implementing them in the day-to-day operations. If you don't have a particular format that you've used before, here's an example that I've found helpful.

"Best Practice" Example SOP Structure

This is the structure we use here at Veterinary Care Logistics, and we have found it to be successful!

PREREQUISITES: what information does the person completing need to know or have access to prior to starting the procedure?

- Here are some questions to consider: Do they need access to specific reports? What about certain modules or access levels in your practice management system? Do they need a particular login for a specific website? What might they need in order to complete this task successfully? How can you set them up for success?

PURPOSE: why does this SOP matter? Why is it important? What purpose does it serve?

POLICY: what principles or practice policies are involved with this SOP? Policies are rules or guidelines that are followed by your practice. It's essentially saying, "This is how we do things at our practice."

- As examples: Medication returns are not accepted by Tank's Animal Hospital, only those team members who are authorized to handle controlled substances should do so, or new medications shouldn't be added to the formulary without prior approval from the practice owner.

PROPERTY: who is ultimately responsible for this SOP?

- As an example, for an ordering or reorder point SOP, the person ultimately responsible might be the inventory manager.

PARTY: who is involved in this SOP? Are there other team members who might be involved but not ultimately responsible for its success? For a task that includes multiple people, it can be helpful to outline each person and what they are ultimately responsible for. But the "party" involved could also just be the person ultimately responsible.

PROCESS: what is the high-level process for this procedure? This should outline the different steps but not necessarily dive into the step-by-step details of how. The process section should be a quick overview for someone to review on the go. For instance, the process for calculating reorder points for all items could look like the example below. When reading this, you get an idea of the steps that should be taken but it doesn't break down exactly how to do it. The process is more of the "what" whereas the procedure is the "how."

To calculate the reorder points (ROP) and reorder quantities (ROQ) for all items:

1) access and export the "quantity sold" report for the necessary date range
2) export the report as an Excel file
3) remove all "extra" rows or columns – anything that is not the item ID, item description, and quantity sold
4) copy and paste all the data and information into the reorder point calculator
5) update the calculated ROP and ROQ in the practice management system.

PROCEDURE: this section should outline step by step how to complete the process. It should include all pertinent details. If a team member were to grab this SOP, they would have no problem finishing the process after following the instructions. This is much more detailed than the quick process above. I also like to include screenshots or a screen recording of the process so the person watching thoroughly understands the steps. An example procedure for calculating reorder points is below.

To calculate the ROP and ROQ for all items:

1) in the menu bar of the practice management system, click the reports button
2) then, select the "item sold summary" report. Once that has been selected, select the item to be calculated and enter the date range for the last six months. If calculating ROPs for all items, leave the item ID selection blank
3) click "run" to preview the report
4) if calculating for a single product, find the six-month usage and set aside (and skip to step XX). If calculating ROPs for all items, export the file as an Excel spreadsheet and follow the following steps
5) open the Excel spreadsheet and remove any blank rows and any column besides the item ID, description, and quantity sold columns. Delete any row totals or other data that are not necessary (see linked screen record video for reference – not actually included in this example)
6) select all items in the spreadsheet and include the item ID, the description, and the quantity sold. Click control+c to copy
7) then, open the reorder point calculator (located on the Server → Inventory → Calculators → Reorder Point Calculator) and paste the data into the appropriate spreadsheet
8) the two-week and 30-day supply for each item should be calculated
9) once the ROP and ROQ have been calculated, return to the practice management system
10) go to the inventory list and select the first item to be updated. Then, click the "Purchasing" tab and enter the new ROP, and ROQ if it has changed
11) continue to enter all the updated ROPs and ROQs.

13.3.1 Example Fill-in-the-Blanks SOPs

Below is an example fill-in-the-blanks SOP for end-of-year inventory counts. The italicized text should be changed or updated for your unique practice.

PREREQUISITES

Prior to completing the end-of-year counts, team members will need access to the following report and permissions in the practice management system:

- _____ *(Report used for counting in software)*
- _____ *(Report used for viewing quantity on hand)*

Software permissions:

- Making a quantity on-hand adjustment
- Viewing above reports
- _____ *(any other specific permissions for your software)*

PURPOSE

The purpose of this SOP is to complete an end-of-year count for tax and inventory purposes.

POLICY

End-of-year counts will be completed each year by _____ *(date or specific goal)*. The goal is to remain *open/closed* during these counts. Each item in the practice will be counted, and the accurate quantity on hand will be updated in the practice management system so that the inventory report can be sent to the accountant for tax purposes.

For hospital supplies, only unopened containers will be counted. Whereas for anything that is sold or dispensed, each unit will be counted. *(Note: revise this statement according to your practice's policy.)*
Add any additional specific practice policies.

PROPERTY

_____ *(Person responsible)*, _____ *(title)*

PARTY

_____ will be responsible for overseeing the end-of-year counts, and the following people will be involved:

- *Team Member A – counting only*
- *All team members will help count*
- *All team members, except ____ department, will help count*

PROCESS

Prior to counting, the inventory list will be prepped and includes the following steps.

1) Print the inventory list *(report name)*.
2) Review the inventory list to see if any products need to be inactivated, changed, or added.
3) Make any adjustments or alterations necessary prior to counting.

Prior to counting (if closing):

- *the practice owner and management team will decide which time and day the practice will be closed for the counting process*
- *clients will be alerted by email and social media of the closure.*

For counting:

- print the count sheets by category
- assign each category to different team members
- inventory will be counted
- *after/while* inventory is counted, update the quantity on hand.

Once the inventory has been counted and adjusted, save three different copies of the inventory report: One for the inventory manager's records, one for the practice owner's records, and one for the accountant.

PROCEDURE

To prep the inventory list:

- access the inventory list *(report name)*. To access, go to _____ → _____ → *(add very clear step-by-step instructions)*
- review each item on the list to check for any products that are no longer carried, products that need to be added, or any products that need a unit of measure adjustment
- to inactivate an item, _____ *(process)*
- to add a product, _____ *(process) OR see "Adding a New Item" SOP*
- to change the unit of measure, _____ *(process)*
- make any adjustments necessary
- once all the adjustments have been made, run the report again and review it once more.

For counting:

1) print the count sheets by category. To access, go to _____ → _____ → *(add very clear step-by-step instructions)*
2) print a PDF of each category *(add very clear step-by-step instructions)*
3) after each category is printed, assign one or two (or more) team members to each category. Provide instructions on what to count, what to do if any issues arise, and what to do once each page or category is complete
4) once all the counts/a specific category has been counted:
   - start at the top of the counts sheet and make an adjustment for each item
   - go to _____ *(add very clear step-by-step instructions)*
   - continue making adjustments for each item on the count sheet
5) once all the items have been adjusted, view the inventory list and review for any errors
6) then, save three different copies *(add step-by-step process)* and:
   - *send one copy to:* _____
   - *save one copy on the server (add step-by-step instructions/location)*
   - _____.

Creating SOPs in your inventory is an asset. First, all the processes for your unique practice are documented so that tasks can be easily delegated if the inventory manager is unavailable. Not only that, but you always have a reference for how something is done. So, if you don't perform a task often (like end-of-year counts), you always have step-by-step instructions and a framework to refer back to.

Another excellent method for maintaining your inventory and making sure everything is on the right track is monitoring key performance indicators.

13.4   Introduction to Key Performance Indicators

Key performance indicators, also shortened to KPIs, are measurable metrics and insights into how well your practice is achieving a specific goal. When you are creating your inventory cycle, how will you know if you are successful? How will you know if you are getting closer to your goals? Answering these questions signals if you are on the right track or if you need to make small adjustments, perform additional "diagnostics," or are lost in the weeds. KPIs help answer these questions.

Think of KPIs like lab work for your practice. They are specific data pieces that are being measured, whether it's the number of new clients per month or a white blood cell count. Determining whether you are above or below the "reference range" can signal if that metric is within normal limits or if you need to dig further.

Similar to lab work, it's not the full picture. You still want to physically examine the patient, get a history from the owner, and look at other clinic signs. It's the same with your inventory. You don't want to look solely at KPIs; you also want to look at how your systems and processes are functioning. For example, you might want to explore how often you're running out of an item, how up to date and accurate the controlled substance log is, or how often products are expiring. Although KPIs don't paint the entire picture of your inventory, they do provide valuable data and insights.

"Best Practice" KPI Questions

Whenever you're looking at your KPIs or deciding which metrics to track, consider the following factors.

- Why is this metric important to me? What am I hoping to learn by measuring this?
- What does success look like? Will measuring this help me understand if we're moving closer to or further away from this goal?
- Once the KPIs are measured or calculated, how will this information be used? How will it inspire action in our inventory or our practice?

Your KPIs should measure information that is relevant and valuable to your practice. What are your practice's values and goals? What's a priority for you this quarter or year? Does your hospital want to monitor how many new patients are seen per month? What about the average transaction charge? Or the number of dentals performed versus how many dental procedures were recommended? Before deciding on what KPIs to track, it's helpful first to understand your goals and priorities and then select metrics to monitor how well you are moving toward that goal.

Common KPIs include:

- gross revenue
- revenue per DVM
- average transaction charge
- new clients per month
- active clients
- total visits per DVM
- expense category breakdown
- surgical or dental procedures per DVM.

As an example, let's say that in the next quarter, the goal of Tank's Animal Hospital is to increase its revenue by 7% over last quarter. They know from experience that they'd like to increase new patient visits, market to current clients with overdue services, and increase the number of dental procedures. So they decide to track gross revenue, new clients per month, average client compliance, percentage of pets with overdue services, and the number of dental procedures during the month.

Once they've chosen which metrics to track, they also decide on what success looks like for each metric and create a "reference range." Alton, who is a whiz at spreadsheets, creates a dashboard to track these metrics month over month. One of their metrics is how many dental services per month they usually book versus their current bookings. They decide that a range of 30–35 dentals per month is ideal. Going forward, they'll be able to track how many dentals are completed per month (among others) and how they're making progress.

Key performance indicators can be a great way to track the overall health and performance of the practice, but they can also help to track the success of certain goals, initiatives, and priorities. After all, who doesn't love a good set of diagnostics giving them more information?

These quantifiable measures of success provide clear data on how your practice is doing. Even more important, though, is what we do with this information. *Key performance indicators are only helpful and meaningful if they inspire action.* Otherwise, it's just another thing on the to-do list and you're just "tracking to track." When defining and outlining your KPIs, it can be helpful to think through what your objectives are with these metrics, how the information will be gathered, and who will be responsible for acting upon the information.

How will you know if a KPI is low or high compared to your benchmark? What corrective steps or actions will need to be taken to correct or impact the metric? Who will be in charge of following through with the improvements?

"Best Practice" KPI Identification

The following questions are helpful when identifying and defining your practice's KPIs.

- What is your desired outcome and what does success look like? Why is this important to you or your practice?
- How are you going to measure progress? What is the "reference range" or target goal for this KPI?
- What steps will need to be taken if this metric is too high or too low? What "corrective actions" might need to be taken?
- Who is responsible for the impact and who has influence on the outcome?
- How will you know you've achieved your goal or have moved closer to success?
- How often will you review this KPI and the progress of any associated tasks or projects?

After you've decided on and established the metrics for your practice, brainstormed how you'll utilize the data and information, and considered the various questions above, it's time to make a dashboard listing all your KPIs, the desired benchmark or reference range, and where you currently stand.

A KPI dashboard doesn't have to be super complex or have a lot of fancy graphics (but go you, if you want to!). A good KPI dashboard functions like a lab test result page after you've run a panel. It should list the metric or KPI (the lab test name), the desired benchmark or result (the reference range), and the current result. How often you "run the lab tests" on your practice depends on your goals and what you're striving for – some metrics may be reviewed weekly, monthly, quarterly, or yearly. If you're not sure, monthly is always a great place to start (Figure 13.1, Table 13.1).

Keep in mind that it doesn't have to be perfect! Start small and expand and improve from there.

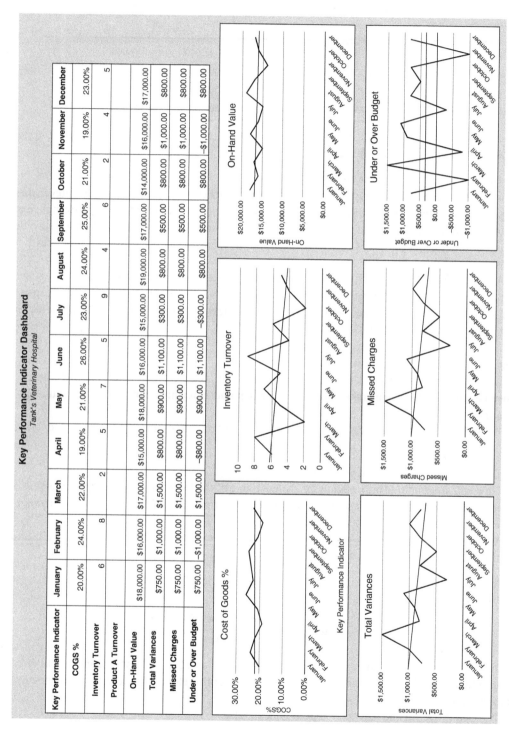

Figure 13.1 An example of a more complex dashboard with a table, graphs for each metric, and a trend line. Nicole Clausen.

Table 13.1 A simple table that can be used to track key performance indicators.

Key performance indicator	January	February	March	April
COGS %	20.00%	24.00%	22.00%	19.00%
On-hand value	$18,000.00	$16,000.00	$17,000.00	$15,000.00
Total variances	$750.00	$1,000.00	$1,500.00	$800.00
Missed charges	$750.00	$1,000.00	$1,500.00	$800.00

13.4.1 Creating a KPI Dashboard

13.4.1.1 Step 1: Determine the Metrics to Track

How do you determine if you are moving closer to or further away from success (whatever that might be)? What metrics would you like to track to keep a check on the health and performance of your practice? Are there any goals or priorities you're working on that you'd like to track specific KPIs for? Choose metrics that will provide information but also inspire action or prompt a further "investigation" into why.

Tip: If your practice doesn't currently track any KPIs, here's your permission to take baby steps! Begin by getting comfortable by tracking just one or two inventory metrics. Then, you can expand and start to track more variables. Remember, we want the data to inspire action and be useful for you, not just add another thing to your to-do list!

13.4.1.2 Step 2: Determine how to Calculate each Metric

Once you've determined what metrics you want to track, the next step is to determine how to calculate these KPIs. Then, take it one step further and determine how or where you'll find information.

For example, if you want to calculate and track your cost of goods sold (COGS), you could follow the steps below.

1) Determine the formula that you'll use.
2) How will you find this information for each variable of the formula (COGS and revenue)? Will it be a report from QuickBooks^{TM} or your accounting software? Your practice management system?
3) Write all the information down so you don't have to remember each month where you'll find the information and how to access it.

Continuing with the COGS example, your outline might look like this.
Formula to calculate:

$$Cost\ of\ Goods\ Sold\left(as\ \%\ of\ Revenue\right) = \frac{Cost\ of\ Goods\ Sold}{Revenue} \times 100$$

To find the cost and revenue variables, access the profit and loss statement from QuickBooks. Note: Make sure the book-keeper has finalized the month before using the cost and revenue information.

To access the profit and loss statement in Quickbooks:

1) go to www.yourexamplesoftware.com
2) on the left-hand side of the screen, click on "Reports" and then "Profit and Loss"

3) change the date filers to the month range you are calculating
4) find the lines "Total Cost of Goods Sold" and "Total Income" and make a note of those numbers for the formula
5) use the formula above to calculate the COGS as a percentage of revenue.

13.4.1.3 Step 3: Next Steps

After determining the metrics you want to calculate and how to calculate them, the next step is to determine what you will actually do with the information. How often will you calculate each metric – monthly, quarterly, or yearly? What makes the most sense for your practice and your goals? Who will be calculating the metrics, and who should know the results?

Continuing with our COGS example from above ...

- COGS will be calculated monthly (for the previous month) by Nicole and then added to the inventory KPI dashboard each month.
- It will also be calculated at the end of each year for a 12-month time period.
- The inventory KPI dashboard will be presented each month at the manager's meeting and reviewed with the practice owner and the management team.
- If COGS are elevated, the next steps will be X, Y, and Z.
- If COGS have decreased, the next steps will be P, Q, and R.

Next, let's explore the KPIs specific to inventory management. You'll learn about calculating your COGS as a percentage of revenue, inventory turnover, value of inventory on hand, and the volume of inventory adjustments.

13.5 Inventory Key Performance Indicators: Cost of Goods Sold (as a Percentage of Revenue)

Originally, COGS was an accounting term that refers to the direct costs of manufacturing or producing goods for a company. Of course, in veterinary medicine, we are not in the business of manufacturing or producing a good. We are a service business that has direct costs related to patient care. These can be direct costs such as inventory sold (like a bag of prescription cat food) or costs associated with inventory used or consumed during a procedure (like isoflurane or gauze).

Essentially, there isn't a clear-cut definition for exactly what is included in the cost of goods umbrella term for every practice. Note: Some practices and organizations refer to them as "cost of sales" rather than "cost of goods."

So, what does COGS mean today for us in the veterinary world? COGS is an umbrella term used to categorize the direct costs of patient care. This category doesn't include labor or any facility costs which are different categories. COGS is often used interchangeably with "inventory costs." Many veterinary-specific accounts use the American Animal Hospital Association (AAHA) Chart of Accounts, which is "the standard for classifying and aggregating revenue, expense, and balance sheet accounts in small-animal veterinary practice." The Chart of Accounts breaks down what's included in various revenue and expense categories and provides information on assets, liabilities, and more.

Some items typically fall under the COGS category but there is some nuance. As a general rule, anything purchased that relates to caring for patients is usually included in the COGS category.

- Pharmaceuticals
- Injectables

- White goods and hospital supplies
- Vaccinations
- Flea, tick, and heartworm prevention
- Over-the-counter, retail items, and supplements
- Prescription and retail diets
- In-house lab supplies
- Reference lab costs
- Cremation costs

The following are typically not included in COGS: Janitorial supplies, office supplies, and any labor or payroll costs. If you have specific questions about exactly what is included (or not), I highly recommend reviewing the AAHA/VMG Companion Animal Chart of Accounts Field Definitions on the AAHA website; it's an excellent resource!

Helpful Definitions

- **COGS**: the price a business pays for items it sells. In the case of veterinary practices, we are selling items and performing a service (veterinary care). So, for veterinary practices, this refers to the costs related to patient care and the costs for products sold. Essentially, it's money spent to care for patients and sell any products.
- **Direct cost**: specific expenses that can be directly linked to selling a product or providing a service. These costs are tied to and necessary for providing veterinary care.
- **Valuation**: simply put, valuation is putting a price tag on a business (in this case, a veterinary practice). In this process, a specialist works to estimate the value of the assets, income, and other factors that make up a veterinary practice.

Let's explore a few scenarios of why this information is important.

Scenario 1
You are a practice manager and get your monthly financial statements from your book keeper. After reviewing them, your cost of goods as a percentage of revenue has been significantly higher this quarter than ever before. You keep going over the financial reports, trying to figure out where the huge increase is coming from. After you think about it, you realize that you had a new specialty surgeon start almost three months ago. You dig into what expenses were categorized under COGS and realize that some equipment purchases and the specialty surgeon's wages (she's an independent contractor) are wrongly classified in the COGS category. You immediately call your book keeper to go over what you discovered. She reclassifies the expenses and your COGS are now much more aligned with what they should be. Yay!

What this means for you: I often see expenses that should be categorized as COGS in that category. This makes your COGS look much higher than they actually are! Knowing what should be included and not included in this category is very important. It's also why I recommend working with veterinary-specific book keepers and/or accountants; veterinary medicine is such a unique industry!

Scenario 2
You are a practice owner who dreams of retiring in the next five years to embark on your next great adventure. You are considering selling your practice but you're not exactly sure how much your practice is worth and what the valuation would be. You talk to a veterinary practice sales and appraisal specialist and have a valuation done. After getting the results back, you realize that your COGS are much higher than you'd like. Knowing that you want to retire soon, you want to decrease your inventory costs to have your practice valued much higher.

You meet with your practice manager and inventory manager to review goals and projects, and make new ones. After looking at your profit and loss statement with the COGS expense category breakdown, you realize that your reference lab costs are almost the same as your reference lab income. Reviewing the reference lab category gets moved to the top of the list!

What this means for you: It's important to focus on and streamline your COGS before you're ready to sell your practice. Reviewing your expense and income subcategories on your profit and loss statement can be revealing!

Scenario 3

Let's say you are reviewing your KPI dashboard and notice that your COGS has risen by four percentage points (from 22% to 26%) in just one month. Panic and distress arise because you aren't sure why or how there was an increase, and you've been working so hard at bringing your costs down. But, after reviewing the subcategories in your profit and loss statement, you realize that the "Therapeutic Diet" costs doubled last month. When you look at your "Therapeutic Diet" revenue, you see it didn't increase. This information quickly pinpoints where and how you should start to investigate why your COGS might have gone up.

13.5.1 What Should Your COGS Be?

Cost of goods sold is probably the most commonly used metric for measuring success when it comes to your inventory. COGS is most often represented as a percentage of revenue. Your practice's ideal COGS percentage will depend on your unique situation and your product-to-service mix. As an example, livestock, equine, and mixed animal practices will typically have a higher cost of goods than small/companion animal practices. Specialty and emergency hospitals will have lower COGS than their general practice counterparts.

A commonly accepted COGS as a percentage of revenue benchmark for small animal general practice facilities is 20%. When comparing your practice to any "benchmark," it's important to compare your practice to similar practices to ensure that you are comparing apples to apples and not apples to octopi. A rural cattle practice is going to have a significantly different goal COGS from a metropolitan specialty and 24/7 emergency practice. Not only that but if your product sales are largely from low-margin products (like diets or preventatives), your COGS may naturally be higher.

Specialty and emergency hospitals typically have lower COGS because they don't carry as much inventory (i.e., vaccinations, heartworm or flea and tick preventatives, many prescription diets, etc.) They also typically generate much more revenue from services than from product sales. On the flip side, equine and livestock practices often have higher COGS for a number of reasons. First, the markup and profit margin percentages are typically lower than those in companion animal practices. Second, they often generate more revenue from product sales (such as vaccines and deworming for large-scale cattle or other livestock operations) and have a different product-to-service revenue mix.

Here are some general COGS range recommendations I most often see.

- Small animal general practice: 18–22%.
- Livestock/large animal practice: 22–24%+.
- Emergency/specialty practice: 5–15%.

There are many factors to consider when determining what the COGS should be for your practice. It can do more harm than good to hyper-focus on an arbitrary goal COGS percentage instead of setting goals for your unique situation.

13.5.2 Formulas for Calculating Your COGS as a Percentage of Revenue

There are two ways to calculate your COGS as a percentage of revenue. The first method is much less common because it involves knowing the exact value of inventory on hand at the beginning and end of every month. This isn't realistic for many practices because it requires a full inventory count each month.

This is the formula for the first method.

$$Cost\ of\ Goods\ Sold = Starting\ Inventory + Purchases - Ending\ Inventory$$

The second method is much more common, and it compares your costs to your revenue. Essentially, this method divides your costs by the revenue in the same time period. The most accurate way to find these numbers is with your accounting software, often using a profit and loss statement. Your practice management system might not be as accurate and likely won't show the full "cost picture."

$$Cost\ of\ Goods\ Sold = \frac{Cost}{Revenue} \times 100$$

The first step is to determine what time-frame to use to calculate your COGS as a percentage of revenue. Would you like to look at your COGS for the past month? The past year? Next, find the total costs of goods sold (in dollars) from your profit and loss statement (Figure 13.2). Then, find your total revenue or income from the same time period. Once you have the two figures, divide the cost of goods by the revenue. Next, multiply by 100 to find the percentage.

Let's explore an example. Tank's Animal Hospital wants to calculate its COGS as a percentage of revenue for the last quarter. After reviewing their profit and loss statement, Dr Tank found that his total COGS was $68,417 and his total revenue was $192,863.

$$Cost\ of\ Goods\ Sold\ (\%) = \frac{Cost}{Revenue} \times 100$$

$$Cost\ of\ Goods\ Sold\ (\%) = \frac{\$68,417}{\$192,863} \times 100$$

$$Cost\ of\ Goods\ Sold\ (\%) = .3547 \times 100$$

$$Cost\ of\ Goods\ Sold\ (\%) = 35.5\%$$

Dr Tank calculated that for the last quarter, their COGS was 35.5%, which was quite a bit higher than their goal.

Once the COGS is calculated, the next step is to interpret this percentage.

- What is your COGS percentage in comparison to the previous time period? Has it increased or decreased?
- What is your COGS percentage in comparison to what's normal or typical for you?

	TOTAL
▸ Income	$25,411.46
▸ Cost of Goods Sold	$4,473.85

Figure 13.2 An example of a profit and loss statement from QuickBooks Online that shows the "Total Income" and "Cost of Goods Sold". Nicole Clausen.

- Where is your COGS percentage in comparison to similar practices?
- Is it higher or lower than you'd like it to be?

The last question is most important! As we discussed earlier in the chapter, once you've calculated and reviewed this metric, will it inspire action? What next steps will you or your management team take if it's higher than you'd like? Even decreasing your COGS as a percentage of revenue by a small amount can greatly impact your profitability.

13.6 Inventory Key Performance Indicators: Inventory Turnover

The next inventory-specific KPI is inventory turnover. This calculates how often a product arrives and is then sold (the number of "turns") in a specific period. This metric is incredibly helpful because it measures the efficiency of your inventory. It can also help you uncover items that are on the shelf for far too long, collecting dust. Overall, inventory turnover measures how well your inventory is performing and how well you are generating revenue from it.

An easy way to remember this is that the healthiest turnover is one that matches your billing cycle. That way, you aren't sitting on piles of excess inventory (that you paid for but hasn't been sold or used). If you are on statement billing and pay for your items once per month, your ideal turnover is once every 30 days or 12 times per year.

While this is a great general rule, there are some exceptions and other factors to consider. For example, if an item takes up a lot of storage space or you don't have a lot of room for a particular item, you might want a higher turnover rate (it comes in and leaves more often). Suppose you have a more compact, inexpensive item (like cotton balls or cotton swabs). In that case, you might have a lower turnover (it's on the shelf for longer) because it's not worth the labor time to constantly be ordering the item.

Take the inventory calculator formula one step further and calculate the average number of days on the shelf. I find that figure to be more helpful than just reviewing the "turns."

Tip: You can also use the circle dot challenge as a way to visualize turnover if that's more applicable to you. Remember, a KPI is only helpful if it inspires action or you can use the number somehow.

How to use this metric: If your COGS are high, calculating the inventory turnover for your entire inventory can be helpful to understand if you are stocking too much and your items are selling slower than you'd like. It's also a good idea to calculate the turnover for individual items you suspect are collecting dust.

13.6.1 Formula for Calculating Inventory Turnover

The formula for calculating inventory turnover is a multi-part equation and is a common measure of efficiency in inventory across many industries. Some practice management systems, like Cornerstone, have an "Inventory Turnover" report. So, if your software has one, it saves you a step! If your PiMS doesn't have a way to calculate turnover, you can calculate the ratio of your entire inventory or an individual product.

When calculating inventory turnover for a specific product, it's important to remember that the variables (starting inventory, ending inventory, and total inventory purchases) should all be in the same units, whether that's bottles, pills, capsules, milliliters, etc. If you're calculating turnover for your inventory as a whole, the variables should be in terms of the value of your inventory.

Helpful Definitions

- **Starting inventory**: either the number of units on hand on the beginning day of that time period or, if you are calculating the turnover for your entire inventory, the value of inventory on hand on the beginning day of that time period.
- **Ending inventory**: the ending inventory is either the number of units on hand on the ending day of that time period or, if you are calculating the turnover for your entire inventory, the value of inventory on hand on the ending day of that time period.
- **Total inventory purchases**: this number should be either the total units you've purchased over the timeframe or the total value of inventory purchases during that time period.

Step 1: Calculate your average inventory on hand.

$$Average\ Inventory = \frac{\left(Starting\ Inventory + Ending\ Inventory\right)}{2}$$

Step 2: Use the above calculation to calculate your inventory turnover ratio. This number will give you the average number of turns per year.

$$Turnover = \frac{Total\ Inventory\ Purchases\ During\ the\ Period}{Average\ Inventory}$$

Once you have calculated your turnover ratio, you can use this number to calculate the average days your entire inventory (or individual product) is on the shelf.

Step 3: Calculate the inventory turnover period (the average days on the shelf).

$$Average\ Days\ on\ Shelf = \frac{365\ Days\left(or\ Days\ in\ Time\ Period\right)}{Inventory\ Turnover}$$

If your inventory turnover is less than ideal, this means your inventory items sit on the shelf for longer and have higher holding costs. To increase your inventory turnover and improve efficiency, you can decrease the quantity purchased at a time. Work out the last time reorder points were calculated and if they should be recalculated or adjusted. Alternatively, suppose your inventory turnover is too high, and it's on the shelf for a very short period. In that case, this means that you are purchasing the same item numerous times throughout the month, and you might be spending unnecessary extra time and labor hours ordering.

Helpful Definitions

- **Holding cost**: the expenses related to keeping an item on the shelf. Holding costs include all the expenses associated with keeping products in inventory until they are sold and can include rent, utilities to keep the area temperature or humidity controlled, insurance, security (like cameras or other technology), taxes on the inventory, and other factors.

13.6.2 Putting Inventory Turnover into Practice

Once you've calculated the turnover for your inventory as a whole or for an individual item, the next step is to interpret the data and understand what it means for your practice or for a product. Let's explore some examples together.

Example 1: Individual Product

In this example, mirtazapine's inventory turnover is being calculated over the last 365 days.

- Starting inventory: 409 units on January 1st.
- Ending inventory: 783 units on December 31st.
- Total inventory purchases: 8900 units purchased between January 1st and December 31st.

Step 1: Calculate the average inventory on hand.

$$Average\ Inventory = \frac{(Starting\ Inventory + Ending\ Inventory)}{2}$$

$$Average\ Inventory = \frac{(409\ Units + 783\ Units)}{2}$$

$$Average\ Inventory = 596\ Units$$

Step 2: Use the above answer to calculate your inventory turnover ratio.

$$Turnover = \frac{Total\ Inventory\ Purchases\ During\ the\ Period}{Average\ Inventory}$$

$$Turnover = \frac{8,900\ Units}{596\ Units}$$

$$Turnover = 14.9$$

In this example, mirtazapine has an inventory turnover of 14.9 or 15 times per year. This means that this item comes into and leaves the practice on average 15 times per year. As a reminder, a good starting point is that your inventory turnover should match your billing cycle. So, if you're on statement billing, an inventory turnover of 12–14 times per year is an effective number to strive for.

The example of 15 times per year is pretty close to the range, so I would classify mirtazapine as having a healthy turnover. If the product had higher turns, this means that it might be coming in and leaving too quickly, potentially increasing labor and ordering costs associated with it. On the other hand, if the inventory turnover was lower, it means the product was sitting on the shelf for longer periods of time before selling. The longer an item sits on the shelf, the more holding costs it incurs.

We can take the turnover calculation one step further by calculating the average days on the shelf.

Step 3: Calculate the average days on the shelf.

$$Average\ Days\ on\ Shelf = \frac{365\ Days\ (or\ Days\ in\ Time\ Period)}{Inventory\ Turnover}$$

$$Average\ Days\ on\ Shelf = \frac{365\ Days}{14.9}$$

$$Average\ Days\ on\ Shelf = 24.5\ Days$$

In this example, mirtazapine is on the shelf for 24.5 days before it's either used or sold. If you were on statement billing, you would likely sell this product before you had to pay for it.

Example 2: Entire Inventory

In this example, Tank's Animal Hospital's inventory turnover is being calculated over the last 365 days.

- Starting inventory: value of inventory on hand on January 1st: $47,139.54.
- Ending inventory: value of inventory on hand on December 31st: $52,801.67.
- Total inventory purchases: $458,206.45.

Step 1: Calculate the average inventory on hand.

$$Average\ Inventory = \frac{\left(Starting\ Inventory + Ending\ Inventory\right)}{2}$$

$$Average\ Inventory = \frac{\left(\$47,139.54 + \$52,801.67\right)}{2}$$

$$Average\ Inventory = \frac{\$99,941.21}{2}$$

$$Average\ Inventory = \$49,970.61$$

Step 2: Use the above calculation to calculate your inventory turnover ratio.

$$Turnover = \frac{Total\ Inventory\ Purchases\ During\ the\ Period}{Average\ Inventory}$$

$$Turnover = \frac{\$458,206.45}{\$49,970.61}$$

$$Turnover = 9.2$$

In this example, Tank's Animal Hospital's inventory turnover was calculated at 9.2. This means that their entire inventory "turns" or comes in and leaves 9.2 times per year. In this example, this number is lower than the recommended range, so inventory might be sitting on the shelf for too long and not efficiently generating an income. I would recommend that Dr Tank evaluate his inventory products (see Chapters 9 and 10 for more information) or "spot check" a few suspected slow-moving inventory items and calculate the turnover rate for those items.

We can take the turnover calculation one step further by calculating the average days on the shelf.

Step 3: Calculate the average days on the shelf.

$$Average\ Days\ on\ Shelf = \frac{365\ Days\ \left(or\ Days\ in\ Time\ Period\right)}{Inventory\ Turnover}$$

$$Average\ Days\ on\ Shelf = \frac{365\ Days}{9.2}$$

$$Average\ Days\ on\ Shelf = 39.7$$

In this example, Tank's Animal Hospital's entire inventory sits on the shelf for an average of 39.7 days before being used or sold. This is only slightly over the recommended range of 25–30 days. It would be smart to investigate further to see if inventory efficiency could be improved.

Calculating your inventory turnover rate and the average number of days a product is on the shelf is a great way to measure your inventory efficiency. This can help you understand if you are effectively generating income from your inventory or if products are moving too slowly.

13.7 Inventory Key Performance Indicators: Value of Inventory On Hand

Measuring the value of your inventory that's "on hand" or on the shelf is an important KPI and can give you a lot of clues on the health of your inventory. Knowing the value of your inventory on hand, or inventory carry, can identify if you have too much inventory on the shelf or if you have excess cash flow locked up in products. It helps you understand how on track (or off track) you are in finding the balance between having enough on hand and too much.

Generally speaking, a good range that I like to aim for with the value of inventory on hand is $15,000–$20,000 per full-time equivalent (FTE) veterinarian. There are a couple of considerations and exceptions to this.

- If you've just made a large or bulk promotional purchase, the value of inventory on hand will be much higher than normal.
- If you're a large or mixed animal practice, this number might be slightly higher, again due to the fact that often more inventory is carried for herd health management.
- This number assumes fairly consistent demand over the year. If your practice has significant seasonal swings, the value of inventory on hand will increase during your busy seasons and decrease in the slower seasons.
- If you're a specialty or emergency practice, you will probably be on the lower end of the spectrum as you typically will carry less inventory than general practice counterparts.

13.7.1 Formula for Calculating Value of Inventory On Hand

$$Value\ of\ Inventory\ On\ Hand = \frac{Total\ Inventory\ Value}{\#\ of\ FTE\ Equivalent\ DVMs}$$

Keep in mind that the total value of your inventory should be accurate before using this formula! Otherwise, the value per veterinarian could be falsely elevated or decreased.

Tip: If you have a part-time veterinarian and aren't sure how to calculate their "FTE," you can divide the number of hours they work per week by 40 hours (considered full time).

As an example, Dr Ollie works a total of 15 hours per week and you want to calculate their "FTE."

$$Full\ Time\ Equivalent = \frac{Number\ of\ Hours\ Worked\ per\ Week}{40}$$

$$Full\ Time\ Equivalent = \frac{15}{40}$$

$$Full\ Time\ Equivalent = 0.375$$

Dr Ollie would be considered 0.375 FTE. Let's now say three other veterinarians work full time at this practice. This particular practice would have 3.375 FTE veterinarians.

Let's explore two examples of calculating the value of inventory on hand.

Example 1

Tank's Animal Hospital has five full-time doctors and one doctor who works about 25 hours per week. Their total value of inventory on hand is $194,258.00. Before we calculate the inventory value on hand per FTE veterinarian, we need to calculate the total number of FTE veterinarians.

$$Full\ Time\ Equivalent = \frac{Number\ of\ Hours\ Worked\ per\ Week}{40}$$

$$Full\ Time\ Equivalent = \frac{25}{40}$$

$$Full\ Time\ Equivalent = 0.625$$

We now know that Tank's Animal Hospital has a total of 5.625 FTE veterinarians, and we can calculate the value of inventory on hand.

$$Value\ of\ Inventory\ On\ Hand = \frac{Total\ Inventory\ Value}{\#\ of\ FTE\ Veterinarians}$$

$$Value\ of\ Inventory\ On\ Hand = \frac{\$194,258.00}{5.625}$$

$$Value\ of\ Inventory\ On\ Hand = \$34,534.76$$

Tank's Animal Hospital has $34,534.76 on hand per FTE veterinarian. This is much higher than the recommended range of $15,000–$20,000. This result shows that they have too much inventory on hand and are likely experiencing negative financial impacts.

When the value of inventory on hand is high, we might experience the following.

- High COGS.
- It might feel like the practice is bringing in revenue, but the bank balance doesn't seem to reflect that.
- Products expire more often than we'd like and there is low product turnover.
- Cash flow might be impacted and, depending on the situation, it can be a challenge to stay current on our monthly bills and expenses

Example 2

In this example, Ollie's Pet Hospital has a total of four veterinarians: two full time and two part time. The first part-time veterinarian works 20 hours a week and the second works 30 hours a week. The total value of inventory on hand is $101,836.00.

The first step will be to calculate the number of FTE veterinarians. Because Ollie's Pet Hospital has two part-time DVMs, calculate both and then add them together.

$$Full\ Time\ Equivalent = \frac{Number\ of\ Hours\ Worked\ per\ Week}{40}$$

$$Full\ Time\ Equivalent = \frac{20}{40} + \frac{30}{40}$$

$$Full\ Time\ Equivalent = 0.5 + 0.75$$

$$Full\ Time\ Equivalent = 1.25$$

Ollie's Pet Hospital therefore has a total of 3.25 FTE veterinarians. Now, we can calculate the value of inventory on hand.

$$Value\ of\ Inventory\ On\ Hand = \frac{Total\ Inventory\ Value}{\#\ of\ FTE\ Veterinarian}$$

$$Value\ of\ Inventory\ On\ Hand = \frac{\$101,836.00}{3.25}$$

$$Value\ of\ Inventory\ On\ Hand = \$31,334.15$$

Ollie's Pet Hospital has $31,334.15 on hand per FTE veterinarian. They are also outside the recommended range of $15,000–$20,000.

There are two main reasons I typically see why the value of inventory might be high for a practice.

- Too many types of products and too many stock-keeping units (SKUs).
- Some products are overstocked, and there's too much on the shelf for a particular item.

If the inventory on-hand value is more than average or is outside the reference range, the first step is to examine your turnover. If your turnover is too low, that means the products are sitting on the shelf for longer than ideal. Let's imagine that instead of purchasing for a veterinary practice, you are buying for a restaurant. If you purchase too much of an item and it sits on the shelf for too long, it will get moldy or spoil. Alternatively, if you have too many types of produce or other items, the kitchen team will only reach for those ingredients needed for their recipes and the rest will spoil.

Although your pharmaceuticals and supplies don't expire as quickly as produce, you can think of inventory similarly. If you have too many types of products, you can have an overflowing pharmacy or central storage. Your team will still reach for their "go-to" products and the rest won't sell as frequently. If some of your products are overstocked, you might end up with expired products, theft, or other types of waste.

The goal is to optimize your turnover. You want to intentionally stock what you are going to use or sell and eliminate or move those items that are infrequently sold to an online pharmacy.

You can troubleshoot or investigate a high value of inventory on hand by:

- reviewing your reorder points. When was the last time reorder points were calculated? Are there any products that have fallen "out of favor" and are sold much less frequently? How much is being purchased at a time? Were there any recent bulk or promotional purchases?
- reviewing your formulary. Take a look at the different products you currently stock. Do you have nine types of ear cleansers? Is there a certain category that has multiple different options with similar products? How many different types of flea, tick, and heartworm prevention are currently on the shelf? How many redundancies do you have?

Helpful Definitions
- **Formulary**: a "menu" or list of medications available at the practice to treat patients.
- **Redundancies**: this means having multiple versions or brands of the same type of medication. An example could be keeping seven different types of canine joint supplements on the shelf.

Having a high inventory value on hand can signal that you have too many "stale" inventory products or that you have excess cash tied up in inventory.

13.8 Inventory Key Performance Indicators: Number of Adjustments or Variances in a Time Period

Although monitoring the number of adjustments or variances during a particular time period isn't a traditional KPI, it can give you a helpful insight into your inventory. Measuring how many and the amount of each adjustment can determine how much inventory went "missing" during the time period.

When cycle counting or performing inventory counts, if there is a difference between what is on the shelf versus what your practice management system says, it's considered shrinkage. This could be related to theft, waste, errors, and expirys, among other reasons. Measuring the "shrink" or what has gone missing and monitoring trends can identify if you have significant missed charges, suspected theft, or if you simply aren't charging appropriately for your inventory.

For example, if you made an adjustment for six tablets one month and the following month, you needed to adjust the same item for 360 tablets, that should be an immediate red flag and prompt an inquiry into what might have happened. After monitoring the adjustments made each month and identifying several medication errors, you might consider: What systems or processes could I add that could help? Is the pharmacy too distracting? Do we need to institute a "no rush zone" in the pharmacy areas? What else could be the "root cause" for excessive medication errors or missed billing?

Helpful Definitions
- **Root cause**: the original source of a problem or the main reason something happens (or goes wrong). Identifying and solving the root cause can help keep problems from recurring. For example, if a pet has multiple chronic urinary tract infections, a veterinarian would likely want to find out and treat the root cause rather than just constantly prescribing antibiotics.

It's also helpful to monitor the total value of adjustments each month. Let's say that one month you have $437 in adjustments and the next month you have $12,586; that's a critical situation you'd want to know about early and get to the bottom of.

Armed with that information, you can make data-informed decisions and investigate why that might be happening. Are there errors in how the item is entered into the practice management system? Is there theft? Was there an error with receiving? Were there missed charges? Did an item expire or was wasted and never removed out of your software? Monitoring the number and value of adjustments can help identify a number of problems with your inventory that need to be immediately addressed and corrected. Remember that any adjustment due to theft, missed charges, waste, and expiry is a loss of revenue for your practice.

The number of adjustments or variances made in a time period should be monitored on a regular basis, at least monthly. This can be done by utilizing an adjustment report in your practice management system or by entering the product, adjustment amount, and value of the adjustment in a spreadsheet.

13.9 Putting It All Together

Key performance indicators tend to all work together and can be used to help diagnose larger problems or areas of opportunity in your inventory. For example, if you realize your COGS as a percentage of revenue (referred to as COGS in this section) are high, you can use the other inventory KPIs to try and get a clearer picture of why that might be. Often, I find that if your COGS are high, your inventory turnover is low (meaning that products are sitting on the shelf for too long), and the value of inventory on hand is usually also high (you have a lot of cash tied up on the shelf). Additionally, if your variances and adjustments each month are also high, it might mean that you are missing charges or, for some reason, not appropriately selling your inventory.

Monitoring your inventory KPIs on a regular and recurring basis is great "lab work" for your practice and can help diagnose challenges as well as catch smaller problems before they escalate into major problems.

"Best Practice" Questions to Consider

- How will I maintain my inventory? What tasks or processes need to happen regularly so our inventory doesn't become a mess again?
- What SOPs should be created for our inventory (and our practice as a whole)? How can I make these SOPs and guidelines as accessible and helpful as possible for the team?
- Are we currently tracking any KPIs? What about any inventory-specific KPIs? What metrics should we start tracking? What steps need to be taken to start tracking and creating a KPI dashboard?

Appendices

A.1 Frequently Asked Questions and Scenarios

A.1.1 What If I Do Not Use a Software?

If your practice does not use a practice management system, there are still ways in which you can effectively manage your inventory. You might not have as many features readily available to you, but there are certainly ways to leverage what you do have in your practice for inventory. Thinking back to the flow of inventory in our practice and our coral reef ecosystem metaphor, the foundation and the important rock formations that our inventory cycle is built upon are the reorder points (ROP) and demand forecasting.

Even if you do not have a practice management system, there are ways to both calculate ROPs and estimate what you'll sell in the future based on historical information. First, think about how you invoice clients. Is it through the practice's accounting software or another electronic method? If so, are there reports available that outline the quantity sold of each product? If that is the case, you can use that information to help calculate your ROPs. If not, you could use the purchase history from your distributor to calculate your ROPs.

It's important to keep in mind that if you are using your purchase history to estimate future demand and calculate your ROPs, any overordering will be perpetuated. It's beneficial to regularly review your turnover to ensure there aren't any products sitting on the shelf for too long. It might be a slightly more iterative process after calculating ROPs and setting up different reorder flags. You might find that you'll need to adjust order points more frequently in the beginning.

It will also be important to monitor your turnover and expiry dates and keep track of items that run out on a regular basis so you can make adjustments if necessary.

If you use another type of inventory management or warehouse management software, what are its capabilities? What features are available to you that could help you manage the flow of inventory in your practice?

Additionally, if your practice has a spreadsheet program like Google Sheets (which is free for Gmail users) or Microsoft Excel, it might be helpful for you to create a spreadsheet. You can use spreadsheets to keep track of your ROPs, commonly used items, expiry dates, and more. Here are some examples of and inspiration for spreadsheets that you could create.

Inventory Management for Veterinary Professionals, First Edition. Nicole I. Clausen.
© 2024 John Wiley & Sons, Inc. Published 2024 by John Wiley & Sons, Inc.
Companion website: www.wiley.com/go/clausen/inventory

A.1.1.1 Reorder Form Tracker

Table A.1 An example spreadsheet to keep track of the various products in your practice and their reorder points. Additional columns could be added to keep track of product sales and usage.

Vendor item number	Description	Minimum quantity	Maximum quantity	or	Reorder quantity	Physical count	Qty to order

A.1.1.2 Product Expiry Date Tracker

Table A.2 A spreadsheet that can be used to track a product's lot number and expiry date. Having a database of all upcoming expiry dates can be beneficial for easy reference.

Category	Product	Lot number	Expiration date

A.1.1.3 Commonly Used Items in Treatments Report

In addition to creating a top product list, you could create a spreadsheet tracker that lists common treatments or procedures and the common inventory items used. Keeping this information in a spreadsheet can be another tool in your toolbox for estimating future demand.

Just because you do not have a practice management system or other inventory software does not mean that all hope is lost! As you are reading through this book, think about the different concepts presented and consider the following questions.

- How can I modify this strategy or tactic to fit the technology I currently use in my practice?
- What system will I need to put in place if my software system does not have the functionality for this?
  - For example, if you aren't able to leverage your software to increase prices as your costs go up, what process or system could you implement so price adjustments can happen when appropriate?
- Even if you do not have a practice management system or specific inventory software, what functionality does your current technology offer that you could use?
  - For example, if you use an accounting software system, does it have any reports that would be helpful?

Table A.3 An example spreadsheet that can be created to keep track of commonly used hospital supplies, white goods, pharmaceuticals, or other inventory items used during procedures.

Treatment	Commonly used items	Amount used

A.1.2   What If I Manage Inventory at an ER or Specialty Clinic?

Managing inventory for an emergency or specialty veterinary practice can look a little different from a general practice facility. Overall, the foundations of how to manage inventory remain consistent. ROPs and demand forecasting will still serve as the basis of your inventory management strategy. It will be advantageous to have systems and workflows for ordering, receiving, pricing, selling, and using your inventory appropriately, as well as optimizing your inventory.

The biggest difference between an ER or specialty practice and a general practice veterinary clinic is typically the size and scale of the facility. Often, an ER or specialty practice will have more veterinarians and multiple departments. I find that, in this instance, it works well to have a central storage area and potentially even a centralized pharmacy. With a centralized storage area, this is where all or most of the inventory and supply backstock will be stored and organized. Then, other areas and departments of the practice can be restocked from the main central storage location. Depending on the practice and the type of reorder flags that are used, it could make sense that once an item leaves the central storage area, that item is considered taken out of inventory and "gone." This means that for ROPs and reorder flags, it often makes sense to base them on what's in central storage rather than the entire practice.

Let's return to Tank's Animal Hospital and their recently opened second location – Dr Tank's Animal ER and Urgent Care. At their practice, Dr Tank has a large dedicated room for central storage and backstock. Within the practice, there is also a centralized pharmacy. Only pharmacy team members fill prescriptions for the rest of the team. In addition to the emergency department, there are also internal medicine, surgery, cardiology, and oncology departments, among others.

Once the inventory arrives in the practice, it immediately gets unpacked and organized into the central storage location or the pharmacy. The central storage is set up with physical ROPs, mainly reorder tags, shelf labels listing the minimum and maximum for each supply, and indicator reorder bins. As an example, for 3 ml syringes, the minimum quantity is 10 boxes and the maximum is 25 boxes.

Once a week, a member of the inventory team restocks each department in the practice. Alternatively, each department leader can also request specific supplies or an early restock if needed. Once boxes of 3 ml syringes leave the central storage area, they aren't considered to be in the on-hand inventory amount for ROPs. So, once there are only 10 boxes in central storage, the syringes would be considered "low" and need to be replenished.

Depending on the practice management system or other inventory software used, there are capabilities to track pharmaceuticals and other items that are sold within the software. If a medication, injectable, or other item tracked in the software needs to be restocked or moved to a different location, it can be transferred to the new location in the software.

Although there are many similarities between ER and specialty or general practice facilities, one of the biggest differences is the scale and size of the practice. The same inventory management principles still apply, but they often need to be implemented or set up differently to accommodate the practice's size and scale.

A.1.3   What If I Manage Inventory at a Large or Mixed Animal Clinic with Mobile Vehicles?

One of the unique challenges for inventory managers at a practice with mobile vehicles is keeping them appropriately stocked, trying to keep track of which inventory is where, and selling products from the appropriate truck. Let's explore the main categories of inventory: Products that are sold and products that are consumed (like supplies or white goods).

A.1.3.1 Products That Are Sold

The intricacies of how this will work for your practice will depend heavily on the type of practice management software you use, its functionality, and the processes that you currently have in place at your practice. As an example, Dr Tank's Animal Hospital has two different mobile vehicles. When Dr Tank goes on an outcall, he will add items to an invoice in the field. In the practice management system, he'll select that he's selling the product from his particular truck. So, the quantity on hand for the items sold will be deducted from his specific truck.

If your practice management system has the functionality for multiple locations and can track the quantity on hand for each truck, that's often a best-case scenario. But sometimes that's not possible with the limitations of your software. If you are not able to have specific locations in your software, what's an alternative that might work for your practice and team? With the functionality of your software, how could you ensure inventory is sold and clients are billed appropriately?

A.1.3.2 Products That Are Consumed

There are a few considerations for products consumed, like white goods, hospital supplies, and other items used during procedures and treatments. For practices with mobile vehicles, I find it works well to have a central storage design similar to that of ER or specialty practices. Once a truck needs to be restocked, the inventory is either transferred to a different location or considered "used" and not counted toward ROPs. Additionally, I would only set ROPs for the main central storage area for hospital supplies and white goods.

Another unique consideration is how the trucks will be restocked. Here are a few ideas that have worked for other practices.

- Each truck and veterinarian has a specific veterinary technician who always works with them. This team member is in charge of keeping track of the inventory on their specific truck and making sure it's restocked as needed.
- A "stock checklist" will be created and used for each truck. The checklist will list each item that's on the truck, the ideal quantity, and other pertinent information. Then, the checklist can be used to restock the truck each week.
- Each veterinarian can request stock from the inventory manager or pharmacy team. The team will prep what was requested and make the transfer in the practice management system. The veterinarian will then pick up their request and restock their truck.

In addition to a bricks-and-mortar facility, practices with mobile vehicles are incredibly diverse, with different patient populations, current billing processes, practice size, and other unique factors. As a result, there is no "one size fits all" system. Your practice will likely have to do a little more trial and error to find a system that works best for you.

A.1.3.3 What If I'd Like More Help and Assistance with My Inventory?

I'm happy to help! I have a full suite of courses and free inventory guides, and I'm the host of the Inventory Nation Podcast. All can be found on my website at www.vetlogic.co/education. Additionally, I also offer bespoke remote inventory consulting. You can learn more at www.vetlogic.co/consulting.

A.2 Formula Quick Reference Guide

A.2.1 Chapter 3: Demand Forecasting, Purchasing Planning, and Reorder Points

A.2.1.1 Average daily use formula

$$Average\ Daily\ Use = \frac{Annual\ Usage\ or\ Purchases}{Number\ of\ Days\ Open\ per\ Year}$$

A.2.1.2 Economic order quantity formula

$$Economic\ Order\ Quantity = \sqrt{\frac{2 \times A \times F}{H \times UC}}$$

A.2.1.3 Lead time method for reorder points

$$Reorder\ Point = \left(Average\ Daily\ Use \times Lead\ Time\right) + Safety\ Stock$$

A.2.1.4 Maximum level formula

$$Maximum\ Level = Reorder\ Point + Reorder\ Quantity$$

A.2.1.5 Reorder quantity formula (two-week supply)

$$Reorder\ Quantity = \frac{Units\ Sold\ or\ Purchased\ in\ Time\ Period}{Number\ of\ Two\text{-}week\ Periods\ in\ Time\ Period}$$

A.2.1.6 Reorder quantity formula (30-day supply)

$$Reorder\ Quantity = \frac{Units\ Sold\ or\ Purchased\ in\ Time\ Period}{Number\ of\ Months\ in\ Time\ Period}$$

A.2.1.7 Reorder quantity formula (specific days of stock)

$$Reorder\ Quantity = Average\ Daily\ Use \times Number\ of\ Days\ Worth\ of\ Stock$$

where

$$Average\ Daily\ Use = \frac{Annual\ Usage}{Number\ of\ Days\ Open\ per\ Year}$$

A.2.1.8 Safety stock: daily use method

$$Safety\ Stock = Average\ Daily\ Use \times Number\ of\ Days$$

A.2.1.9 Safety stock: maximum use minus average use calculation method

$$Safety\ Stock = \left(Maximum\ Daily\ Usage \times Maximum\ Lead\ Time\right) - \left(Average\ Daily\ Usage \times Average\ Lead\ Time\right)$$

A.2.1.10 Time-frame method for reorder points (two-week supply)

$$Reorder\ Point = \frac{Units\ Sold\ or\ Purchased\ in\ Time\ Period}{Number\ of\ Two\text{-}week\ Periods\ in\ Time\ Period}$$

A.2.1.11 Time-frame method for reorder points (two-week supply with annual sales)

$$Two\text{-}week\ Supply = \frac{Annual\ Usage\left(or\ Purchases\right)}{26}$$

A.2.2 Chapter 4: Efficient Ordering

A.2.2.1 Bulk order quantity

$$Bulk\ Order\ Quantity = Average\ Daily\ Use \times Billing\ Terms\left(in\ Days\right)$$

where

$$Average\ Daily\ Use = \frac{Annual\ Usage}{Number\ of\ Days\ Open\ per\ Year}$$

A.2.2.2 Days of stock formula

$$Days\ of\ Stock = \frac{Total\ Quantity}{Average\ Daily\ Use}$$

A.2.3 Chapter 6: Strategic Inventory Pricing

A.2.3.1 Markup percentage calculation formula

$$Markup\ Percentage = \frac{\left(Selling\ Price - Unit\ Cost\right)}{Unit\ Cost} \times 100$$

A.2.3.2 Markup pricing formula

$$Selling\ Price = Cost + \left(Cost \times Markup\%\right)$$

A.2.3.3 Margin pricing formula (with no indirect costs included)

$$Price = Total\ Product\ Cost + Margin(\$)$$

A.2.3.4 Margin pricing formula (with indirect cost included)

$$Price = Total\ Product\ Cost + \left(Total\ Product\ Cost \times Indirect\ Cost\%\right) + Margin$$

A.2.3.5 Overhead cost formula

$$Product\ Cost + \left(Product\ Cost \times 40\%\right) = True\ Product\ Cost +$$
$$\left[True\ Product\ Cost\left(Profit\% + DVM\ Pay\right)\right] = Price$$

A.2.3.6 Standard pricing formula

$$Product\,Cost + \left[Product\,Cost \left(Labour\% + Facility\% \right) \right] = True\,Product\,Cost +$$
$$\left[True\,Product\,Cost \left(Profit\% + DVM\,Pay \right) \right] = Price$$

A.2.4 Chapter 13: Maintaining Your Inventory and Key Performance Indicators

A.2.4.1 Cost of goods sold formula

$$Cost\,of\,Goods\,Sold \left(as\%\,of\,Revenue \right) = \frac{Cost\,of\,Goods\,Sold}{Revenue} \times 100$$

A.2.4.2 Cost of goods sold formula (accounting for purchases)

$$Cost\,of\,Goods\,Sold = Starting\,Inventory + Purchases - Ending\,Inventory$$

A.2.4.3 Inventory turnover formula

Step 1: calculate the average inventory

$$Average\,Inventory = \frac{\left(Starting\,Inventory + Ending\,Inventory \right)}{2}$$

Step 2: calculate the inventory turnover

$$Turnover = \frac{Total\,Inventory\,Purchases\,During\,the\,Period}{Average\,Inventory}$$

Step 3: calculate the average days on the shelf

$$Average\,Days\,on\,Shelf = \frac{365\,Days \left(or\,Days\,on\,Time\,Period \right)}{Inventory\,Turnover}$$

A.2.4.4 Value of inventory on-hand

$$Value\,of\,Inventory\,On\,Hand = \frac{Total\,Inventory\,Value}{\#\,of\,FTE\,Equivalent\,DVMs}$$

A.3 Example Standard Operating Procedure for Calculating Reorder Points

Below is an example of a standard operating procedure (SOP) on how to calculate ROPs in a veterinary practice.

SOP No. 123	Date of last revision: 19 May 2023
Author: Nicole Clausen	Implemented date: 27 May 2023
Date created: 19 May 2023	Approved by: Dr Tank

A.3.1.1 Prerequisites

Prior to calculating ROPs, a team member will need access to the following reports from XYZ software.

- Quantity Sold Report (for calculating all items).
- Item Sold Report (for calculating individual items).

In addition, a team member will need the ROP Calculator spreadsheet.

A.3.1.2 Purpose

The purpose of this SOP is to calculate ROPs and reorder quantities (ROQs) for all inventory items. The ultimate goal is to calculate ROPs so that "low" is quantified and a flag can be created for when to order. Then, once a product is considered low, the ROQ can be used to order the appropriate amount.

A.3.1.3 Policy

Reorder points and ROQs should be reviewed and recalculated (if necessary) every six months (or three months after a doctor leaves or joins the practice). Once implemented, the ROPs and ROQs calculated should be used to ensure proper inventory turnover and maintain appropriate inventory cost levels.

Generally speaking, ROPs and ROQs are calculated with six months of sales data. For seasonal products, two ROPs and ROQs should be calculated, one for the peak time and one for the lull time. Emergency medication ROPs and quantities will be set by the medical director. As a general rule, ROPs will be calculated as a two-week supply of the product and the ROQ will be a 30-day supply.

A.3.1.4 Property

Georgia, lead inventory manager.

A.3.1.5 Party

Georgia will ultimately be responsible for calculating the ROPs, but the following team members will be involved in the process.

- Ollie – maintaining reorder tags on consumables and hospital supplies.
- Mackenzie – updating ROPs, ROQs, and overstock levels in the practice management system.
- Amelia (medical director) – calculating and relaying ROPs and ROQs for emergency medications.

A.3.1.6 Process

To calculate the ROPs and ROQs for a single item.

1) Access and export the Item Sold Summary for that item for the necessary date range.
2) Find the six months' usage for the item.
3) Use the following formula for ROPs: six months' usage/13. Note: 13 represents the number of two-week periods within six months.
4) Use the following formula for reorder quantity: six months' usage/6. Note: 6 represents the number of 30-day periods within six months.
5) Update the ROP and ROQ in the practice management system.

To calculate the ROPs and ROQs for all items.

1) Access and export the Quantity Sold Report for the necessary date range.
2) Export the report as an Excel file.
3) Remove all "extra" rows or columns – anything that is not the Item ID, Item Description, and Quantity Sold.
4) Copy and paste all the data and information into the ROP Calculator.
5) Update the calculated ROPs and ROQs in the practice management system.

A.3.1.7 Procedure

To calculate ROPs and ROQs for all items

1) In the menu bar of the practice management system, click the Reports button.
2) Then, select the Item Sold Summary Report. Then, select the item to be calculated and enter the date range for the last six months. If calculating ROPs for all items, leave the Item ID selection blank.
3) Click "Run" to preview the report.
4) If calculating for a single product, find the six-months usage and set aside (and skip to step XX). If calculating ROPs for all items, export the file as an Excel spreadsheet and follow the steps below.
5) Open the Excel spreadsheet and remove any blank rows and any column besides the Item ID, Description, and Quantity Sold columns. Delete any row totals or other data that are not necessary (see linked screen record video for reference – not actually included in this example).
6) Select all items in the spreadsheet and include the Item ID, Description, and Quantity Sold. Click control + c to copy.
7) Then, open the ROP Calculator (located on the Server → Inventory → Calculators → ROP Calculator) and paste the data into the appropriate spreadsheet.
8) The two-weeks and 30-days supply for each item should be calculated.
9) Once the ROPs and ROQs have been calculated, return to the practice management system.
10) Go to the Inventory List and select the first item to be updated. Then, click the "Purchasing" tab and enter the new ROP, and the ROQ if it has changed.
11) Continue to enter all the updated ROPs and ROQs.

A.4 Emergency Preparedness Inventory Management Plan

It can be helpful to craft an emergency preparedness inventory plan in case there's a natural disaster, extreme weather event, or other scenario that can cause significant supply chain disruptions. The plan can outline critical supplies to your practice and how you'll approach or manage any shortages.

A.4.1 Example: Emergency Preparedness Inventory Management Plan – Critical Supplies for ABC Veterinary Hospital

List the supplies, medications, and equipment that are critical to your operation as a practice. Include a list for each location if they differ.

A.4.1.1   Critical Supplies and Medications for ABC Veterinary Hospital Include:

1) List critical supplies, medications, or other inventory items that are critical to the function of your practice. This could include vaccinations, medications necessary for surgical procedures, euthanasia solution, medications for emergent/critical care patients, syringes, needles, etc.

A.4.1.2   Critical Supplies Necessary during (Situation, i.e., Viral Outbreak)

1) Catheters – preferred brand:
   a) If unavailable – alternatives include:
2) Catheter caps
3) Rescue (or other disinfectant)
   a) If unavailable – alternatives include:
4) Masks
5) _____

A.4.1.3   Critical Supplies Necessary during (Situation, i.e., Natural Disaster)

1) Pain management – preferred medications include:
   a) Hydromorphone
   b) Fentanyl
2) Bandaging supplies and white goods – preferred products and amounts
   a) 4×4″ gauze – 20 sleeves
   b) _____
3) _____

Note: List all the critical or important supplies depending on the category of emergency situation or crisis – the goal is to be prepared whatever the situation!

A.4.1.4   Stock Levels During an Emergency Situation

List all your ideal or recommended stock levels for critical items during an emergency or crisis situation.

1) Personal protective equipment:
   a) Gloves – two months' stock level (6 boxes)
   b) Masks – three months' stock level (8 boxes)
   c) Disposable gowns – two months' stock level (10 medium and 5 large gowns)
2) Etc.

A.4.1.5   Alternative and Contingency Plans

Alternative and Contingency Plans for ABC Veterinary Hospital:

1) In the event of backorder or unavailability of _____, _____ should be used as an alternative.
2) Etc.

A.4.1.6   Important Contacts during an Emergency or Crisis

Important contacts for ABC Veterinary Hospital during an emergency:

1) Contact #1
2) Contact #2

A.5 Glossary

ABC analysis A method for sorting and prioritizing products based on their sales volume or quantity sold. Helps to focus time and effort on the most critical and important items.

Allocation When a product has limited availability, the vendor or company tries to limit how much can be purchased at a time to avoid it being completely out of stock. It helps manage limited stock and ensures the product is distributed fairly.

Average daily use The amount that your practice uses or consumes in a typical day. For example, among all my dogs, they eat about four cups of food a day. Their average daily use of dog food would be four cups.

Backorder A product that is not available for purchase for a variety of reasons. Sometimes, you can place an order to go on a "Backorder List," and as soon as it's in stock, the order will be shipped out to you.

Biological products Medications or products made from living organisms or their parts. This umbrella term can include vaccines, blood products, gene therapies, or other medications derived from cells or tissues.

Carrying cost The cost of keeping an item on the shelf.

Cash flow The amount of money moving in and out of a business. Money flows in from income and payments collected from clients. It flows out for expenses like facility costs, payroll and labor costs, inventory costs, and other expenses. When there is more money coming in than going out of a practice, that creates a positive cash flow.

Chart of accounts In accounting, a chart of accounts is like a map that organizes all the financial transactions of a practice. It's a list of all the different types of accounts where the money, assets, debts, and expenses are recorded. Each account has a specific code or number (specifically called a general ledger code) that helps keep everything organized and easy to find. Think of it as a directory that helps accountants track and manage the practice's finances effectively.

Cost The amount the practice pays for an item. Also called "direct cost."

Cost-based pricing Involves setting the price based on the cost of the item, plus any indirect costs, plus the desired level of profit.

Cost multiplier Takes the cost and multiplies it by the factor to arrive at the selling price.

Cycle counting Counting small amounts of inventory throughout the year on a rotational basis.

Demand How much was used or sold.

Demand forecasting The process of using data and information to predict how much inventory you'll sell or use in the future. Essentially, it's looking at the past to make an educated guess about the future.

Demand shift A change in what products are needed. This can be due to changes in medication preference, seasonality, changes in the care team, an increase or decrease in overall patient visits, or a change in a specific kind of case (for example, if you see eight cases of pancreatitis in one week whereas you normally see two a month), among other factors.

De novo practice A brand new practice that is starting from scratch. Instead of buying an existing practice, a veterinarian builds or establishes their own practice independently.

Discrepancy When there is a difference between what is on the shelf and what your practice management system says you have.

Dispensing fee A service charge for filling the prescription. With this fee, the client is paying for the service and expertise that come with filling the prescription.

Distributor A distributor is an intermediary entity between the producer or manufacturer of a product and a veterinary practice (examples include MWI Animal Health, Covetrus, Patterson Veterinary, and Midwest Veterinary Supply). They are essentially like Dunder Mifflin in vet med.

Diversion When someone with authorized access to medications misuses the medications for personal gain or nonmedical purposes. Motives for diversion can include personal use or selling the drugs.

Electronic dispensing cabinet A sophisticated (and expensive) piece of technology used in veterinary practices (and other healthcare facilities) to manage and dispense medications and occasionally medical supplies efficiently.

Ending inventory The ending inventory is either the number of units on hand on the ending day of that time period or, if you are calculating the turnover for your entire inventory, the value of inventory on hand on the ending day of that time period.

Formulary A "menu" or list of medications that are available at the practice to treat patients.

Handling fee A service charge for extra care, expertise, and work involved in managing certain medications or products. This fee often covers additional effort, specialized storage, or any special precautions taken for that medication.

Holding costs Include costs such as rent, opportunity cost, insurance, temperature controls, and insurance, among others, to keep that inventory item safe and protected until it's sold.

Indirect costs The costs, outside the direct cost of the inventory item, related to purchasing and keeping the item in stock.

Injection fee A service charge for administering an injection. With this fee, the client is paying for the team's time, expertise, and equipment to administer the injection safely and properly.

Inventory Inventory is an essential list of all the items in your practice related to caring for a patient, including pharmaceuticals, prescription or retail diets, injectables, in-house reference lab supplies, white goods, syringes and needles, and more.

Inventory manager This text refers to a veterinary professional who is tasked with inventory management in some way as an inventory manager.

Inventory turnover A measure of how quickly an item comes in and leaves a business; it is a great measure of inventory efficiency. High turnover means items are not just sitting on the shelf, whereas low turnover means they are on the shelf for long periods before they are used or sold.

Inventory turns How many times a practice sells and purchases inventory in a given time period. High inventory turns are generally better because it's a sign that a practice is efficiently selling or using its products and not letting them sit on the shelves for too long.

Labor costs The inventory team's time to place, receive, enter, and manage orders.

Lead time Lead time is the time between when you realize a product is low and when it's received and ready to be sold. It's essentially the waiting time after you have discovered the item is low.

Lean management This is the business version of minimalism! It's about minimizing waste – whether it's time, resources, or extra steps in a process – to make everything work smoothly and save money.

Low-margin product When a practice only keeps a small portion of the revenue for a particular product as profit after covering the costs.

Manufacturer A company that makes goods for sale (examples: Nutramax Laboratories Inc., Zoetis, Elanco Animal Health, Boehringer Ingelheim Vetmedica, Ceva Animal Health, Hill's Pet Nutrition).

Margin The amount of money a business makes after subtracting all its costs and expenses from the revenue it generates.

Markup percentage An amount that needs to be added to the cost of the item to find the selling price.

Maximum inventory level The maximum amount you'd want on the shelf. Note: this is different from the reorder quantity.

Mindset A set of beliefs, notions, or assumptions that shape how you view yourself and the world around you.

Minimum inventory level Typically the reorder point for that item or the lowest inventory level you would want to have on hand.

Planogram A diagram of where items should be placed in the zone.

Prescription fee An additional fee added on top of an inventory item, in addition to the price of the item. These fees can include prescription dispensing fees, injection fees, handling fees, and controlled substance fees.

Prescription monitoring program A system that helps track the prescriptions people and animals receive for certain medications. It's a database that healthcare and veterinary professionals and authorities submit to and use to monitor the prescribing and dispensing of controlled substances.

Price The amount the client pays for an item.

Profitability How well a business is making money or earning a profit. A profitable business is one that ends up with more money left over after paying any expenses.

Profit margin The amount of money a practice (and a business, in general) makes after subtracting all its costs and expenses from the revenue it generates.

Purchase order (PO) A receipt in your practice management system that is essentially a list of all the things ordered from a particular supplier with the quantity ordered and the cost of an item +/− additional information like expiry date, lot number, etc.

Redundant products Multiple versions or brands of the same type of medication. An example could be keeping seven different types of canine joint supplements on the shelf.

Reorder bin Each bin is assigned to a specific product and when the quantity of that product drops to a certain level, it's time to reorder.

Reorder flag A flag or signal to indicate when an item is running low. I classify them into three major categories or buckets. The first type of reorder point is electronic. The second is a manual or visual reorder point and the third is a physical reorder point.

Reorder point (ROP) The level of inventory at which a particular item should be ordered. This is also considered the minimum inventory level.

Reorder tag A physical flag used as a reminder that it's time to order and replenish an inventory item. They are typically small cards or tags placed on shelves or products that indicate when it's time to order more of a particular item.

Replenishment Adding or ordering more stock to replace what has been used or sold.

Root cause The original source of a problem or the main reason something happens (or goes wrong). Identifying and solving the root cause can help to prevent problems recurring. For example, if a pet has multiple chronic urinary tract infections, a veterinarian would likely want to find out and treat the root cause rather than just constantly prescribing antibiotics.

Safety stock A backup supply or extra "cushion" of inventory, just in case. It's additional inventory beyond what you would normally keep which is "insurance" against any unexpected situations.

Shrinkage A term used to describe when an item goes missing without a clear explanation and cannot be accounted for. This can be due to theft, missed charges, errors, or other causes.

Standard operating procedures (SOPs) A set of rules or instructions for doing something the same way every time. Essentially, they are guidelines that explain how to perform tasks or handle certain situations consistently and efficiently.

Starting inventory Either the number of units on hand on the beginning day of that time period or, if you are calculating the turnover for your entire inventory, the value of inventory on hand on the beginning day of that time period.

Stockout Running out of a product or item.

Supply chain The journey a product takes from individual raw components to a final finished product in your practice. Disruptions can happen anywhere along the supply chain, impacting the availability of a product.

Valuation The estimated value of the business. During a valuation, a specialist looks at things like revenue, profit, assets (like buildings or equipment), debts, and other factors. The number can change over time, just like the value of a car or a house.

Value-based pricing Involves setting the price of an item based on how much the perceived value is to clients.

Variance The difference between the actual amount of a medication or item and what was supposed to be there according to records or expectations.

References

5S – What are The Five S's of Lean? (n.d.). https://asq.org/quality-resources/lean/five-s-tutorial (accessed 6 April 2024).

Ackerman, L. (2020). *Blackwell's Five-Minute Veterinary Practice Management Consult*. Wiley.

Docherty, P., Kira, M., and Shani, A. (2008). *Creating Sustainable Work Systems: Developing Social Sustainability*. Routledge.

Drug Enforcement Administration (2023a). Gabapentin (Neurontin®). www.deadiversion.usdoj.gov/drug_chem_info/gabapentin.pdf (accessed 6 April 2024).

Drug Enforcement Administration (2023b). *Practitioner's Manual*. Drug Enforcement Administration.

Grissinger, M. (2010). The five rights: a destination without a map. *P & T: A Peer-reviewed Journal for Formulary Management* 35 (10): 542.

Heinke, M.L. (2014). *Practice Made Perfect: A Complete Guide to Veterinary Practice Management*. American Animal Hospital Association.

Seibert, P.J., Jr (n.d.). Controlled Drug Logs: Documenting the 'Ins' and 'Outs.' www.isvma.org/wp-content/uploads/2023/02/Controlled_Drug_Logs_Documenting_the_Ins_and_Outs.pdf (accessed 6 April 2024).

Sharkey, L. (2023). Is gabapentin a narcotic or controlled substance? www.healthline.com/health/is-gabapentin-a-narcotic#state-regulations (accessed 6 April 2024).

Simplilearn (2023). What is lean management? www.simplilearn.com/what-is-lean-management-article (accessed 6 April 2024).

Teitelman, J. (n.d.). Ep. 78 | Busting Controlled Substance Myths with Retired DEA Jack Teitelman. Inventory Nation Podcast. https://vetlogic.co/ep-78-busting-controlled-substance-myths-with-retired-dea-jack-teitelman (accessed 6 April 2024).

Index

Note: Page numbers in *italic* and **bold** refers to figures and tables, respectively.

Inventory Management for Veterinary Professionals, First Edition. Nicole I. Clausen.
© 2024 John Wiley & Sons, Inc. Published 2024 by John Wiley & Sons, Inc.
Companion website: www.wiley.com/go/clausen/inventory